Digitization in Dentistry

Priyanka Jain • Mansi Gupta
Editors

Digitization in Dentistry

Clinical Applications

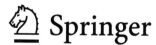 Springer

Editors
Priyanka Jain
Department of Endodontics
National University College of Dentistry
Manila
Philippines

Mansi Gupta
Department of Prosthodontics
Indraprastha Dental College
Ghaziabad
Uttar Pradesh
India

ISBN 978-3-030-65171-8   ISBN 978-3-030-65169-5   (eBook)
https://doi.org/10.1007/978-3-030-65169-5

This Springer imprint is published by the registered company Springer Nature Switzerland AG
The registered company address is: Gewerbestrasse 11, 6330 Cham, Switzerland

Foreword

We are in the digital age, and apparently we have been there since the mid-1970s according to the experts in that field. I graduated from dental school in 1970, and I can assure you that our education and experiences were entirely analog. Our preclinical laboratory was equipped with belt-driven handpieces, and we were just introduced to air-driven "high-speed" handpieces for patient care shortly thereafter. Our patient charts consisted of various sizes and colors of paper with (mostly) legible variations of written words, along with sometimes not fully processed radiographic films, some of which had come loose from their cardboard mountings. Our patient communication was either face-to-face, a hand-delivered letter, or a telephone call. There usually was no reliable way to leave a message since answering machines were seldom available or reliable. Our oral hygiene instructions consisted of the patient, sitting in our chair, holding a large mirror in one hand while we showed them how and where to brush with their other hand (the concept of flossing was coming in a few years). They dutifully followed our promptings, in between their drooling and awkwardness; and then they were sent home to try and comply. As a student, our only clue as to some form of digital information was large green bar pages and somewhat washed-out type showing our clinical progress. Those pages were somehow produced from our carbon-copied coupons that were signed off by an instructor when we completed the procedure. That transformation was mysterious, and I can only picture a clerk sitting at a console, inputting that information into an expensive mass of whirling discs and flashing lights, which then spit out the green bar paper.

My first several years in practice during the 1970s were equally analog, although we did produce some simple bulky videotapes about home care that we could playback for the patient, followed by some beautiful photographs of a sample of our restorative dentistry. Of course, the final single photo was the result of perhaps an entire roll of film. Our radiographs were still being processed in the darkroom with chemicals of questionable safety, and our diagnostic methods were based on our observations and semi-accurate measurements on plaster models. Our treatment planning used wax to approximate a recontoured tooth surface or to simulate restoring the space of a missing tooth.

Fast forward to the present day—dentistry and digitization have a happy relationship. The bits and bytes of our digitized dental information allow us easy storage and availability. It is now such a pleasure to record our examination findings: such items as periodontal data, hard and soft tissue images, pulp vitality tests, and radiographs are all instantly searchable and then displayed in organized areas of our computer's monitor. Gone are the days of trying to ensure the date and accurate number and of a pocket depth, our only remembering a possible enamel crack, or looking at a poorly developed radiograph.

In this book, you will read about the aspects of digitization in dentistry. Using the quality and detail of digitized examination categories, we can more easily decide on a diagnosis and then present treatment plan options to our patients. One example is our ability to use three-dimensional radiograph imaging to discover pathology as well as to analyze the site of an implant fixture placement. Another significant development is the digital impression. In the past, you waited several minutes while your less than relaxed patient tries to tolerate an awkward tray filled with runny material, with you both hoping for a usable impression. Now, in a few seconds, you can quickly analyze an optical impression with its remarkable detail, and your patient is comfortable. Dental surgical procedures, endodontic, orthodontic, periodontic, and restorative procedures all have digital components to aid in the delivery of those therapies. Esthetic procedures can be planned using digital aides on an image of the patient's own teeth, as well as capturing the various contours and shading to produce excellent and satisfying restorative results. Occlusion and temporomandibular joint function can be digitally analyzed, and then tooth surface modification and muscular therapy can be planned and further studied for stability.

Our digital instrumentation continues to improve and advance. Clearly computers are the primary example with increased speed, storage, touch screens, and wireless technology. Indeed, all our data can be accessed that information can be quickly, securely, and easily shared. Our patients could download their records, treatment recommendations, and our instructions; moreover, specialists can understand our referrals. Various other devices are enhanced with digital technology: measurement of endodontic canal lengths is very accurate, and dental lasers are calibrated and their emission energy is precisely controlled.

As in any book, the chapters and their authors have labored to produce the most current information available. However, the development, engineering, design, and manufacture of digital products and services will add to what we know and what we use. For example, three-dimensional non-radiologic imaging using lasers is being studied, and research into nanotechnology will certainly improve our dental materials as well as the pharmacological components of our medications. I can imagine having robotic assistance for some dental surgical procedures, such as gingival grafting or endodontic canal shaping. Moreover, I can dream about using virtual reality in our treatment proposals for esthetic procedures, where the patient actually "sees" the new smile before we proceed. In other words, this book is not the final version of our knowledge, but it is comprehensive for the present.

Looking back over my 50 years in dentistry, I know that our personal touch and communication still is relevant. Digitization has and will continue to aid us in delivering excellent dental care, enhancing our knowledge and experiences. This book will give you that information that will help you become a better dentist. Enjoy!

Donald J. Coluzzi
Department of Preventive and Restorative
Dental Sciences
University of California
San Francisco School of Dentistry
San Francisco, CA, USA

Preface

Dentists with decades of experience can clearly look back at the advances in dentistry, since the turn of the millennium, and state that the dental profession has experienced a tremendous amount of technological growth in the digital era. Digital dentistry could be defined as any dental technology or device that comes with digital or computer-controlled components in contrast to mechanical or electrical alone. This broad definition can range from the most common area of digital dentistry—CAD/CAM (computer-aided design/computer-aided manufacturing)—to the new treatment protocols that challenged the traditional methods like the invention of the turbine handpiece and dental implants.

The majority of the areas of dentistry (not exhaustive) which incorporate some type of digital components are as follows: caries diagnosis; CAD-CAM; Computer-aided implant dentistry—including design and fabrication of surgical guides; Digital radiography—intraoral and extraoral, including cone beam computed tomography (CBCT); Lasers; Occlusion and TMJ analysis and diagnosis; Digital Smile Designing; and Shade Matching. In order to be fully advantageous, digital dentistry should include improved efficiency (both cost and time), improved accuracy when compared to traditional methods, and a high level of predictability of positive outcomes. Digital intraoral impressions, digitally fabricated dentures, use of AI, storage of patient data, and the virtual patient are no longer fiction, but, in fact, is now a reality.

This new discipline of digital dentistry is now integrated in educational curriculum in dental schools and in routine clinical practice. Therefore, this comprehensive textbook on *Digitalization in Dentistry* details the digital technology available and describes its indications, contraindications, advantages, disadvantages, limitations, and clinical applications in all aspects of dentistry. The main focus of this textbook is the practical and clinical application of digital technology covering all aspects of dentistry. Available technologies, equipment, and devices are discussed in detail and explained on how they are incorporated in routine clinical practice.

The target audience for this book is a broad group of professionals and includes dental students, general dental practitioners, and specialists of all the dental disciplines. It may also be useful for dental technicians, dental assistants, dental radiographers, and hygienists interested in recent digital advances in the dental field. We hope that the reader will gain a comprehensive understanding of digital applications in dentistry. However, technology changes rapidly, and although every attempt has been made to discuss both the available and the developing technologies expected to be on the market in the future, the scope and list of areas are ever evolving.

There are many other areas of digital dentistry available, and many more are further being researched. Digital dentistry, when properly implemented and fully educated, can bring increased joy in practicing dentistry, and better care for the patients can be delivered.

Manila, Philippines   Priyanka Jain
Ghaziabad, India   Mansi Gupta

Acknowledgments

We would like to start by thanking and acknowledging the contributors to this book who dedicated their expertise, time, and talents to this project. Without their support, this project would not have been successful. Thank you for your hard work and patience.

Working with a talented, patient, and highly professional team at Springer has been an enriching experience. Some of the many people that we'd like to express our gratitude to include:

Alison Wolf

Niveka Somasundaram

And to the many more who helped those named above we extend a heartfelt *"Thank You"!*

We would also like to thank our parents, families, and friends, near and far, who supported us patiently throughout the many hours spent working on this.

We would also like to state that the Editors and authors have made every effort to obtain permission from copyright holders to reproduce material in this book and to acknowledge these sources correctly. However, any omissions brought to our attention are unintentional and will be remedied in future editions.

Contents

Artificial Intelligence and Big Data in Dentistry

1

Priyanka Jain and Catherine Wynne

1.1 Introduction

The profession of dentistry continuously demonstrates innovation and improvement on many fronts such as clinical applications, research, training, and education. This new era includes the broad array of technologies that brings the communication, documentation, manufacture, and delivery of dental therapy under the umbrella of computer-based algorithms. Digital dentistry can be defined as the use of any dental-related technology or device that is built-in digital or computer-controlled elements rather than operated electrically and/or mechanically alone.

Historically, digital advances have three foci: CAD/CAM systems, imaging, and practice/patient management systems. CEREC™, the first commercially available in-office CAD/CAM system made possible, the delivery of same-day restorations. Early drivers in imaging include both the intraoral imaging systems integral to the CERECTM system and evolutions in digital radiography. First introduced in the late 1980s, digital radiography has transformed the dental field, enhancing image quality, evolving from phosphor plates to solid-state detectors, cone beam computed tomography (CBCT), and new generations of digital impression taken with intraoral scanners. The development of cone beam computed tomography (CBCT) heralded a second wave of excitement as three-dimensional images of the craniofacial region offered new advantages in diagnostics and therapy. When iterative improvements in hardware, software, and materials merged in the early 2000s, new accomplishments in clinical dentistry were realized.

P. Jain (✉)
Professor, Department of Endodontics, National University College of Dentistry, Manila, Philippines

C. Wynne
University of Dundee, Dundee, Ireland

Practice management software makes possible capturing patient demographics, scheduling appointments, and generating reports. In parallel, electronic patient records, a digital version of patients' clinical information, motivated changes in tracking patients' health, facilitating quality of care assessments, and proved a resource for research, including evaluation of efficiency and efficacy of clinical procedures. In parallel, other technologies influenced and enabled innovations in digital dentistry, often at a remarkable pace. While not a comprehensive list, these technologies undoubtedly include sensor miniaturization, artificial intelligence, augmented and virtual reality, robotics, 3D printing, telehealth, Big Data, internet of things, nanotechnology, quantum computing, biomedical engineering, cost of data storage, connectivity, and others.

This chapter is an introduction to this book. As stated above, the list of digital technologies is not exhaustive, and every attempt has been made to include the most recent innovations to keep the reader up to date. However, technologies change and new innovations may already be on the market by the time this book goes into printing.

The chapter will review how digital dentistry has influenced different aspects of dentistry in brief. A major part of this introductory chapter will deal with the scope of Big Data and Artificial Intelligence, the two most recent advancements in digital dentistry.

While the scope of digital systems is immense, those discussed in this book focus primarily on those that have implications and opportunities for developments and innovations in clinical dentistry. Digitization, being so significant in the dental practice, needs to be understood well. The book serves as a contemporary reference considering the pros and cons of various technological progresses. The impact of digital technology in dentistry is immense, hence for ease its influence is considered under sections—the clinical aspect, laboratory procedures, training of students, patient motivation, practice management, and dental research (Table 1.1).

1.2   Recent Trends in Digitization

The digital transformation in dental medicine is recognized as one of the major innovation of the twenty-first century. The implementation of mobile technologies into the medical sector is fundamentally altering the ways in which healthcare is perceived, delivered, and consumed. The most recent trends and innovations of this new digital era, with potential to influence the direction of dentistry in the future, are: *(1) rapid prototyping (RP), (2) augmented and virtual reality (AR/VR), (3) artificial intelligence (AI) and machine learning (ML) for diagnostic analysis, (4) Big Data and analytics (personalized (dental) medicine and linkage of health data, mHealth, teledentistry, and development of electronic health records).*

The advancement and increased use of Internet and Communication Technologies (ICT), the rise of Big Data and algorithmic analysis, and the origin of the Internet of Things (IOT) are a multitude of interconnected innovations that are having a significant impact on today's society and affecting almost all spheres of our lives,

Table 1.1 Applications of digitization in dentistry

Aspect	
Role of digitization for training and research	Audiovisual aids
	Virtual simulators for surgical training
	Haptics
	Virtual dental patient (PerioSlim™)
	Digital material testing
Role of digitization in diagnosis and treatment planning	Digital radiography, CBCT
	Radiovisiography (RVG)
	Dental photography
	Diagnosing occlusal errors (T scan)
	Diagnosing TMJ disorders
	Big data analytics
Role of digitization in treatment	Digital impressions
	CAD CAM (restorations, tissue scaffolds, surgical
	Guides)
	Digital shade analysis
	Digital smile design
	Lasers
	Virtual articulators
	Teledentistry
	Research
	Robot-assisted treatments
Role of digitization for patient motivation and practice management	Intraoral camera
	Educational software
	Digital data (electronic health records, radiographs,
	Digital photographs, intraoral scans)
	Patient interactions (consultations, shared decisions, healthy behaviors)
Other activities	Epidemiology research

including medical science [1, 2]. Dentistry, as a branch of medicine, has not remained unaffected by the digital revolution. Research in the dental field on the effect of digitization is focused on both dental clinical practice and research.

Linkages of population health data could prove beneficial for research, such as assisting with the identification of unknown correlations of oral diseases with suspected and new contributing factors and furthering the creation of new treatment concepts [3]. Digital imaging can promote accurate tracking of the distribution and prevalence of oral diseases to improve healthcare service provisions [4]. New possibilities have opened up for automated processing in radiological imaging using artificial intelligence (AI) and machine learning (ML). AI can also be used to enhance the analysis of the relationship between prevention and treatment techniques in the field of oral health [5]. A digital or virtual dental patient, via 3D cone beam computed tomography (CBCT) and 3D-printed models, could be used for precise preoperative clinical assessment and simulation of treatment planning in dental practice [6, 7]. This topic is dealt with in great detail later in the book. With the use of smartphones and wearable technologies, mobile health (mHealth) applications are increasingly gaining popularity and being explored by healthcare providers and companies' provision of healthcare services [8].

It is important to keep in mind that since these technologies are still at the early phases of implementation and trials, technical issues and certain drawbacks might emerge. Basic science, clinical trials, and subsequently derived knowledge for innovative therapy protocols need to be redirected toward patient-centered outcomes, enabling the linkage of oral and general health instead of merely industry-oriented investigations [5]. For example, use of Big Data analytics and its applications and AI must be done systematically according to harmonized and inter-linkable data standards, otherwise issues of data managing and garbage data accumulation might arise [9]. AI for diagnostic purposes is still in the very early phases, and analysis of diverse and huge amounts of EHR (electronic health records) data still remains challenging [10]. In the simulation of a 3D virtual dental patient, dataset superimposition techniques are still in their experimental phase.

It needs to be understood that digital smart data and other technologies will not replace humans providing dental expertise and the capacity for patient empathy. The dental team that controls digital applications remains the key and will continue to play the central role in treating patients. In this context, the latest trend word created is *augmented intelligence*, that is, the meaningful combination of digital applications paired with human qualities and abilities in order to achieve improved dental and oral healthcare ensuring quality of life [11].

1.2.1   Rapid Prototyping (RP)

In dental medicine, several digital workflows for production processing have already been integrated into treatment protocols, especially in the rapidly growing branch of computer-aided design/computer-aided manufacturing (CAD/CAM), and rapid prototyping (RP) [12]. RP is a type of computer-aided manufacturing (CAM) and is one of the components of rapid manufacturing. RP is a technique to quickly and automatically construct three-dimensional (3D) models of a final product or a part of a whole using 3D printers. These 3D physical structures are known as rapid prototypes. RP technique allows visualization and testing of objects [13].

Rapid prototyping may be categorized into *additive method (widely used) and subtractive (less effective)*. The additive manufacturing process allows inexpensive production of complex 3D geometries from various materials and involves minimal material wastage [14]. The frequent technologies that are adopted in dental practice are selective laser sintering (SLS), stereolithography, inkjet-based system (3D printers [3DP]), and fused deposition modelling (FDM).

CAD and RP technologies are being used in various fields of medicine and dentistry. They have had a considerable impact especially on the rehabilitation of patients with head and neck defects, in fabrication of implant surgical guides, zirconia prosthesis and molds for metal castings, maxillofacial prosthesis and frameworks for fixed and removable partial dentures, and wax patterns for the dental prosthesis and complete denture.

In dentistry, one of the main difficulties today is the choice of materials. Commercially available materials (wax, plastic, ceramic, metal) commonly used for RP are currently permitted for short to medium-term intraoral retention only and not yet intended for definitive dental reconstructions [15].

RP has the potential for mass production of dental models, and also for the fabrication of implant surgical guides [16]. Production in large quantities at the same time in a reproducible and standardized way is an advantage in reducing the costs. It can also be used in 3D-printed models for dental education based on CBCT or micro CT. An initial study, however, has revealed that 3D-printed dental models can show changes in dimensional accuracy over periods of 4 weeks and longer. Further investigations comparing different 3D printers and material combinations are however still required [17]. The limitations of RP technology include complicated machinery and dependency on expertise to run the machinery during production in addition to the high cost of the tools.

Further research is currently focused on the development of printable materials for dental reconstructions, such as zirconium dioxide (ZrO_2) [18]. This different mode of fabrication of ZrO_2 structures could allow us to realize totally innovative geometries with hollow bodies that might be used, for example, for time-dependent low-dose release of anti-inflammatory agents in implant dentistry [19].

From a futuristic point, synthesis of biomaterials to artificially create lost tooth structures using RP technology could prove to be revolutionary [20]. Instead of using a preformed dental tooth databank, a patient-specific digital dental dataset could be acquired at the time of growth completion and used for future dental reconstructions. Furthermore, the entire tooth can be duplicated to serve as an individualized implant. RP technology can provide customized and tailored solutions to suit the specific needs of each patient. While the future looks promising from a technical and scientific point of view, it is not yet clear how RP and its products will be regulated.

1.2.2 Big Data

Information is the key for better practice and new innovations. The more information we have, the more we can arm and organize ourselves to deliver the best outcomes. Data collection plays an important role in this regard. In today's modern age, we produce and collect data about almost everything in our lives such as social activities, science, work, health etc., and this is increasing at a rapid pace. In a way, we can compare the present situation to a data deluge. The technological advances have helped us in generating more and more data, but we have seemed to reach a level where it has become unmanageable with currently available technologies. However, as the data has been getting bigger, our ability to transform and translate the data has also improved, and allowed us to move from reporting what has happened in the past (data reports or "descriptive analytics") to learning what is going to happen in the future (data science or "predictive analytics") [21].

This has led to the creation of the term "big data" to describe data that is large and unmanageable. In order to meet our present and future social needs, we need to develop new strategies to organize this data and to extract the information contained and transform the raw data into knowledge and derive meaningful information. One such need is healthcare. Like every other industry, healthcare is producing data at a tremendous rate that presents many advantages and challenges at the same time. "Big Data" begins to form when a group of data sets brought together become so large and complex that it begins to challenge contemporary data processing and analytical approaches. More data does not let us see more of the same but it allows us to see better, to see different, and to see something new.

Health data can be gathered from routine care and other sources such as social determinants of health, posts by patients on internet forums, surveys and questionnaires from patient support groups and patient diaries. Big Data collaborations involve interactions between a diverse range of stakeholders with varying analytical, technical, and political capabilities. Medical data has its uses in many areas of applications in healthcare, such as prognostic analysis and predictive modelling, identification of unknown correlations of diseases, clinical decision support, treatment concepts, public health surveys, and population-based clinical research, as well as the evaluation of healthcare systems [22].

Even though a number of definitions exist for Big Data, the most accepted is given by Douglas Laney who observed that (big) data was growing in three different dimensions, namely, volume (the amount of collected data), velocity (the speed of generated data), and variety (the source and type of data) (known as the 3 Vs) [23]. The "big" part of "big data" is indicative of its large volume. In addition to volume, the Big Data description also includes velocity and variety. These three Vs have become the standard definition of Big Data. Another accepted fourth V is "veracity" (the quality of incoming data) [24] (Table 1.2).

Table 1.2 What creates Big Data?

Data accumulation matters (velocity)	Indicates the speed or rate of data collection and making it accessible for further analysis Data accumulates expansively
Data quality matters (veracity)	Indicates the quality, authenticity, "trustworthiness" of data [25]. More data does not always give us more "value" Information from data becomes more valuable when the data is more reliable Data-driven decision-making requires accurate and reliable data
Data size matters (volume)	At its most elementary level, big data is about bringing datasets together There is no critical mass of data alone needed to make it "big."
Data complexity matters (variety)	Variety indicates the different types of organized and unorganized data that any firm or system can collect, such as video, audio files A mix of varying types and sources of data is needed to make it complex and large Data linkages are important

Biomedical Big Data amasses from different sources such as electronic health records, health research, wearable devices, and social media. The delay in reaping the benefits of biomedical Big Data in dentistry is mainly due to the slow adoption of electronic health record systems, unstructured clinical records, tattered communication between data silos, and perceiving oral health as a separate entity from general health. Recent recognition of the complex interaction between oral and general health has acknowledged the power of oral health Big Data on disease prevention and management.

This section will introduce the reader about the basics of Big Data and data analytics in dentistry related to different applications such as population data linkage, personalized medicine and electronic health records (EHRs), and mobile health (mHealth) and teledentistry.

1.2.2.1 Electronic Health Records (EHR) and Data Analytics

The electronic health record is a rich source of data that helps dentists monitor the health data of their patients and promote the sharing of information between various members of the healthcare team. EHRs have introduced many advantages for handling modern healthcare-related data. Dental professionals have access to the medical and dental history of the patient. This enables an improved care coordination and communication among healthcare providers and patients. Healthcare professionals have also found access over web-based and electronic platforms to improve their practices significantly using automatic reminders and prompts regarding follow-ups and appointments, and other periodic checkups. EHR enables faster data retrieval and helps provide access to millions of health-related medical information. EHR is further covered in Chap. 13. Table 1.3 gives its uses in dental practices.

National Institutes of Health (NIH) recently announced the "All of Us" initiative that aims to collect one million or more patients' data such as EHR, including medical imaging, socio-behavioral, and environmental data over the next few years [26].

Similar to EHR, an electronic dental record (EDR) stores the standard medical, dental, and clinical data gathered from the patients. EHRs, EDRs, personal health record (PHR), medical practice management software (MPM), and many other healthcare data components collectively have the potential to improve the quality, service efficiency, and costs of healthcare. The Big Data in healthcare includes the healthcare payer-provider data (such as EHR, EDR, pharmacy prescription,

Table 1.3 Uses of EHR

Uses of EHR in dental settings
• Maintain patient documentation and records
• Integration of digital technologies
• Clinical support tools
• Identification of gaps in care
• Access and storage of digital images
• Support for administrative tasks
• Evaluation of practice-based treatment outcomes

insurance records) along with the gene expression data and other data acquired from the smart web of Internet of things (IoT). The management and usage of such healthcare data is, however, dependent on information technology.

By analyzing Big Data, dentists can help patients improve health, diagnose the disease at an early stage, and also provide them with personalized dental care. But analyzing huge amounts of patient data manually is impossible. Big Data analytics help in analyzing this data, including personal patient data and demographic data, to identify which oral health problems recur repeatedly, thus helping the dental professionals in diagnosing and treatment planning. Also, by examining the medical and dental records, Big Data analytics can give dentists accurate insights into the oral health problems that are likely to occur in the future. In a nutshell, by analyzing real-time data, Big Data analytics help in revolutionizing the oral health of the population, thereby paving the way to precision medicine. Falling costs (per record) of digital data storage and the spread of low-cost and powerful statistic tools and techniques to extract patterns, correlations and interactions, are also making data analytics more usable and valuable in dental medicine. However, there remains barriers to its universal adoption and integration that still needs to be overcome.

Recent research has focused on the implementation of EHRs both in private practices and in dental education [27–29]. Cederberg and Valenza [28] argue that the use of digital records might compromise the doctor–patient relationship in the future, as easy access to all relevant information through digital means and forced focus on the computer screen could accustom both dentists and students to becoming more detached from patients. Big Data in the field of biomedical research is also useful as researchers analyze a large amount of data obtained from multiple experiments to gain novel insights. However, this poses issues of informed consent for both patients and research participants [30, 31].

Other ethical issues that arise from its use are data security, resulting in a breach of patient privacy and confidentiality [28, 32]. The legal issues surrounding health privacy, for example, sharing of data across national borders, creates hurdles for both individuals trying to access their own personal information as well as for biomedical researchers attempting to establish randomized controlled clinical trials. Therefore, dental biobanks with sensitive patient material, such as saliva, blood, and teeth, must be clarified, as these samples could be used for genetic analysis [33]. Data anonymization is a type of information sanitization where privacy protection is the single most intent. It is the process of either encoding or removing personally identifiable information from datasets. Anonymization methods include encryption, hashing, generalization, and pseudonymization. De-anonymization is the reverse engineering process used to detect the source data. The most common technique of de-anonymization is cross-referencing data from multiple sources [34].

The concept of "blockchain" is also gaining popularity in data sharing. It is a distributed ledger technology implemented in a decentralized manner used to record transactions [35]. Therefore, dentists can store their patients' records on a decentralized ledger, helping them save their money and time in having paper-based records. The records are kept across many computers such that data cannot be changed retroactively without the alteration of all subsequent blocks and collusion with the entire network [36]. Additionally, dentists and patients can reap the advantage of blockchain being "immutable," helping their records to be secure by offering distributed database, peer-to-peer transmission, transparency with pseudonymity, irreversibility of records, and computational logic [37].

Challenges associated with Big Data should also be considered at the same time, apart from data sharing. Storing large volume of data is one of the main challenges, and an on-site server network can be expensive to scale and difficult to maintain. The data needs to cleansed or scrubbed to ensure the accuracy, correctness, consistency, relevancy, and purity after acquisition. This cleaning process can be manual or automatized. Patients produce a huge volume of data that is not easy to capture with traditional HER format, as it is not easily manageable. It is too difficult to handle Big Data especially when it comes without a perfect data organization. A need to code all the clinically relevant information is required. As a result medical coding systems like International Classification of Diseases (ICD) code sets were developed. However, these come with their own limitations. Studies have observed various physical factors that can lead to altered data quality and misinterpretations from existing medical records [38]. Images often suffer technical barriers that involve multiple types of noise and artefacts. Improper handling of medical images can also cause tampering of images which may lead to delineation of anatomical structures.

1.2.2.2 Personalized Medicine and Data Linkages

Personalized medicine can change how dental research is conducted. Genomic sequencing and recent developments in medical imaging and regenerative technology have redefined personalized medicine to perform patient-specific precision healthcare [39, 40]. An interdisciplinary approach to dental patient sample analysis in which dentists, physicians, and nurses can collaborate to understand the interconnectivity of disease in a cost-effective way can be made possible [41]. Examining large population-based patient groups could detect unidentified correlations of diseases and create prognostic models for new treatment. Linkage of population-based data has changed the way epidemiological surveys in public health are conducted and will play a predominant role in future dental research. The linkage of individual patient data gathered from various sources enables the diagnosis of rare diseases, and completely novel strategies for research [32] helps to identify unknown correlations of diseases, prognostic factors, and newer treatment concepts, and to evaluate healthcare systems [42].

Register-based controlled (clinical) trials (RC(C)T) is a relatively new approach in dental research. These trials can provide comprehensive information on hard-to-reach populations and allow observations with minimal loss to follow-up. However, they require large sample sizes and generate high level of external validity. In the context of data linkage in dental practices and personalized medicine, research has shown that consent might be a significant issue concerning data usage as the patient cannot be completely informed about the ways in which the collected data is/will be used [43]. Data anonymization [44] and patient confiden-tiality [45] are other issues of data linkage. Therefore, the use of linked biomedi-cal data to support register-based research presents the challenge of disclosing sensitive information about individuals whose consent cannot be easily obtained in retrospect.

Individual dental disciplines (Prosthodontics, Restorative Dentistry, Periodontology, Oral Surgery, and Orthodontics) usually tend to work in isolation in academic dental institutions or large dental service providers. This can result in non-standardized diagnostics within the different departments. An integrated approach with standardized dental diagnostic protocols could enhance better patient flows and reduced overall treatment time and support interdisciplinary linked-therapy planning with improved quality, higher efficiency, and increased patient satisfaction [46]. Additionally, linking this standardized dental diagnostics with biomedical patient-level data could provide the information needed to better understand the epidemiology and etiological pathogenic pathways of oral diseases [47].

The collected data and information of population-based register-based controlled clinical trials RC(C)Ts can also provide an understanding of current and future applications of personalized dental medicine and help to improve prevention and rehabilitation concepts of oral diseases. In the future, private dental professionals together with academic dental institutions will increasingly generate digital data. A major challenge will be the compliance with quality standards in data acquisition, storage, and safe transfer. This will have an impact on the daily routine for the gen-eral dental practitioner [46].

1.2.2.3 Mobile Health (mHealth) and Teledentistry

Digital technologies are altering the ways in which healthcare is delivered and consumed. Tele-healthcare enables a convenient way for patients to increase self-care while potentially reducing office visits and travel time [48]. Considering the growing number of the elderly population with reduced mobility and/or nursing homestay, special-care patients, as well as people living in rural areas, these patient groups benefit significantly from teledentistry [49, 50]. Internet is the basis of modern systems of teledentistry, being able to transport large amounts of data. All new systems of teledentistry are internet-based. Changes within the past decade in the speed and method of data transfer have prompted clinicians and information technology experts to re-evaluate teledentistry as a highly valuable healthcare tool.

The practice of medicine using digital mobile devices, known as mHealth or mobile health, pervades different degrees of healthcare by finding ways to utilize mobile technologies for remotely measuring health and delivering healthcare and preventive health services. Newer mHealth technologies with embedded sensors require little attentional effort from the user and allow the unobtrusive collection of objective, high-resolution data on "real-world" health indicators and health behav-iors [51, 52].

The capabilities of mHealth have led to the development of personalized healthcare delivery models that shift the responsibility for personal health away from health systems toward the individuals. By allowing individuals to conveniently track and manage everything about their health, from blood pressure to glucose, the mHealth technology encourages individuals to be actively responsible for their own health, helps them understand their health status, and engages them in preventive behaviors while being guided by input from their health professionals. Furthermore, the remote monitoring abilities of mHealth technologies allows the professionals to proactively identify those at risk for an adverse health event and intervene in a timely manner.

The application of mHealth technology is of great relevance to dentistry. Most often, a patient's non-adherence to toothbrushing techniques recommended by dental professionals is misunderstood, forgotten, or even completely ignored [53]. The variety of brushing techniques recommended by dentists and dental associations also adds to the confusion among patients [54]. The gap between quality oral hygiene routines and what is actually practiced by individuals is further increased by the dentist's inability to monitor actual brushing behaviors and good oral hygiene practices at home. Newer mHealth-based technology platforms being developed allow unobtrusive, remote monitoring of toothbrushing behaviors in real-world settings and provide customized, titrated feedback (Fig. 1.1).

The Remote Oral Behaviors Assessment System (ROBAS) utilizes commercially available electronic toothbrushes and/or smart watches as data collection devices and captures key details of toothbrushing behaviors (when used, for how long, pressure applied, dental quadrants covered) in the home setting. The ecologically accurate data is collected and securely transmitted to a cloud server for subsequent analyses by appropriate statistical tools. Such a mHealth platform could serve as the basis of a scalable, interactive ecosystem that passively monitors OHRs, infers and predicts improper OHRs, and delivers engaging and timely personalized feedback to support quality OHRs by individuals [21].

Currently, brushing and flossing behaviors are recorded by measuring traditional oral hygiene indicators (i.e., dental plaque, periodontal inflammation, and caries) during a clinic visit in addition to patient self-reports of their toothbrushing practices. However, they become difficult when involving larger groups or populations, particularly those without regular access to dental services. Low-touch mHealth systems could help clarify the precise relationships between toothbrushing behaviors captured in the home environment and the health outcome (i.e., plaque and dental disease) assessed in the dental setting. By utilizing mHealth's real-time monitoring and feedback capacities, dental professionals would be better armed to stress upon the importance of correct and long-term adherence to oral hygiene practices and understand the determinants/predictors of why individuals do or do not engage in the prescribed oral hygiene practices [21]. Using mHealth systems in combination with oral hygiene practice measurement and feedback devices (i.e., electronic toothbrushes, smartphones) and back-ended by risk prediction and personalized

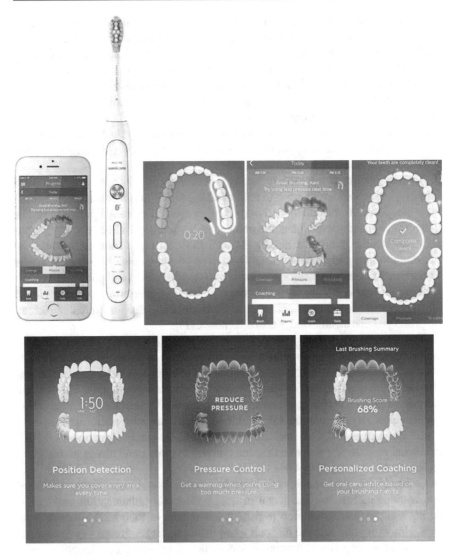

Fig. 1.1 Smart toothbrush and its working

intervention algorithms, digitally engaged patients would exert more control of their own oral health while providers would be able to provide quality patient-centered and value-based care.

As discussed previously for other Big Data clinical applications, issues of data security, patient anonymity [55, 56] and confidentiality [57] are primary concerns, as networked transfer through unsecure means could enable unwarranted third parties to obtain easier access to sensitive patient data. Cvkrel [56] argued that mHealth creates additional vulnerability as smartphones gather additional data that are usually not collected by healthcare practitioners (e.g., fitness data, sleep patterns), and, as it is an object of everyday use, it might be easily accessible to unauthorized people. Also, easy access through the smartphone to raw data including data related to dental care could be counterproductive and harmful for patients who might self-adjust the prescription given by the practitioner. mHealth can also have an impact on the patient's consent if not appropriately informed about all of the risks that teledentistry implies [57]. A 2015 WHO global survey revealed affordability, legal issues, evidence of cost-effectiveness, and lack of legislation or regulation as key barriers to mHealth adoption [58]. Beyond digital literacy and affordability, the ability of digital approaches to improve oral health practices and self-care ultimately depends on patient adoption and sustained engagement.

1.2.3   Artificial Intelligence (AI)

What is AI? AI can be seen as the intelligence of machines, that is, work performed by machine, in difference with the natural intelligence performed by humans [59, 60]. The term AI is mostly associated with robotics. It describes how intelligent systems (i.e., artificial intelligence) technology is used to develop a software or a machine that can easily mimic human intelligence and cognitive skills and perform specific activities like problem solving and learning. John McCarthy, a mathematician who coined the term artificial intelligence in 1955, is known as the father of artificial intelligence. He explained the potential of machines to perform tasks that can fall in the range of "intelligent" activities [61]. Therefore, AI can be defined as "a field of science and engineering concerned with the computational understanding of what is commonly called intelligent behavior, and with the creation of artefacts that exhibit such behaviour" [62]. Hence, this field deals with computational models that can think and act intelligently, like the human brain, and construct algorithms that can learn from data to make predictions.

With a significant increase in the patient data, electronic health records, its documentation and introduction of Big Data, AI in dentistry or medicine has started gaining popularity with the advent of data computing as well as cloud computing ability and availability of vast amount of data collected.

1.2.3.1 How Are Artificial Intelligence (AI) and Big Data Intertwined?
One of the advantages of AI is the ability for computers to "read" and "analyze" large amounts of data in a fraction of the time as opposed to a human. Having more reliable and current data to reference, dentists will soon be able to streamline decision-making in treatment while reducing errors. Specifically, AI can

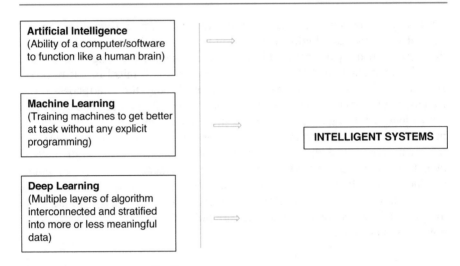

Fig. 1.2 Important aspects of intelligent systems

scan all records in a single practice to look for trends in the patient population and can further be integrated with electronic health systems already available.

In the field of dentistry, artificial intelligence is becoming important in radiology due to its ability to detect abnormalities in radiographic images that are unnoticed by the naked human eye, with more emphasis on diagnostic records in terms of digital IOPAs (Intraoral periapical), three-dimensional (3D) scans, and cone beam computed tomography (CBCT). Information can be gathered and computed to create an AI for aiding quick diagnosis and treatment planning. The existing literature reveals that intelligent systems have served as useful adjunctive tools for radiologists in the analysis of large quantities of diagnostic images with improved speed and accuracy [63–70]. They have the ability to detect abnormalities within images that may go unnoticed by the naked eye or to solve problems not resolved by human cognition.

To understand AI, it is important to know few of these key terminologies (Fig. 1.2). Basic introduction will be given to the principle behind AI. For detailed understanding of the mechanisms of AI, the reader may refer to a previously published literature.

1. Machine learning is a subfield of AI, which depends on algorithms to predict outcomes based on unseen data and without actually being programmed. Machine learning refers to the ability of machines to gain human-like

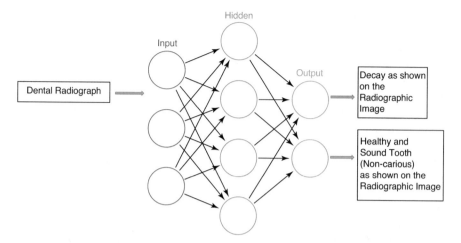

Fig. 1.3 Application of deep learning to detect caries on a radiographic image. The x-ray is imported to the computer as the input, and through the hidden layers the algorithms will classify the x-ray image as carious/sound tooth (as the output), based on AI

intelligence without explicit programming; that is, decisions are mostly data-driven rather than being strategically programmed for a certain task [71]. This helps to resolve issues without human input. For example, a machine learning (ML) algorithm can recognize or detect a lymph node in the head-and-neck image as normal or abnormal by analyzing thousands of such images which are labelled as normal or abnormal [72, 73].

2. A popular type of ML model are neural networks (NNs), artificial neural networks (ANNs). Neural networks are a set of algorithms that compute signals via artificial neurons. The purpose of neural networks is to create neural networks that function like the human brain, but with networks which are created on a computer. Hence, they can be engineered to solve a specific task like radiographic image showing a decayed tooth (Fig. 1.3).

3. Deep learning is a component of machine learning that utilizes the network with different and multiple layers (hence "deep") in a deep neural network to analyze the input data. The purpose of deep learning is to construct a neural network that automatically identifies patterns to improve feature detection [74]. In a more recent innovation, deep learning programs comprise convolutional neural networks that utilize self-learning back-propagation algorithms to learn directly from the data via end-to-end processes to make predictions [75]. These programs are mainly used for processing large and complex images such as 2D radiographs or 3D CT. This differentiates deep learning from machine learning, which builds algorithms directed by the data [76].

1.2.3.2 AI and its Applications in Dentistry

In diagnosis and treatment, neural networks (NNs) can be significant, particularly in diseases and conditions with multifactorial cause or without any precise etiology. An example is recurrent aphthous ulceration where clinical diagnosis is usually made on the basis of exclusion of other factors. In a study, data from 86 participants were used to construct and train a neural network to predict the factors appearing to be related to the occurrence of recurrent aphthous ulcers such as gender, hemoglobin, serum Vitamin B12, serum ferritin, red cell folate, salivary candidal colony count, and further retested with untrained data of 10 participants, to test the predictions [77]. AI can also be used for screening and classifying suspicious altered mucosa undergoing premalignant and malignant changes. Minute changes at single pixel level which might go unnoticed by the naked eye can also be detected.

Artificial intelligence can be used to predict a genetic predisposition for oral cancer for a large population [78]. Artificial neural networks (ANNs) are a promising tool for predicting the sizes of unerupted canines and premolars with greater accuracy in the mixed dentition period [79] and can also be optimized for predicting the tooth surface loss, which is a universal problem that involves an irreversible, multifactorial, non-carious, physiologic, pathologic, or functional loss of dental hard tissues [80].

In orthodontics, AI models have been used to assess the craniofacial skeletal and dental abnormalities in cephalometry followed by comparison with an expert opinion. The assessments were found to be equivalent. In addition, the model pointed out contradictions presented in the data that were not noticed by the orthodontists [81]. It can also be used to provide orthodontic consultations to general practitioners for the alignment of crowded lower teeth [82].

A study was conducted to construct an artificial intelligence expert system for the diagnosis of extractions using neural network machine learning and to evaluate the performance of this mode. This study suggested that artificial intelligence expert systems with neural network machine learning could be useful in orthodontics and can be used as a tool for making decisions in clinical practice [83].

Other studies have also demonstrated the application of AI technologies in interpretation of cephalometric radiographs and identifying the landmarks. Studies conducted by Kunz et al. [84] and Hwang et al. [85] showed great accuracy in identifying the landmarks similar to the trained human eye using a specialized artificial intelligence (AI) algorithm and deep learning-based automated identification system, respectively. Furthermore, Choi et al. reported the use of new artificial intelligence model to decide the case for surgery/non-surgery using the lateral cephalometric radiographs. The results showed that the AI system was effective with 96% success rate in diagnosing the surgery/non-surgery cases [86].

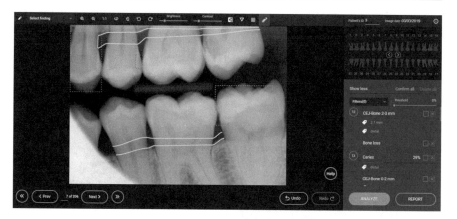

Fig. 1.4 Bitewing analysis with AI highlighting bone loss >2 mm as well as a line highlighting the bone ridge and between CEJs *(Reproduced with permission from Denti.AI)*

In prosthetic dentistry, use of AI can guide the dental professional during the procedure of making a digital impression [87]. Factors such as facial measurements, ethnicity, and patient preferences need to be taken into account while creating an esthetic prosthesis. All these factors (and more) can be integrated by the use of a design assistant, which uses AI (RaPid). RaPiD integrates computer-aided design (CAD), knowledge-based systems and databases, and recruits a logic-based information as a unifying medium [88].

In the field of periodontics, Lee et al. developed an architecture and predicted that the accuracy of detecting periodontitis in premolars and molars was 81.0% and 76.7%, respectively [63]. A model which successfully distinguishes between inflamed and healthy gingiva has also been demonstrated [83]. ANN can also effectively be used in classifying patients into aggressive periodontitis and chronic periodontitis group based on their immune response profile by using parameters, like leukocyte counts in peripheral blood [89]. Yauney et al. used an AI-based system based on CNNs for correlating poor periodontal health with systemic health outcomes and reported that AI can be used for automated diagnoses and for screening other diseases [90]. Figure 1.4 shows the use of AI in the estimation of bone loss.

In endodontics, AI assessments can be used to detect vertical root fractures on CBCT images and radiographs. A study by Johari et al. using probabilistic neural network (PNN) displayed excellent performance with an accuracy of 96.6% for the diagnosis of vertical root fractures [91]. Saghiri et al. used artificial neural network (ANN) system in determining the working length [92] and for location of minor apical foramen [93]. The results showed accuracy of 96% and 93%, respectively. Figure 1.5 shows the use of AI for endodontic visualization.

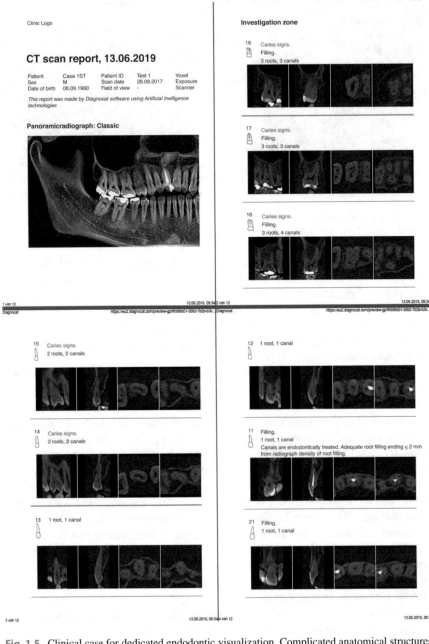

Fig. 1.5 Clinical case for dedicated endodontic visualization. Complicated anatomical structures of root canal systems in endodontics require careful studying of the image. A 32-year-old male patient was referred for undefined pain in the maxillary anterior. The medical and dental history was without pathological findings. Uploading the dataset to the AI software, defining the region of interest (ROI), by selecting tooth #11, all images (roots, canals, periapical region) were visualized accordingly. A hyperdense tooth-like structure could be visualized apical to tooth 11. The diagnosis of supernumerary tooth (mesiodens) could be made. The patient received the medical report and was sent back to the referring clinic for further treatment (*Courtesy Oral Health and Dr Jörg Mudrak*)

With respect to treatment planning, the neural networks when optimally trained with respect to lower third molars were found to have high specificity and sensitivity equivalent to specialist consultation in categorizing tooth to "gold standard" [94].

Other ingenious applications of AI include "bioprinting" where living tissue and even organs can be constructed in consecutive thin layers of cells, which in the future may be used for reconstruction of oral hard and soft tissues which are lost due to pathological or accidental reasons and robotic surgery, where robotic surgeons perform semiautomated surgical tasks with increasing efficiency under the guidance of an expert surgeon [72].

Most of the published literature and research on AI is focused on models that rely on convolutional neural networks (CNNs) and artificial neural networks (ANNs). These AI models have been used in detection and diagnosis of dental caries, vertical root fractures, apical lesions, salivary gland diseases, maxillary sinusitis, maxillofacial cysts, cervical lymph nodes metastasis, osteoporosis, cancerous lesions, alveolar bone loss, predicting orthodontic extractions, need for orthodontic treatments, cephalometric analysis, age and gender determination. These studies indicate that the performance of an AI-based automated system is excellent. They mimic the precision and accuracy of trained specialists; in some studies, it was found that these systems were even able to outmatch dental specialists in terms of performance and accuracy [95].

Despite all the potential, AI solutions have not by large entered routine medical and dental practice, education, and research in its full capacity. In dentistry, convolutional NNs have been adopted in research settings only from 2015 onwards, mainly on dental radiographs, and the first applications involving these technologies are now entering the clinical arena [96]. As with every technological advancement, AI also has its own sets of limitations such as the complexity of the mechanism, the cost involved, and the large amount of data required for training and precision. Medical and dental data are not as easily available and accessible as other data, due to data protection concerns. Datasets lack structure and are often relatively small, at least when compared with other datasets in the AI realm. Data on each patient are complex, multidimensional, and sensitive, with limited options for triangulating or validating them. Medical and dental data from electronic medical records show low variable completeness with data often missing systematically and not at random. Moreover, questions toward responsibilities and transparency remain. Figure 1.6 shows AI technology in use for caries detection, while Fig. 1.7 depicts the smart margin. Figures 1.8 and 1.9 show the use of AI and its clinical applications in other areas of dentistry.

Digital dentistry, like any other new innovation, also comes with its own share of risks, as we have already seen in this chapter. It is only by finding the solutions to these challenges can the technologies be fully accepted and integrated in the field for long-term use. Table 1.4 addresses these challenges and provides some recommendations.

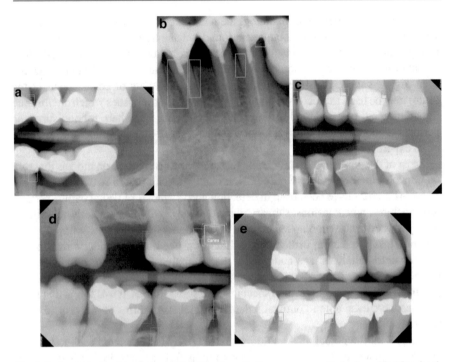

Fig. 1.6 (**a–e**) Caries detection and identification of other common pathologies with AI technology (*Image Courtesy- Pearl Inc.*)

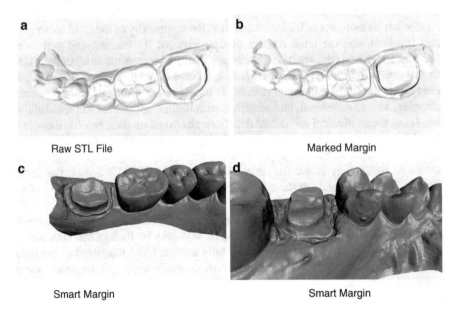

Fig. 1.7 AI for crown preparation—Smart Margin (*Image courtesy- Pearl Inc.*). (**a, b**) Automated margin marking done **by AI in seconds.** It provides better margin accuracy and clinical outcome with minimal to no human interaction required for laboratories or in-house milling and has the potential for hundreds of thousands of margins completed each day automatically. (**c, d**) Margin detection using AI technology. AI can be used to mark a margin before sending to the laboratory

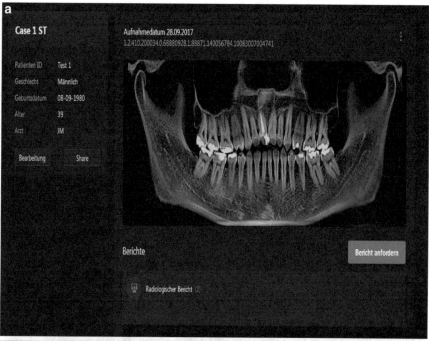

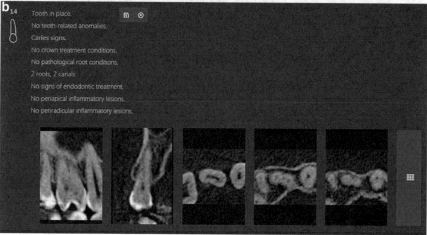

Fig. 1.8 Oral structures description including differential diagnoses. Selection of dedicated images to support individualized therapeutic planning (AI technology can be used for differential diagnosis in its generated description. This limits the time spent for analysis and provides hints to possible pathological processes, even if those where not primarily indicated. (**a**) Diagnocat—an AI software—analyzes the acquired CBCT in DICOM format (a standard format in medical imaging) enabling a smooth data transfer. (**b**) A neural network, while processing DICOM files of CT images, finds and segments the main anatomical regions (jaws, teeth, periapical lesions). Diagnocat identifies various conditions and disorders by assessing 50 signs (normal appearance, filling, crown, treated root canal, implant, sign of periapical lesion, etc.) and selects dedicated images to support an individualized therapeutic planning) (***Courtesy Oral Health and Dr Jörg Mudrak***)

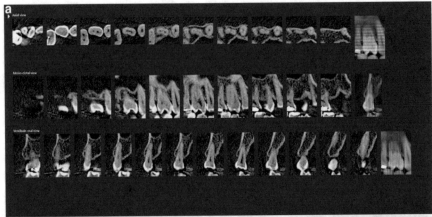

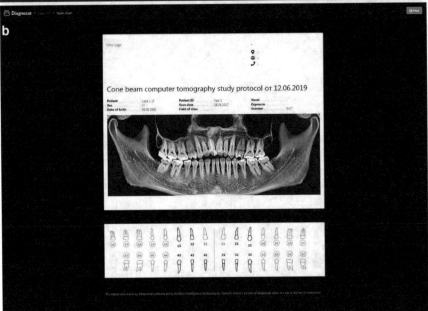

Fig. 1.9 (**a, b**) Using AI Software (Diagnocat) for clinical cases. Apart from a panoramic image, the patient report contains the dental chart with annotation in color on the teeth with findings requiring the patient's attention marked in red. (***Courtesy Oral Health and Dr Jörg Mudrak***). (**a**) Panoramic view of various thicknesses. (**b**) Set of slices in three planes for each tooth

Table 1.4 Digital dentistry: ethical challenges and implications

Challenges	Issues	Issues addressed
Big data	Data security (sharing, storage, and use) Risk of data manipulation (digital double) [97] Falsification of data (e.g., digital dental radiographs)	Data privacy guidelines must be observed Data storage should be compatible with data privacy laws [98, 99]
Dental professional–patient relationship	Threats to the traditional direct two-way relationship	Maintain interaction and empathy with the patient Other opportunities, i.e., decision-making systems help make fewer misjudgments, electronic records reduce the administrative work, and thereby can concentrate more on the patient, teledentistry can increase access to care [100, 101], improved communication via aids, and patient education
Digital literacy	Dental professional (need for continuous willingness to learn about the technology to be used) Patient (need for a sufficient understanding of the technology to be used)	Both practitioners and patients must be able to cope with the digital technology to be applied, whether as users or recipients
Clinical evidence (or lack of)	Lack of clinical trials in many digital technologies in dentistry (evidence gap) replacement/upgrading of systems and software by follow-up systems before completion of ongoing trials [97]	Research should focus on randomized controlled trials Which assess comprehensively the advantages and disadvantages of the digital technology and its protocols

1.3 Conclusion

The usage of digital technology in dentistry is growing rapidly. Ongoing and further research should be integrated with clinical practice for better results. It should not be implied that digital smart data technologies will replace humans and their capacity for patient empathy. The collection, storage, and analysis of digitized biomedical patient data poses several challenges. In addition to technical aspects for the handling of huge amounts of data, an ethical and meaningful policy must ensure the protection of patient data for safety and management.

However, the benefits of digital applications will complement human qualities and abilities in order to achieve improved and cost-efficient healthcare for patients. Augmented intelligence based on Big Data will help to reduce the incidence of misdiagnosis and provide other more useful insights quickly, accurately, and easily. This is all achievable without losing the human touch.

References

1. Lynch C. How do your data grow? Nature. 2008;455:28–9.
2. Boyd D, Crawford K. Critical questions for big data. Info Commun Soc. 2012;15:662–79.
3. Joda T, Waltimo T, Pauli-Magnus C, Probst-Hensch N, Zitzmann NU. Population-based linkage of big data in dental research. Int J Environ Res Public Health. 2018;15:2357.
4. Hogan R, Goodwin M, Boothman N, Iafolla T, Pretty IA. Further opportunities for digital imaging in dental epidemiology. J Dent. 2018;74:S2–9.
5. Joda T, Waltimo T, Probst-Hensch N, Pauli-Magnus C, Zitzmann NU. Health data in dentistry: an attempt to master the digital challenge. Public Health Genomics. 2019;22:1–7.
6. Vandenberghe B. The digital patient—imaging science in dentistry. J Dent. 2018;74:S21–6.
7. Joda T, Wolfart S, Reich S, Zitzmann NU. Virtual dental patient: how long until It's here? Curr Oral Health Rep. 2018;5:116–20.
8. Nilsen WJ, Kumar S, Shar A, Varoquiers C, Wiley T, Riley WT, Pavel M, Atienza AA. Advancing the science of mHealth. J Health Commun. 2012;17:5–10.
9. Brodt ED, Skelly AC, Dettori JR, Hashimoto RE. Administrative database studies: goldmine or goose chase? Evid Based Spine Care J. 2014;5:74–6.
10. Liang H, Tsui BY, Ni H, Valentim CCS, Baxter SL, Liu G, Cai W, Kermany DS, Sun X, Chen J, et al. Evaluation and accurate diagnoses of paediatric diseases using artificial intelligence. Nat Med. 2019;25:433–8.
11. Joda T, Bornstein MM, Jung RE, Ferrari M, Waltimo T, Zitzmann NU. Recent trends and future direction of dental research in the digital era. Int J Environ Res Public Health. 2020;17:1987.
12. Wataha JC, Messer RL. Casting alloys. Dent Clin N Am. 2004;48:vii–viii. 499-512
13. Winder J, Bibb R. Medical rapid prototyping technologies: state of the art and current limitations for application in oral and maxillofacial surgery. J Oral Maxillofac Surg. 2005;63:1006–15.
14. Joda T, Ferrari M, Gallucci GO, Wittenben J-G, Bragger U. Digital technology in fixed implant prosthodontics. Periodontol. 2017;73:178–92.
15. Azari A, Nikzad S. The evolution of rapid prototyping in dentistry: a review. Rapid Prototyp J. 2009;15:216–25.
16. Dawood A, Marti B, Sauret-Jackson V, Darwood A. 3D printing in dentistry. Br Dent J. 2015;219:521–9.
17. Lech G, Nordström E. Dimensional stability of 3D printed dental models. Master's Thesis, Malmö University Electronic Publishing, Malmö, Sweden 2018.
18. Galantea R, Figueiredo-Pinaa CG, Serro AP. Additive manufacturing of ceramics for dental applications: a review. Dent Mater. 2019;35:825–46.
19. Zocca A, Colombo P, Gomes CM, Gunster J. Additive manufacturing of ceramics: issues, potentialities, and opportunities. J Am Ceram Soc. 2015;98:1983–2001.
20. Bose S, Ke D, Sahasrabudhe H, Bandyopadhyay A. Additive manufacturing of biomaterials. Prog Mater Sci. 2018;93:45–111.
21. Shetty V, Yamamoto J, Yale K. Re-architecting oral healthcare for the 21st century. J Dent. 2018;74(Suppl 1):S10–4. https://doi.org/10.1016/j.jdent.2018.04.017.
22. Lee CH, Yoon HJ. Medical big data: promise and challenges. Kidney Res Clin Pract. 2017;36(1):3–11.
23. Laney D. 3D data management: controlling data volume, velocity, and variety, application delivery strategies. Stamford: META Group Inc; 2001.

24. Mauro AD, Greco M, Grimaldi M. A formal definition of big data based on its essential features. Libr Rev. 2016;65(3):122–35.
25. McAfee A, Brynjolfsson E. Big data: the management revolution. Harv Bus Rev. 2012;90:60–6. 68, 128
26. https://allofus.nih.gov/.
27. Boden DF. What guidance is there for ethical records transfer and fee charges? J Am Dent Assoc. 2008;139:197–8.
28. Cederberg RA, Valenza JA. Ethics and the electronic health record in dental school clinics. J Dent Educ. 2012;76:584–9.
29. Szekely DG, Milam S, AKhademi J. Legal issues of the electronic dental record: security and confidentiality. J Dent Educ. 1996;60:19–23.
30. Ioannidis JP. Informed consent, big data, and the oxymoron of research that is not research. Am J Bioeth. 2013;13:40–2.
31. Martani A, Geneviève LD, Pauli-Magnus C, McLennan S, Elger BS. Regulating the secondary use of data for research: arguments against genetic exceptionalism. Front Genet. 2019;10:1254.
32. Cederberg R, Walji M, Valenza J. Electronic health records in dentistry: clinical challenges and ethical issues. Cham, Switzerland: Springer Science and Business Media LLC; 2014. p. 1–12.
33. Benitez K, Malin B. Evaluating re-identification risks with respect to the HIPAA privacy rule. J Am Med Inform Assoc. 2010;17(2):169–77.
34. Kelman CW, Bass AJ, Holman CD. Research use of linked health data—a best practice protocol. Aust N Z J Public Health. 2002;26(3):251–5.
35. Cunningham J, Ainsworth J. Enabling patient control of personal electronic health records through distributed ledger technology. Stud Health Technol Inform. 2017;245:45–8.
36. Till BM, Peters AW, Afshar S, Meara J. From blockchain technology to global health equity: can cryptocurrencies finance universal health coverage? BMJ Glob Health. 2017;2(4):e000570.
37. Angraal S, Krumholz HM, Schulz WL. Blockchain technology: applications in health care. Circ Cardiovasc Qual Outcomes. 2017;10(9):e003800.
38. Belle A, et al. Big data analytics in healthcare. Biomed Res Int. 2015;2015:370194.
39. Garcia I, Kuska R, Somerman MJ. Expanding the foundation for personalized medicine: implications and challenges for dentistry. J Dent Res. 2013;92:3–10.
40. Marrazzo P, Paduano F, Palmieri F, Marrelli M, Tatullo M. Highly efficient in vitro reparative behaviour of dental pulp stem cells cultured with standardized platelet lysate. Stem Cells Int. 2016;2016:7230987.
41. Di Sanzo M, Borro M, La Russa R, Cipolloni L, Santurro A, Scopetti M, Simmaco M, Frati P. Clinical applications of personalized medicine: a new paradigm and challenge. Curr Pharm Biotechnol. 2017;18:194–203.
42. Jorm L. Routinely collected data as a strategic resource for research: priorities for methods and workforce. Public Health Res Pract. 2015;25:e2541540.
43. Zijlstra-Shaw S, Stokes CW. Learning analytics and dental education; choices and challenges. Eur J Dent Educ. 2018;22:e658–60.
44. Day PF, Petherick E, Godson J, Owen J, Douglas G. A feasibility study to explore the governance processes required for linkage between dental epidemiological, and birth cohort, data in the UK. Community Dent Health. 2018;35:228–34.
45. Eng G, Chen A, Vess T, Ginsburg GS. Genome technologies and personalized dental medicine. Oral Dis. 2011;18:223–35.
46. Glick M. Taking a byte out of big data. J Am Dent Assoc. 2015;146:793–4.
47. Aldridge RW, Shaji K, Hayward AC, Abubakar I. Accuracy of probabilistic linkage using the enhanced matching system for public health and epidemiological studies. PLoS One. 2015;10:e0136179.
48. Wang S, Parsons M, Stone-McLean J, Rogers P, Boyd S, Hoover K, Meruvis-Pastor O, Gong M, Smith A. Augmented reality as a telemedicine platform for remote procedural training. Sensors. 2017;17:2294.
49. Jampani ND, Nutalapati R, Dontula BS, Boyapati R. Applications of teledentistry: a literature review and update. J Int Soc Prev Community Dent. 2011;1:37–44.

50. Estai M, Kruger E, Tennant M, Bunt S, Kanagasingam Y. Challenges in the uptake of telemedicine in dentistry. Rural Remote Health. 2016;16:3915.
51. Kumar S, Nilsen W, Pavel M, Srivastava M. Mobile health: revolutionizing healthcare through transdisciplinary research. Computer. 2013;46:28–35.
52. Nilsen W, Kumar S, Shar A, Varoquiers C, Wiley T, Riley WT, Pavel M, Atienza AA. Advancing the science of mHealth. J Health Commun. 2012;17:5–10. https://doi.org/10.1080/1081073 0.2012.677394.
53. Weinstein P, Milgrom P, Melnick S, Beach B, Spadafora A. How effective is oral hygiene instruction? Results after 6 and 24 weeks. J Public Health Dent. 1989;49:32–8. https://doi.org/10.1111/j.1752-7325.1989.tb02017.x.
54. Wainwright J, Sheiham A. An analysis of methods of toothbrushing recommended by dental associations, toothpaste and toothbrush companies and in dental texts. Br Dent J. 2014;217:E5. https://doi.org/10.1038/sj.bdj.2014.651.
55. Da Costa ALP, Silva AA, Pereira CB. Tele-orthodontics: tool aid to clinical practice and continuing education. Dental Press J Orthod Rev. 2012;16:15–21.
56. Cvrkel T. The ethics of mHealth: moving forward. J Dent. 2018;74:S15–20.
57. Nutalapati R, Boyapati R, Jampani ND, Dontula BSK. Applications of teledentistry: a literature review and update. J Int Soc Prev Community Dent. 2011;1:37–44.
58. World Health Organization. From innovation to implementation, eHealth in the WHO European Region. 2016.
59. Deshmukh SV. Artificial intelligence in dentistry. J Int Clin Dent Res Organ. 2018; 10:47–8.
60. Park WJ, Park JB. History and application of artificial neural networks in dentistry. Eur J Dent. 2018;12:594–601.
61. Rajaraman V. John McCarthy father of artificial intelligence. Reson. 2014:198e207.
62. Ramesh AN, Kambhampati C, Monson JRT, Drew PJ. Artificial intelligence in medicine. Ann R Coll Surg Engl. 2004;86:334–8.
63. Lee JH, Kim DH, Jeong SN, Choi SH. Diagnosis and prediction of periodontally compromised teeth using a deep learning- based convolutional neural network algorithm. J Periodontal Implant Sci. 2018;48:114–23.
64. Lee JH, Kim DH, Jeong SN, Choi SH. Detection and diagnosis of dental caries using a deep learning-based convolutional neural network algorithm. J Dent. 2018;77:106–11.
65. Vinayahalingam S, Xi T, Bergé S, Maal T, de Jong G. Automated detection of third molars and mandibular nerve by deep learning. Sci Rep. 2019;9:9007.
66. Hiraiwa T, Ariji Y, Fukuda M, Kise Y, Nakata K, Katsumata A, et al. A deep-learning artificial intelligence system for assessment of root morphology of the mandibular first molar on panoramic radiography. Dentomaxillofac Radiol. 2019;48:20180218.
67. Tuzoff DV, Tuzova LN, Bornstein MM, Krasnov AS, Kharchenko MA, Nikolenko SI, et al. Tooth detection and numbering in panoramic radiographs using convolutional neural networks. Dentomaxillofac Radiol. 2019;48:20180051.
68. Krois J, Ekert T, Meinhold L, Golla T, Kharbot B, Wittemeier A, et al. Deep learning for the radiographic detection of periodontal bone loss. Sci Rep. 2019;8:8995.
69. Ariji Y, Fukuda M, Kise Y, Nozawa M, Yanashita Y, Fujita H, et al. Contrast-enhanced computed tomography image assessment of cervical lymph node metastasis in patients with oral cancer by using a deep learning system of artificial intelligence. Oral Surg Oral Med Oral Pathol Oral Radiol. 2019;127:458–63.
70. Kim DW, Lee S, Kwon S, Nam W, Cha IH, Kim HJ. Deep learning-based survival prediction of oral cancer patients. Sci Rep. 2019;9:6994.
71. Das S, Dey A, Pal A, Roy N. Applications of artificial intelligence in machine learning: review and prospect. Int J Comput Appl. 2015;115:31–41.
72. Khanna SS, Dhaimade PA. Artificial intelligence: transforming dentistry today. Indian J Basic Appl Med Res. 2017;6:161–7.
73. Hwang JJ, Sergei A, Efros AA, Yu SX. Learning Beyond Human Expertise with Generative Models for Dental Restoration. CoRR abs/1804.00064; 2018.

74. Akst J. A primer: artificial intelligence versus neural networks. Inspiring Innovation: The Scientist Exploring Life, 2019: 65802.
75. Hopfield JJ. Neural networks and physical systems with emergent collective computational abilities. Proc Natl Acad Sci U S A. 1982;79:2554–8.
76. Doi K. Computer aided diagnosis in medical imaging: historical review, current status, and future potential. Comput Med Imaging Graph. 2007;31:198–211.
77. Dar-Odeh NS, Alsmadi OM, Bakri F, Abu-Hammour Z, Shehabi AA, Al-Omiri MK, et al. Predicting recurrent aphthous ulceration using genetic algorithms-optimized neural networks. Adv Appl Bioinforma Chem. 2010;3:7–13.
78. Majumdar B, Saroda SC, Saroda GS, Patil S. Technology: artificial intelligence. BDJ. 2018;224:916.
79. Moghimi S, Talebi M, Parisay I. Design and implementation of a hybrid genetic algorithm and artificial neural network system for predicting the sizes of unerupted canines and premolars. Eur J Orthod. 2011;34:480–6.
80. Al Haidan A, Abu-Hammad O, Dar-Odeh N. Predicting tooth surface loss using genetic algorithms-optimized artificial neural networks. Comput Math Methods Med. 2014;2014:1–7.
81. Mario MC, Abe JM, Ortega NR. Paraconsistent artificial neural network as auxiliary in cephalometric diagnosis. Artif Organs. 2010;34:E215–21.
82. Williams JS, Matthewman A, Brown D. An orthodontic expert system. Fuzzy Sets Syst. 1989;30:121–33.
83. Chen YC, Hong DJ, Wu CW, Mupparapu M. The use of deep convolutional neural networks in biomedical imaging: a review. J Orofac Sci. 2019;11:3–10.
84. Kunz F, Stellzig-Eisenhauer A, Zeman F, Boldt J. Artificial intelligence in orthodontics: evaluation of a fully automated cephalometric analysis using a customized convolutional neural network. J Orofac Orthop. 2020;81:52e68.
85. Hwang HW, Park JH, Moon JH, et al. Automated identification of cephalometric landmarks: part 2-might it be better than human? Angle Orthod. 2020;90:69e76.
86. Choi HI, Jung SK, Baek SH, et al. Artificial intelligent model with neural network machine learning for the diagnosis of orthognathic surgery. J Craniofac Surg. 2019;30:1986e9.
87. Khanna S. Artificial intelligence: contemporary applications and future compass. Int Dent J. 2010;60:269–72.
88. Alexander B, John S. Artificial intelligence in dentistry: current concepts and a peep into the future. Int J Adv Res. 2018;6:1105–8.
89. Papantonopoulos G, Takahashi K, Bountis T, Loos BG. Artificial neural networks for the diagnosis of aggressive periodontitis trained by immunologic parameters. PLoS One. 2014;9:e89757.
90. Yauney G, Rana A, Wong LC, Javia P, Muftu A, Shah P. Automated process incorporating machine learning segmentation and correlation of oral diseases with systemic health. EMBC 2019:3387e93.
91. Johari M, Esmaeili F, Andalib A, Garjani S, Saberkari H. Detection of vertical root fractures in intact and endodontically treated premolar teeth by designing a probabilistic neural network: an ex vivo study. Dentomaxillofac Radiol. 2017;46:20160107.
92. Saghiri MA, Asgar K, Boukani KK, et al. A new approach for locating the minor apical foramen using an artificial neural network. Int Endod J. 2012;45:257e65.
93. Saghiri MA, Garcia-Godoy F, Gutmann JL, Lotfi M, Asgar K. The reliability of artificial neural network in locating minor apical foramen: a cadaver study. J Endod. 2012;38:1130e4.
94. Brickley MR, Shepherd JP, Armstrong RA. Neural networks: a new technique for development of decision support systems in dentistry. J Dent. 1998;26:305–9.
95. Khanagar SB, et al. Developments, application, and performance of artificial intelligence in dentistry- a systematic review. J Dent Sci. https://doi.org/10.1016/j.jds.2020.06.019.
96. Schwendicke F, Golla T, Dreher M, Krois J. Convolutional neural networks for dental image diagnostics: a scoping review. J Dent. 2019;91:103226.
97. Gross D, Gross K, Wilhelmy S. Digitalization in dentistry: ethical challenges and implications. Quintessence International 2019. General Dentistry. Volume 50; number 10.

98. Leake N, Baxter T. Big data: storage, sharing and usage. In: Rekow D, editor. Digital dentistry. A comprehensive reference and preview of the future. Berlin: Quintessence Publishing; 2018. p. 335–53.
99. Goertz D. Digital practice: curse or blessing [in German]? DZW Spec. 2016;1:38–9.
100. Schweikardt C, Gross D. Technologized medicine- dehumanized medicine? Introductory thoughts [in German]. In: Brukamp K, Laryionava K, Schweikardt C, Gross D, editors. Technologized medicine- dehumanized medicine? Ethical, legal and social aspects of new medical technologies [in German]. Kassel: Kassel University Press; 2011. p. 7–11.
101. Kumar S, editor. Teledentistry. Cham: Springer; 2015.

Digital Diagnosis and Treatment Planning

2

Mansi Gupta

2.1 Introduction

It is very important to form diagnosis, if we want to manage a problem accurately. Over the years, there has been tremendous advancement that help to make the diagnosis and then design our treatment plan. Now is the age of virtual reality. The "godfather" of digital dentistry is the French Professor Francois Duret, who invented dental CAD CAM in 1973. The new image reconstruction techniques provide a faster and more accurate workflow.

Conventional techniques in dentistry have worked successfully for decades and is still being used effectively. However, to keep with the changing technologies and for a faster, more accurate, and more efficient workflow, there is a large potential in digital dentistry. There are many areas of digital dentistry available, and many more are being researched. Some (but not limited to) of the commonly used techniques are as follows:

1. Digital radiography.
2. Intraoral imaging and computer-aided design/computer-aided manufacturing (CAD/CAM).
3. Shade matching and digital smile designing.
4. Virtual articulators and digital face bows.
5. Lasers.
6. Occlusion and temporomandibular joint (TMJ) analysis and diagnosis.
7. Digital diagnosis for orthodontic treatment.
8. Digital photography.
9. Patient's data storage and transfer.
10. Patient's education and communication.

M. Gupta (✉)
Department of Prosthodontics, Indraprastha Dental College, Ghaziabad, India

© Springer Nature Switzerland AG 2021
P. Jain, M. Gupta (eds.), *Digitization in Dentistry*,
https://doi.org/10.1007/978-3-030-65169-5_2

Currently, digital dentistry is an umbrella topic that covers almost all the areas of dental specialties ranging from diagnosis, record keeping, surgical aspects, and computer-aided design or computer-aided manufacturing (CAD/CAM), and 3D printers. While each aspect is important in its own way, it is their incorporation as a whole that makes dental care effective and successful. Most of the topics mentioned above will be covered separately in great detail as individual chapters in this book. This chapter will only deal in detail about topics that are not covered elsewhere in the book. Others will be introduced and touched upon briefly.

2.2 Caries Detection Methods

It is important to detect caries as early as possible to reverse/halt the carious process or to restore the tooth in a most conservative manner. While the explorer is still widely used in routine practice, there are a lot of new technologies and methods which are more accurate and sophisticated for caries detection than the conventional tactile and radiographic methods (Tables 2.1 and 2.2).

Some of the caries detection units have lasers that cause fluorescence of tooth, while others use transillumination to see through enamel. While some of these technologies are standalone units, a few may also be integrated into intraoral cameras. Some examples include Microlux Dental Caries Detection System, Cam X Spectra Caries Detection System, DOE Transilluminator, LUM G2, Ortek-ECD, and The Canary System. A few are discussed here although the evidence supporting new systems is currently limited.

Table 2.1 Recent caries detection methods

Medium	Types
Radiographic methods	• Digital subtraction radiography • Digital image enhancement • Tuned aperture computed tomography (TACT) • Computerized tomography scan (CT scan) • X-ray microtomography • Transverse microradiography
Visible light	• Electronic caries monitor (ECM) • Fiber-optic transillumination (FOTI) • Quantitative light-induced fluorescence (QLF) • Digital image fiber-optic transillumination (DiFOTI)
Laser light	• Laser fluorescence measurement (DIAGNOdent) • Quantitative light-induced fluorescence (QLF)
Electric current	• Electrical conductance measurement (ECM) • Electrical impedance measurement
Ultrasound	• Ultrasound caries detector
Endoscopy	Videoscope White light fluorescence Endoscopically viewed filtered fluorescence

Table 2.2 Characteristics of advanced caries detection methods

Method	Advantages	Disadvantages
Digital imaging fiber-optic transillumination	• Can detect incipient and recurrent caries • Detects cracks, tooth fractures, and wear • Uses safe white light • Ability to image all coronal surfaces including interproximal, occlusal, smooth surfaces • Determines depth of lesion accurately	• Technique-sensitive • High cost
Fibre-optic transillumination	• Identifies changes in tooth characteristics that are otherwise unobservable in a visual tactile examination	• Uncertainty of the reliability of devices
Quantitative light/laser-induced fluorescence	Provide early caries detection and quantification Parameters measured are lesion depth, size, and severity Image acquired can be stored and transmitted for referral purposes	Cannot detect incipient lesions effectively Cannot differentiate between decay, hyperplasia, or unusual anatomic features Inability to detect interproximal lesions It is limited to measurements of enamel lesions High cost
Laser light DIAGNOdent	Early detection of caries Reliable method [18] Reproducible results The DD device is capable of diagnosing dental caries which are not visible clinically or even radiographically Able to diagnose pit and fissure caries Simple and easy to use Noninvasive and pain-free	False results with plaque and debris Not useful for proximal caries detection Cannot be used for the detection of recurrent caries High cost
Electrical conductance	Early detection of fissure caries in recently erupted molar teeth Predicts probability that a sealant or a restoration will be required Within 18–24 months Good reproducibility	Uncertainty of the reliability of devices particularly due to the necessity to place the probe in an identical location for a reproducible result Detection of caries is limited only to occlusal surfaces of teeth Cannot be used where amalgam filling is present
Ultrasound caries detector	Quick and reliable tool for the detection of caries in enamel Effective in detecting proximal caries that were missed out on radiographs	Not a quantitative method of caries detection

Fig. 2.1 (**a, b**) VistaCam
iX HD Smart with Proof &
Proxy Heads *(Courtesy
Duerr Dental India
Pvt. Ltd.)*

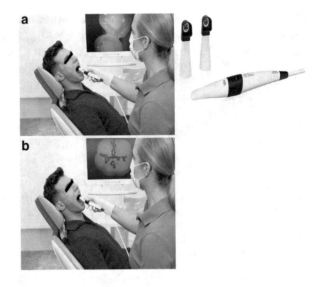

2.2.1 Intraoral Television Camera (IOTV)

The probe or wand of the camera projects a magnified digital image of teeth on the screen of computer. This helps in visualizing the oral cavity better and at the same time the diagnosis can be explained to the patient (Fig. 2.1a, b).

2.2.2 Visible Light

These techniques are based upon the phenomenon of light scattering and utilize different light sources.

2.2.3 Fiber-Optic Transillumination (FOTI)

First designed by Friedman and Marcus in 1970, this technique is based on the principle that carious enamel has a lower index of light transmission than the enamel that is intact [1]. Fibre-optic transillumination (FOTI) uses a light emitted from a handheld device which illuminates the tooth. Any changes in the mineralization of the tooth will appear as shadows in the tooth. FOTI technique is indicated in detecting occlusal and proximal caries. Enamel and optical disruption can occur by penetrating photons of light through densely packed hydroxyapatite crystals.

2.2.4   Digital Imaging Fiber-Optic Transillumination

Digital imaging fiber-optic transillumination (DIFOTI) was developed in an attempt to reduce the disadvantages of FOTI, by combining FOTI with a digital CCD camera. It consists of two handpieces: one for occlusal surface and one for smooth surface and interproximal areas. Its main indications are detection of incipient and frank caries in all tooth surfaces and detecting cracks, and secondary caries around restorations [2–4]. An example of this system is DIAGNOcam.

Other examples of LED-based caries detection system for detecting and quantifying caries include Midwest Caries ID™ (MID) and Vista Proof-VP. In MID, a specific fiber-optic signature captures the resulting reflection and refraction of the light in the tooth. This data gets converted to electrical signals which pass through the software algorithm already installed in the computer and helps to detect the presence of any carious activity [1].

2.2.5   Electrical Caries Monitor (ECM)

Electrical impedance measurement is a measure of degree at which an electric circuit resists electric current flow when a voltage is applied across two electrodes. Caries tissue has a lower impedance than sound tooth. It is also known as electronic caries monitor [5]. ECM measures the electrical resistance of the area of tooth under controlled drying. This method helps in differentiating between sound and carious dental tissues, through electrical conductivity [2].

CarieScan is a device that uses alternating current impedance spectroscopy. Insensitive level of electric current is passed through the tooth to check for the location and presence of any carious lesion. CarieScan provides a qualitative value of diseased tooth as it is not affected by optical factors like discoloration or staining [1].

2.3   Lasers

2.3.1   Quantitative Light-Induced Fluorescence (QLF)

Fluorescence (green and red) is a phenomenon by which an object is excited by particular wavelength of light, and the fluorescent (reflected) light is of a larger wavelength [6]. QLF is based on the principle of fluorescence. It provides a fluorescent image of a tooth surface within yellow-green spectrum of visible light that quantifies mineral loss and size of the lesion. The QLF devices shown in Figs. 2.2 and 2.3 use blue light to illuminate the tooth. This causes the teeth to fluoresce in

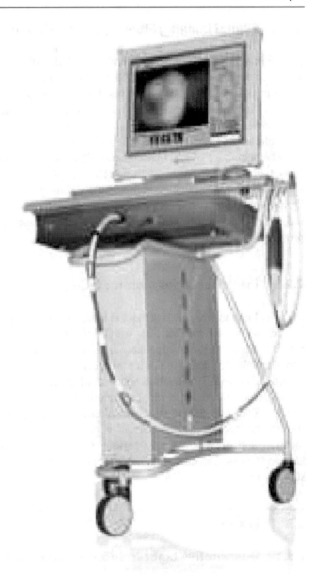

Fig. 2.2 The Inspektor™
Pro QLF camera system
*(Courtesy of Dr. Elbert de
Josselin de Jong and Dr.
Elbert Waller, Inspektor
Research Systems, BV in
Amsterdam, The
Netherlands)*

green (so-called autofluorescence). The resulting QLF images show a higher contrast between sound and demineralized tooth tissue.

It is suitable for detecting early enamel lesions (in clinically inaccessible areas) particularly progression or regression of white spots of smooth surface lesions (Figs. 2.4 and 2.5).

Fig. 2.3 The Inspektor™ QLF-D Biluminator™ 2+ camera system *(Courtesy of Dr. Elbert de Josselin de Jong and Dr. Elbert Waller, Inspektor Research Systems, BV in Amsterdam, The Netherlands)*

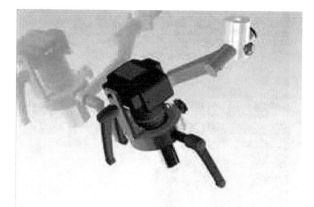

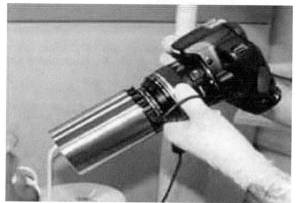

2.3.2 DIAGNOdent Laser System

DIAGNOdent laser was first introduced in 1998 by Hibst and Gal and is a variant of QLF system. It uses infrared laser fluorescence of 655 nm for the detection of occlusal and smooth surface caries by using a simple laser diode to compare the reflection wavelength against a well-known healthy baseline to uncover decay. Unlike the QLF system, the DD does not produce an image of the tooth; instead it displays a numerical value on two LED displays. It has a pen handpiece that is suitable for diagnosis of dental caries without radiographs and any mechanical damage to the tissues. This system uses a low-power laser directed onto the tooth. Healthy tooth structure displays little or no fluorescence resulting in very low-scale readings on the display whereas carious teeth structure displays fluorescence, giving elevated scale readings on the display. Use of laser fluorescence device provides results that are more consistent with tactile examination comparing with other methods.

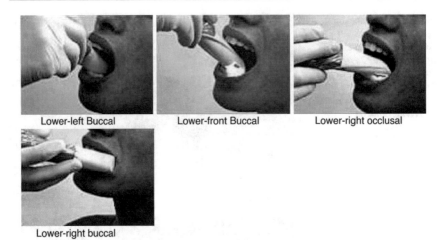

Lower-left Buccal   Lower-front Buccal   Lower-right occlusal

Lower-right buccal

Fig. 2.4 Orientations of the QLF handpiece when taking an image of various surfaces *(Courtesy of Dr. Elbert de Josselin de Jong and Dr. Elbert Waller, Inspektor Research Systems, BV in Amsterdam, The Netherlands)*

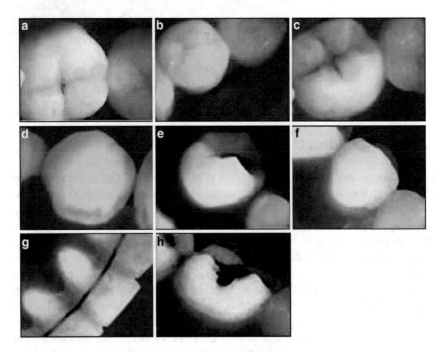

Fig. 2.5 Some examples of QLF images. (**a**) Occlusal view of the upper left second molar with enamel breakdown in the central fossa. (**b**) Sound fissures in the upper right 2nd bicuspid. (**c**) Fissures of the upper right second molar are covered by matured plaque obstructing a clear view. (**d**) Red fluorescence inside a white spot lesion developed during orthodontic treatment (the QLF image was made after professional cleaning). (**e**) Calculus at the proximal area. (**f**) Matured plaque at the proximal area. (**g**) Retention wires are a good retention site for plaque. (**h**) Matured plaque along the gingival margin. *(Courtesy of Dr. Elbert de Josselin de Jong and Dr. Elbert Waller, Inspektor Research Systems, BV in Amsterdam, The Netherlands)*

The device's inability to determine the depth of the carious lesions has been mentioned [7]. Some recent studies claim that fluorescence-based intraoral devices do not contribute to a better detection of early carious lesions [8, 9]. Nevertheless, they can be used in conjunction with the International Caries Detection and Assessment System (ICDAS), a relatively new technique for the measurement of dental caries [10]. DIAGNOdent pen is a latest advancement to the DIAGNOdent technology and is used to detect pit and fissure and smooth surface caries accurately.

2.3.3   Ultrasonography

Ultrasound caries detection method (UCD) was first suggested over 30 years ago; however, it has been used more in the last decade [11] for detecting early carious lesions on smooth surfaces. The principle is that images of tissues can be collected by reflected sound waves. Demineralization of natural enamel is assessed by ultrasound pulse-echo technique. It is observed that there is a definite correlation between the mineral content of the body of the lesion and the relative echo amplitude changes [12].

Studies have shown that UCD could differentiate between cavitated and non-cavitated proximal lesions [13]. It has also been shown that UCD reduces patient exposure to radiation and has higher sensitivity and lower specificity than the radiographs in diagnosis of interproximal caries [14]. Research has also shown UCD can be used successfully in the determination of thickness changes in enamel [15].

2.4   Diagnosis in Endodontics: Pulp Vitality Tests

2.4.1   Laser Doppler Flowmetry (LDF)

LDF was first described, in dentistry, by Gazelius et al. in 1968. LDF helps to measure the true vitality of the pulp (i.e., pulpal blood flow and not the sensory function) using noninvasive techniques like gas desaturation and intravital microscopy. Although the use of LDF is well established in many fields of dentistry (Table 2.3), its use has been limited to dental schools in research studies rather than clinical use due to its cost and complicated procedures.

The technique uses a light beam from a helium-neon (He-Ne) laser emitting at 632.8 nm. Other wavelengths of semiconductor laser have also been used: 780 and 780–820 nm (Fig. 2.6) [16]. Laser light is transmitted to the dental pulp by means of a fiber-optic probe placed against the tooth surface. Backscattered reflected light has a different frequency with respect to the static surrounding tissues and is considered as the output signal. Signal is recorded as the flux (velocity and concentration) in an arbitrary term, perfusion units (PU), for example, 2.5 V of blood flow is equivalent to 250 PU (Fig. 2.7a, b). It should be emphasized that the optical properties of a tooth change when the pulp becomes necrotic, and this can produce changes in the LDF signal that are not due to differences in blood flow [17].

Table 2.3 Uses of LDF in clinical dentistry

Specialty	Uses
Endodontics	To determine the vitality of an injured tooth
	Evaluating replanted tooth pulp vitality at different time periods
	To determine the postsurgical healing of periapical lesions after endodontic surgery
	As an aid in the differential diagnosis of non-odontogenic periapical pathosis
Orthodontics	To check reactions of tooth during orthodontic Treatment
	Used for pulpal blood flow measurement when employing rapid tooth movement
Oral and maxillofacial surgery	Used to determine the vitality of involved teeth by measuring the blood flow in the dental pulp after maxillary or mandibular orthognathic surgery
	Used to evaluate the blood flow in soft tissues where good vascular supply in the flap indicates a reduced chance of infection and the potential for good wound healing
Restorative and prosthodontic treatment	To assess the vascularity of the area of bone planned for implant placement in patients receiving radiation prior to dental implant fixation
Pediatric dentistry	Effective and reliable evaluating dental pulp vitality, in teeth with immature root formation and open apex

Various studies have been performed to investigate the preferred testing parameters for LDF. Gazelius et al. stated that though 750 nm laser penetrated deeper, they were associated with signal contamination of non-pulp origin from surrounding tissues [18]. Later studies showed that the problem of signal contamination was associated with the extensive scattering of light with longer wavelength lasers. The laser beam produced should be low-power beam ranging from 1 to 2 Mw [19].

Calibration of probes is another important criteria to get accurate readings [20]. The probe, when in contact with tooth, contains both receiving and sending optic fibers, with two detectors placed in a triangular arrangement at one end of probe, while the other being the source (Fig. 2.8). It was noted that with larger optical fiber separation distance on the probes, higher was the signal output (as larger area was covered), which increases the chances of blood flow signal contamination from non-plural sources [21]. Hence, 0.5 or 0.025 mm separation distances are preferred [22].

The advantages of LDF are many including being noninvasive in nature, painless, accurate, and reproducible. It is most useful in pediatric and medically compromised patients where their responses may not be relied upon. There are few drawbacks as well, such as high economic cost and the sensor should be completely stable to be able to record accurate reading. Discolored tooth crown may give a false positive response due to blood pigments that may interfere with laser light transmission. This method makes it difficult to measure vitality in teeth with large restorations, such as metal inlay, crown or orthodontic brackets, and requires individual

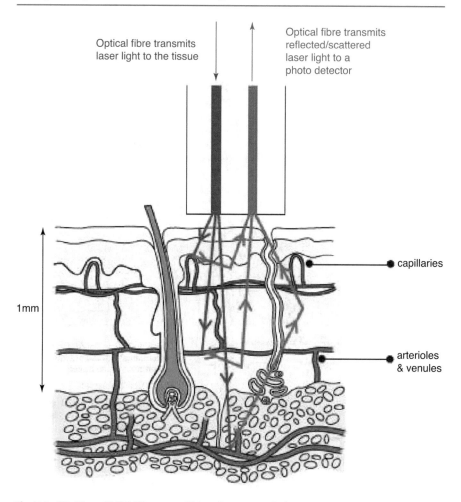

Fig. 2.6 Working of LDF *(Courtesy of Moor Instruments Ltd.)*

stabilizing devices for the probe (such as splint or silicone). Any stimulation or effect of supporting tissues, such as gingival or oral, may interfere with accurate recordings [23].

2.4.2   Pulse Oximetry

Compared to laser Doppler flowmeters, pulse oximeters are relatively inexpensive and commonly used in general anesthetic procedures. The term oximetry means determining the percentage of oxygen saturation of the circulating arterial blood [23]. It helps in differentiating between nonvital and vital tooth. Since oxygenated and deoxygenated hemoglobin have different colors, they absorb different amounts of red and

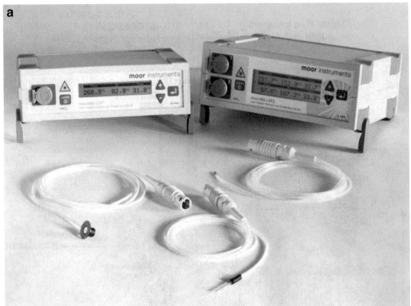

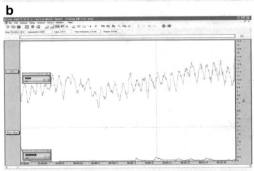

Tooth Vitality is confirmed by examining both the pulsatility and magnitude of the traces.

Trace Characteristics:

Vital: Relatively high blood flow usually with a pulsatile (cardiac frequency) component.

Non Vital: Relatively low blood flow with no clear pulsatility.

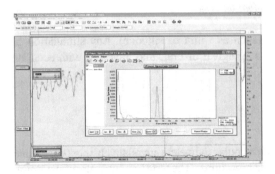

As a further aid to vitality assessment, it is possible to quantify and assess cardiac pulsatility of the tooth blood flow: the flux traces can be transformed with Fourier analysis (FFT using moorVMS-PC software). FFT examples are shown left; note the prominence of the peak at cardiac frequency (here about 60 cycles per minute) indicating pulp vitality.

Fig. 2.7 (**a**) MoorVMS-LDF—single and dual channel modules with Memory Chip probes. (**b**) Tooth Vitality testing using LDF (*Courtesy of Moor Instruments Ltd.*)

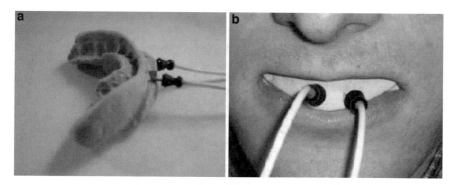

Fig. 2.8 (**a**) Dental Putty probe holder for chronic blood flow pressures. (**b**) Dental putty holder in position with two lase doppler probes *(Courtesy of Moor Instruments Ltd.)*

infrared light. Pulse oximeter, with the help of probes, emit red and infrared light to transilluminate the concerned vascular area. This allows the photodetectors to identify the absorbance peak and hence calculate the pulse rate and oxygen saturation levels [2].

2.4.3   Other Noninvasive Experimental Tests for Pulp Vitality

1. *Transmitted Laser Light (TLL):* This technique is an experimental variation to LDF, aimed at reducing the non-pulp signals. Obstruction and/or interference from within the tooth structure will affect the results [24].
2. *Dual Wave Spectrophotometry (DWS):* This technique uses dual wavelength of visible light to ascertain the contents of pulp chamber that are either empty, filled with fixed pulp tissue, or filled with oxygenated blood. DWS has been tested with positive, but only initial, experimental results [25].
3. *Photoplethysmography:* This is an optical measurement technique that helps to detect blood volume anomalies in the microvascular bed of tissue. It was developed for pulp testing in an attempt to improve pulse oximetry, by adding a light with a shorter wavelength. The results, while promising, were still uncertain and questionable [26].
4. *Transillumination:* This technique uses a strong light source which identifies color changes that may indicate pulp pathosis. This technique may not be useful in large posterior teeth and especially in teeth with large restorations. However, it is a helpful adjunct to conventional pulp tests, and it can help to identify cracks in teeth.

2.5   Diagnosing Periodontal Disease

New innovations in technology in the field of periodontal diagnosis is slowly gaining momentum (Table 2.4). Devices such as periodontal probes, biosensors, nanotechnology, ultrasonography, and optical imaging systems are being encouraged

Table 2.4 Advances in periodontal diagnosis

Clinical diagnosis	Periodontal probes
	Non-periodontal probes
Radiographic diagnosis	Digital radiography
	3D imaging methods
	Other recent techniques
	Implant site imaging
Microbiologic diagnosis	Microscopic identification
	Bacterial culture
	Enzymatic assays
	Immunoassays
	Diagnostic assays based on molecular biology techniques
Characterizing host response	Host response in periodontal disease
	Diagnostic biomarkers in saliva
	Diagnostic biomarkers in GCF

with a view to better determining the health and/or disease status of patients. Few novel methods that are currently being explored as complementary tools in periodontal diagnostics are discussed in this section. However, the reader should keep in mind that some of these techniques are still under research with their clinical potential yet to be validated and interpreted. Despite excellent progress in diagnostic methodology, conventional methods remain the standard for disease evaluation till date. Advancements in clinical and radiological diagnostic techniques for periodontics will be discussed in detail in this chapter. For other methods, the reader is directed to other literature.

2.5.1 Periodontal Pocket Probes

First-generation probes are the conventional or manual periodontal probes such as Williams periodontal probe. Pockets can be assessed using a probe which are thin calibrated (marked in mm) metal instruments. The probe is carefully inserted into the gingival sulcus, and advanced gradually to the base of the pocket until resistance is met by the first intact collagen fiber. Manual periodontal pocket depth measurement is highly variable and are frequently affected by factors such as thickness of the probe, angle of insertion, degree of pressure applied, and degree of periodontal inflammation.

Second-generation periodontal probes, also known as *constant force probes*, were developed to provide constant pressure during periodontal pocket measurement. This reduces the measurement variation. However, probing errors arise due to faulty data readout and estimation of attachment level. Another major disadvantage is the lack of tactile sensation. Examples include True Press Sensitive probe, Armitage probe, and van der Velden probe [27].

Third-generation probes are also known as *constant force-automated probes*. Just like their predecessors, they use controlled or constant force application in combination with automated measurements and computerized storage of data.

Examples include The Foster Miller probe, The Florida probe, The Toronto Automated probe, and the Interprobe. The drawbacks include deeper penetration of the probe beyond the junctional epithelium, thus overestimating the pocket depth, and underestimating it after loss of inflammation, and inability to achieve 3D information about the disease. The accuracy and reproducibility is also affected as the tactile sensation is decreased.

Fourth-generation probes are 3D probes. Currently, they are still under development. The aim is to record the data at sequential probe positions along the gingival sulcus. Despite all the advances in periodontal probe generations, they remain invasive and, the probe tip can cross the junctional epithelium. Fifth-generation probes are being devised to eliminate these disadvantages.

Fifth-generation probes, also known as *ultrasonographic probes*, are noninvasive probes which help to identify the attachment level without penetrating it (Fig. 2.9). An ultrasound or other device is added to a fourth-generation probe which offers the potential for earlier detection of periodontal disease activity, noninvasive diagnosis, and greater reliability of [28]. The ultrasonic (US) probe (only probe available as yet) uses ultrasound waves to assess, image, and locate the upper border of the periodontal ligament and its variation, thus identifying the extent and quality of epithelial attachment to the tooth surface, providing information on health of gingival tissue (Fig. 2.10a, b). However, more research is needed to validate these claims. Drawbacks include high cost and technical expertise [27, 29, 30].

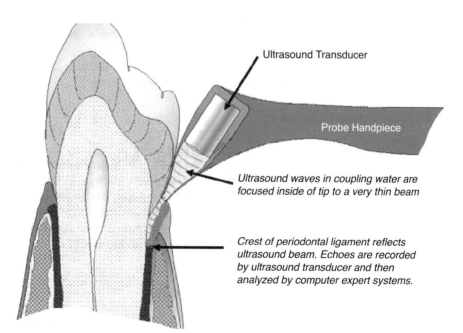

Ultrasound Transducer

Probe Handpiece

Ultrasound waves in coupling water are focused inside of tip to a very thin beam

Crest of periodontal ligament reflects ultrasound beam. Echoes are recorded by ultrasound transducer and then analyzed by computer expert systems.

Fig. 2.9 Probe tip is placed at the gum line with thin ultra sound beam projecting into tissues (*Courtesy of Prof. Mark K. Hinders*)

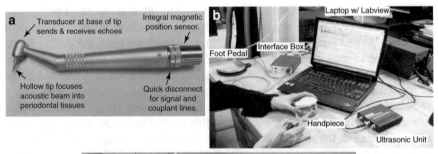

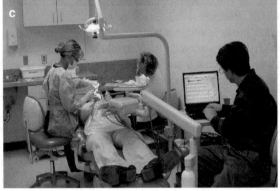

Fig. 2.10 (**a, b**) Ultrasonic Periodontal probe. (**c**) Investigational version of an ultrasonographic periodontal probe in a study performed in Norfolk, VA (*Courtesy of Prof. Mark K. Hinders*)

2.6   Other Devices (Non-periodontal Probes)

2.6.1   Detecting Calculus

Calculus detection probes are useful in detecting subgingival calculus by means of audio readings. For example, the DetecTar probe (DENTSPLY Professional, Des Moines, IL) is a lightweight calculus detection probe which can be autoclaved. It produces an audible beep to signify calculus detection. However, it is expensive and the handpiece is bulky. The probe has a short waterline hookup, which restricts ergonomic placement of the unit. As with many automated probes, there is potential for false positives and false negatives. Further research is still required [27].

2.6.2   Periodontal Disease Evaluation System

Halitosis or bad breadth is caused by byproducts of the metabolic activity of micro-organisms (mainly anaerobic) in the oral cavity. These by-products are mainly volatile sulfur compounds like hydrogen sulfide and methyl mercaptan [31]. Though organoleptic or sniff test still remain the standard tests, their main drawback is that these tests are subjective, that is, they depend on the examiner's interpretation about the quality of the door. Subjective measures are difficult to document in research. Since objective data are more likely to be standardized, instruments were developed to measure the volatile sulfur compounds in the air exhaled through mouth.(C) Examples include Halimeter™ (Interscan Corporation, Chatsworth, CA, USA) and Breath Alert™ (Tanita Corporation, Tokyo, Kantō, Japan). However, not many studies have verified its accuracy and relevance in clinical practice [32].

The Diamond Probe/Perio 2000 System (Diamond General Development Corp, Ann Arbor, MI) can be used during routine dental examinations to detect periodontal disease by measuring relative sulfide concentrations as an indicator of gram-negative bacterial activity. A single-use disposable probe tip with microsensors connected to a main control unit is used [33]. This system detects periodontal disease at an early stage. It can also check an active site that may require treatment. A drawback of this system is that the probing pressure is not controlled. Also, periodontal disease caused by bacteria that does not produce volatile sulfur compounds may not get recorded [34].

2.6.3 Gingival Temperature Detection

Subgingival temperature at diseased sites is increased as compared to normal healthy sites. It helps to detect periodontal disease at an early stage. It is the only indicator that can be evaluated both quantitatively and objectively. An example is the *Periotemp Probe* (Abiodent Inc., Danvers, MA), which is a temperature-sensitive probe [35]. It has two light indicating diodes: red-emitting diode, which indicates higher temperature, and green-emitting diode, which indicates lower temperature. Higher temperature denotes greater risk for future attachment loss. This probe is indicated in detecting initial inflammatory changes. However, breath airflow resulting in surface cooling may cause difficulty in determining even a normal temperature distribution [36].

2.6.4 Periodontal Imaging Technologies

These are used to measure reproducible accurate pocket depth and 3D visualization (Table 2.5). Further details are given in Chaps. 3 and 11 in this book. An example of photo-acoustic ultrasound image is explained in Figs. 2.11 and 2.12.

2.7 Digital Prosthodontics

Digital dentistry includes a broad spectrum of technologies bringing communication, documentation, manufacturing, and delivery of dental treatment under one umbrella. With improvements in hardware, software, and materials in the early 2000s, new accomplishments in clinical dentistry have been realized. Same-day, chairside

Table 2.5 Various imaging technologies for pocket depth measurement

Method of imaging	Benefits	Limitations
CBCT	High resolution Low radiation exposure Broad range of applications Popular and widely used in dental care	Ionizing radiation Metallic image artifacts
OCT (optical coherent tomography)	High resolution and tissue contrast Nonionizing	Cannot be used for deep tissue imaging due to scattering of the light waves
Photoacoustic imaging topography	Nonionizing High resolution and tissue contrast Deep tissue imaging	Thick bones can distort signal Poor penetration of gas cavities
MRI	Nonionizing Soft and hard tissue imaging	Long scanning time Only soft tissue imaging with low resolution is possible with conventional MRI Not enough evidence to show if newer generations of MRI can image periodontal pockets

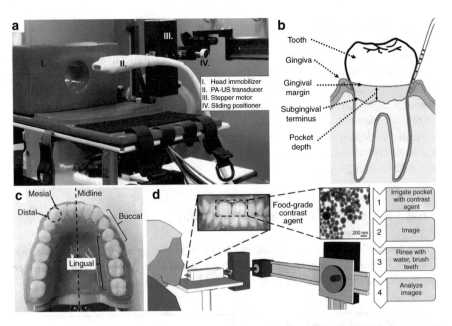

Fig. 2.11 Overview of the imaging setup, periodontal anatomy and workflow. (a) The PA-US transducer was connected to a stepper motor for axial scanning and a sliding positioner for lateral control. The head mobilizer rested on a flat surface (b) Periodontal anatomical features (c) Anatomical terms for reference (d) Experimental workflow—A contrast agent was used to irrigate the pocket of the target tooth followed by photoacoustic imaging. The pocket is then rinsed with water and images analyzed to measure pocket depths. (*Courtesy of Dr. Jesse V. Jokerst, Department of NanoEngineering, University of California, San Diego*)

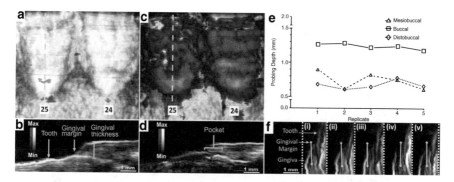

Fig. 2.12 Photoacoustic-Ultrasound (PA-US) images of teeth # 31, 41 before and after administration of contrast agent with demonstrated reproducibility. (**a**) Frontal cross section of 31, 41 prior to administration of the contrast agent. (**b**) Sagittal cross section of 41 (yellow dotted line). (**c**) Frontal cross section of 31, 41 with photoacoustic signal overlaid on ultrasound after administration of the contrast agent. (**d**) Sagittal cross section of 41 (yellow dotted line) shows the soft–hard tissue interface and pocket revealed below the gingival margin (**e**, **f**) Reproducibility of measurements for different probing locations around the tooth. Each PA-US image in (**f**) corresponds to the Mesio buccal probing depth measurement (squares) for its given replicate number on the *x*-axis in (**e**). Light yellow lines show the pocket measurements, white lines depict the ultrasound, and red lines show the photoacoustics. (*Courtesy of Dr. Jesse V. Jokerst, Department of NanoEngineering, University of California, San Diego*)

restorations of dimensional and esthetic accuracy are now a possibility. Guided implant surgeries provided enhanced workflow and safety (Fig. 2.13). Digital technology is driving a significant change in the practice and delivery in prosthodontics.

2.7.1 Assessing Occlusion

2.7.1.1 T-Scan System
In 1987, Maness developed the T-Scan system to analyze relative occlusal force that is recorded intraorally by a sensor in real time [37]. TekScan (T-scan) and MatScan (automated computerized sensor for analyzing dental occlusion) are used to accurately study the occlusal contacts and the forces created, even the slightest occlusal interferences, which are significant in planning full-mouth rehabilitation and implant-protected occlusion (Fig. 2.14).

The system has several advantages such as simple operation, 3D viewing of occlusion, timed analysis of force during various positions of teeth contact, and the documentation and monitoring of the occlusal condition after various treatment (Fig. 2.15). Other benefits include identifying premature contacts and interferences in dynamic occlusion, and demonstration of the contact information through movements in sagittal axis and transverse axis of occlusal plane. The fourth generation of this system exists with many improvements using thin sensors. Limitations include the inability to measure absolute force value, non-reproducibility of data. The thick sensors may inhibit dental proprioception.

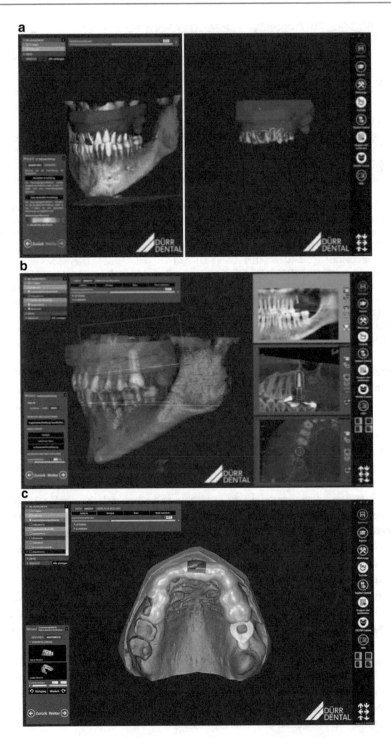

Fig. 2.13 Guided implant planning. (**a**) Automatic expansion of the matching of intraoral impressions and CBCT. (**b**) Intuitive and efficient implant planning. (**c**) User friendly drill template planning *(Courtesy Duerr Vista Soft, Duerr Dental)*

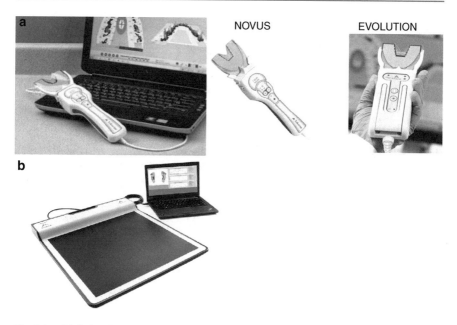

Fig. 2.14 Digital occlusal analysis instrument. (**a**) T scan system with two models of handles. (**b**) Mobile Tek Mat *(Courtesy Dr. Vikas Aggarwal)*

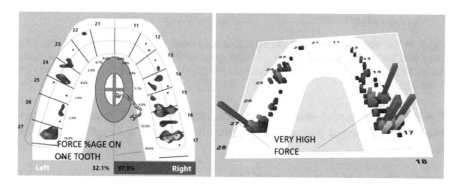

Fig. 2.15 T Scan showing 2D and 3D pictures of records *(Courtesy Dr. Vikas Aggarwal)*. T scan gives first point of contact between upper and lower teeth. It records the timing and duration of contact between teeth. It records the percentage of force existing between all teeth at a particular point of time (it can record up to 500 frames per second)

T-Scan can be used in any dental procedure where articulating paper is used. It helps in evaluating any para-functional mandibular movements occlusal and chewing force before placement of implants [38]. In orthodontics, it helps to achieve the goal of correcting malocclusion and analyzing the proper bite force [39]. It also helps to check and correct any improperly restored tooth in restorative dentistry [40]. It can also help to evaluate occlusion after surgery in cases of mandibular and dentoalveolar fractures. Mat scan helps to identify plantar pressure profile asymmetries between left and right feet. Figure 2.16 shows plantar pressure and body balance in relation to change in occlusal balance. Thus, they are effective in

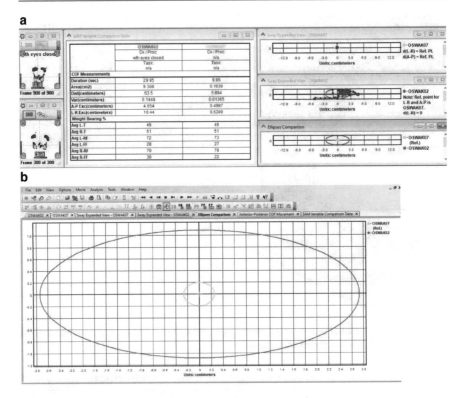

Fig. 2.16 (**a**) Mat scan analysis. (**b**) Difference of body sway. The red circle is showing the body sway with natural bite, the green circle is showing the decrease in body sway after wearing the dental splint, and the small green circle represents better and improved body balance (Courtesy Dr. Vikas Aggarwal)

fabrication of protective mouth guards, which are checked with mobile mat to provide better balance of players' body, especially in sports like rugby, boxing, ice hockey, etc.

2.7.1.2 Virtual Articulators Digital Facebows

Virtual Facebow (VF) was developed as a digital substitute (Research Driven, Komoka, Ontario) to provide an alternative and to overcome the issues associated with the analog Facebow, that is, mounting of casts to an articulator. It prevents and minimizes errors in patient positioning, allows for accurate mounting of casts by reinforcing the various anatomical considerations, and provides for an effective and accessible digital substitute with unlimited use.

The image obtained by VR is transferred to a virtual articulator with CAD CAM systems (Fig. 2.17). In prosthetic dentistry, virtual articulator improves the designing of dental prosthesis by adding virtual reality applications for the analysis of complex static and dynamic occlusal relations. It is mainly used for the simulation of the mechanical articulator requiring digital 3D representations of the jaws. With

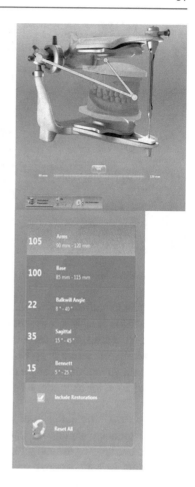

Fig. 2.17   Virtual articulator *(Courtesy of Denstply, Sirona)*

patient-specific data on jaw movements, it simulates them and provides a dynamic visualization of the occlusal contacts. This reduces the error of design and helps in creating an improved prosthesis with simulation of centric relation, protrusion, and laterotrusion (Fig. 2.18). There are currently two types of virtual articulators available:

1. *Mathematically Simulated Virtual Articulator* [41]: This allows the recording and reproducibility of all movements based on mathematical simulation of articulator movements. It is fully adjustable and allows for recording movements such as curved Bennett movement, condylar angle, protrusion, retrusion, laterotrusion, or any other movement required for adjustment. Thus, with this information, the articulator automatically simulates the motion of lower jaw like a mechanical articulator. The main disadvantage is that it is not possible to obtain individualized movement paths of each patient. Examples of this type of articulators include Stratos 200, Szentpetery's virtual articulators.

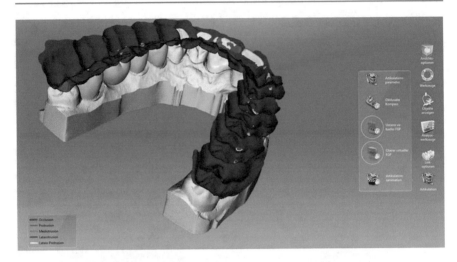

Fig. 2.18 Representation of occlusal contacts *(Courtesy of Denstply, Sirona)*

2. *Completely adjustable virtual articulator (motion analyzer)*: It records and reproduces precise movement paths of the mandible using an electronic jaw registration system called jaw motion analyzer (JMA). It was designed in Greifswald University of Germany by Kordass and Gartner. If the JMA tool is not available, different jaw motions can be defined via parameters as used with the mechanical articulators, for example, Kordass and Gartner virtual articulators.

The virtual articulators provide improved communication between the dentist and the technician, simulating patient-specific data in real time. It provides 3D visualization and allows to navigate, assess, and analyze both static and gnathic joint movements, in both dynamic and static occlusion.

But virtual articulators have high economic cost as it requires scanners, software programs, and sensors. The dentist and his team require high level of knowledge, training, and skill about the CAD-CAM systems.

Recent advances in this field include the 3D virtual articulator system (Zebris Company, D-Isny). In addition to analysis of mandibular movements, this type of articulator also analyzes masticatory movements including force at the points of contact and the frequency of contacts in relation to time [42].

2.7.1.3 Assessing Temporomandibular Joint Disorders

As stated above, use of T-Scan allows to assess any problematic occlusal contacts and helps in effective diagnosis and treatment planning. The study of jaw movements allows detection and assessment of TMJ functional irregularities. Jaw tracking devices (e.g., K6 Diagnostics, K7) are used to study jaw movements and occlusion, which may be a traumatic etiological factor for any type of TMJ disorder [43] (Fig. 2.19a, b). The elevated muscle activity associated with malocclusion can be detected with surface electromyography (EMG). An EMG device, namely, BITE STRIPTM, can record muscle activity for some hours and provide useful information in nocturnal bruxism [44].

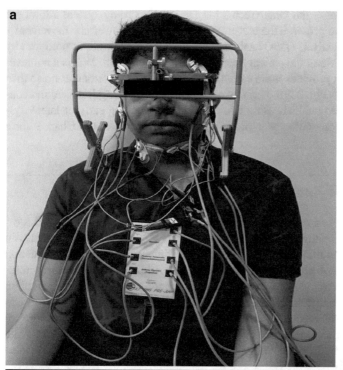

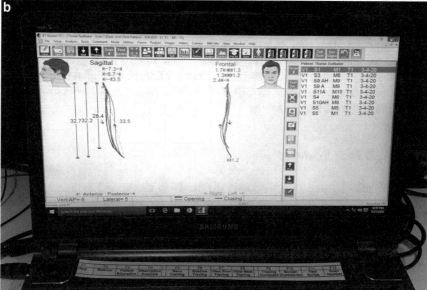

Fig. 2.19 (**a**) TMJ Evaluation (setup on patient) using K7 mandibular tracking device consisting of CMS (computerized mandibular scanning), K7 EMG eight channel surface electromyograph (EMG) and K7 ESG Electrosonograph (TMJ vibration sound) Evaluation system. (**b**) Simple opening and closing of the mouth (sagittal frontal mode). It helps to check whether mandible closes to occlusion without any deviation (from its muscles oriented pathway) or if it has to accommodate to habitual occlusion. Downward arrow shows opening and upward arrow shows closing of mouth (*Courtesy of Dr. Nafisa Khan and Dr. Imthiaz Refayee*)

Another example is the GnathTech TMJ Digital Recording system allows the dentist to record and preserve the real-time trajectory of the lower jaw movement.

Joint vibration analysis (JVA) analyzes and records TMJ vibrations produced by tissues of the joint when the patient opens and closes the mouth. JVA is a noninvasive technique as it provides more essential information of the articular noise than other methods [45] (Fig. 2.20). *Kondrat* conducted a study using Bio JVA and concluded that vibration analysis using Bio JVA allows detecting early or latent dysfunction of temporomandibular joint [46]. The reader is referred to Chap. 9 for a detailed reading.

2.8   Digital Diagnosis in Orthodontics

In this twenty-first century, advancement and development of integrated 3D tools for diagnosis and treatment planning is one of the most exciting developments in dentistry. Computed tomography (CT) and three-dimensional (3D) reconstruction in the 1970s brought about a revolution in diagnostic radiology because cross-sectional imaging became possible. Digital orthodontics has created a paradigm shift in diagnosis and treatment planning with more focus on soft tissue response to treatment. Diagnostic records in orthodontics can be broken into essential and supplement diagnostic aids. Essential aids refer to medical and dental history, intra and extra oral examination, study models, radiographs, and photographs [47]. They also include x-rays [48].

Orthodontic diagnosis includes three components: facial, dental, and skeletal. Most of conventional diagnostic aids provide only 2D representation of the patient [49]. Advanced 3D technological methods gives high-quality diagnostic information in three planes to orthodontist which helps in designing a comprehensive treatment plan. Digital diagnostic aides include (but not limited to) digital study models, radiographic techniques such as CBCT, Lateral Cephalogram, DentaScan, Rapid prototyping, and Sure smile system.

2.8.1   3D Face Scanner

3D facial scan is used in orthodontic diagnosis to assess and measure aesthetic facial parameters, and evaluate the craniofacial growth and development [50]. Clinical evaluation of the facial morphology is still subjective as it prevents accurate measurement and documentation of facial structures over time, due to the changes following various esthetic or reconstructive procedures [51]. Some commonly used 3D photogrammetric imaging systems are 3dMDface System (3dMD, Atlanta, USA), 3D Vectra (Canfield Imaging systems, Fairfield, USA), and Facial Insight 3D (Motion View Software, LLC, TN, USA).

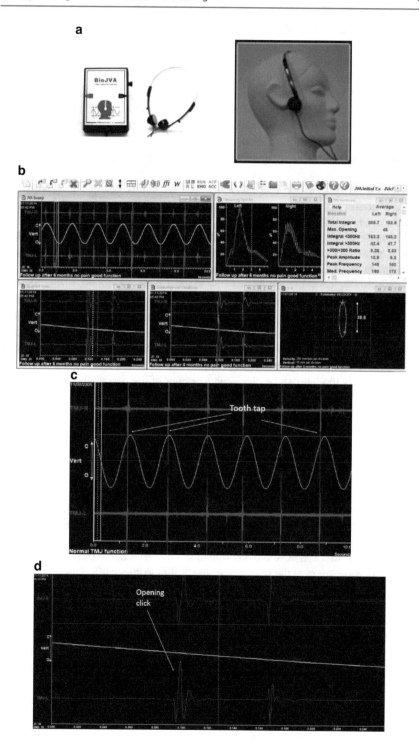

Fig. 2.20 (a) Joint vibration analysis. (b) Appearance of recording, giving objective information about the diseased joint. (c) Normal silent joint. (d) Zoomed image of the vibration *(Courtesy of Dr. Vikas Aggarwal, Bioresearch Inc.)*

2.8.2 Digital Study Models

Study models provide record of malocclusion before treatment, stages of treatment, and final outcome of treatment. They have traditionally been cast out of either plaster or stone but have certain drawbacks such as storage and retrieval, transferability, and longevity. The introduction of digital models offers the orthodontist various advantages over the traditional method, namely, no laboratory procedure needed, the ability to create multiple diagnostic setups, no physical storage space needed, fast and efficient retrieval at any place, no chance of physical damage, can be used to create indirect bracket bonding setups, precision in measurements such as tooth size, arch length and width, space analysis etc., and can be easily shared with other dental practitioners via email to facilitate interdisciplinary treatment planning. These can be acquired by intraoral scan, CBCT, or by scanning an impression or plaster model (Fig. 2.21). But on the other hand, they also suffer from certain limitations such as lack of tactile input, expensive, inability to mount on an articulator, requirement of additional equipment requirement and training.

Currently, digital study models can be viewed from any angle, turned through 360° in all planes of space and even opened to allow upper and lower models to be viewed separately. Scanning can be done via a direct or an indirect method. Direct methods makes the use of intraoral scanners whereas indirect methods are produced by scanning the alginate impressions and plaster models, with either intraoral scanner or computed tomography imaging [52].

Digital study models can be produced by either of the two methods:

1. Destructive imaging where part of casts are removed, little by little, while it is being imaged.
2. Nondestructive imaging which uses laser or structured light, or x-ray to an image while leaving the original cast intact.

An example is the OrthoCAD digital study model by CADENT (computer-aided dentistry, Fairview, NJ, USA). It optically scans the model image from a plaster equivalent. These are then transferred to orthodontist through the patent OrthoCAD software user interface. This software allows both structured and free manipulation of models in virtual space, and data collection through a range of diagnostic tools. OrthoCAD software give the practitioner the ability to rotate, tilt, and section models, and hold them in any position, thus allowing for detailed analysis. Models can be brought up instantly for further chairside clinical information at any/every visit.

Geodigm is another software on the market offering all the advantages of a digital model. Models are constructed through a proprietary laser scanning process that digitally maps the geometry of patient's anatomy into a high dimensional 3D image, with an accuracy of 0.1 mm. In addition, Geodigm also has color bite mapping features and an articulation feature to set the center of rotation. A more recent advancement is the e-plan software, which simulates multiple treatment plans to help determine most effective treatment and gives the patient an opportunity to view their teeth from a posttreatment view [53].

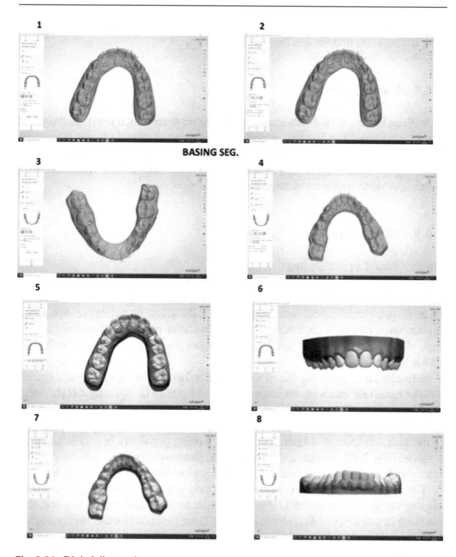

Fig. 2.21 Digital diagnostic casts

2.8.3   Sure Smile

The objective of a Sure Smile system is to use new advanced computerized technology to transition an orthodontic practice to a digital platform, for all aspects of the treatment planning. It is useful for diagnosis, choosing between different treatment plans, and discussing treatment plan with patient. It provides a view of the post treatment which helps the practitioner to plan the best aesthetic smile possible [52]. Benefits include reduced errors in treatment resulting from appliance management such as bracket positioning and arch wire selection, improved patient communication, and reduced undesirable tooth movement.

2.8.4 DentaScan

DentaScan is a computed tomography software program which provides images of maxilla and mandible in axial, panoramic, and cross-sectional planes. It provides improved evaluation of osseous maxilla and mandible and are useful in head and neck surgery. Their main benefit in orthodontics is the reduction in treatment errors, which are due to appliance management.

2.8.5 3D Printing

2.8.5.1 Rapid Prototyping

This was founded by Wilfried Vancraen in 1990 as the first rapid prototype. 3D printing allows the user to create or print 3D objects, prototypes, and parts in any shape from a virtual model in a range of materials. These materials are then joined in succession on top of each other through an additive process by computer control technology. Some of the 3D printing technologies currently available for orthodontic use are mentioned below.

Selective Laser Sintering (SLS) and Selective Laser Melting (SLM) use specific powder materials which are melted and sintered together in layers by a high-energy laser beam. Stereolithography (SLA) was presented by Charles W. Hull in 1986. It is the first "rapid prototyping" process and produces solid items by printing thin layers that is later solidified by a laser light. SLA is gaining popularity in planning implant surgeries (Fig. 2.22). However, this technique is also currently being used for planning cranial and maxillofacial procedures [51] and implant surgeries (Fig. 2.23a, b).

The inkjet-based system consists of a nozzle which propels a liquid adhesive binding agent. This is added to the raw powder material and further bonded, thus resulting in one layer of the model. Layer by layer are built like this until complete fabrication is achieved. Fused Deposition Modelling (FDM) releases a thermoplastic material from a nozzle in layer by layer pattern, which is regulated by temperature. This technique is quick and easy to use, is less expensive, and involves less wastage of material [54]. Others are laminated object manufacturing (LOM) and digital light processing (DLP). Box 2.1 tells us how the method of making impression and then obtaining the prosthesis has changed with time.

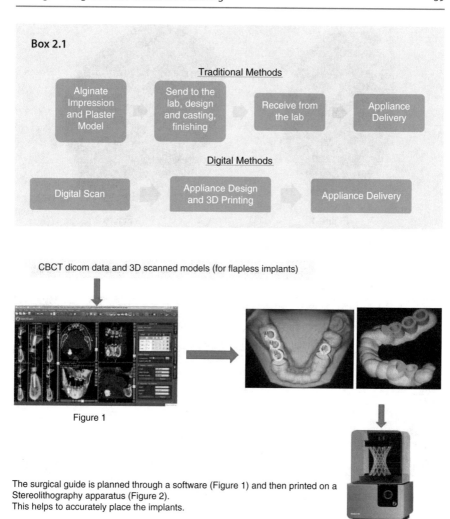

Box 2.1

Traditional Methods

Alginate Impression and Plaster Model ➡ Send to the lab, design and casting, finishing ➡ Receive from the lab ➡ Appliance Delivery

Digital Methods

Digital Scan ➡ Appliance Design and 3D Printing ➡ Appliance Delivery

CBCT dicom data and 3D scanned models (for flapless implants)

Figure 1

The surgical guide is planned through a software (Figure 1) and then printed on a Stereolithography apparatus (Figure 2).
This helps to accurately place the implants.

Figure 2

Fig. 2.22 Workflow for an implant surgical guide *(Courtesy of Sagmarks Pvt. Ltd.)*

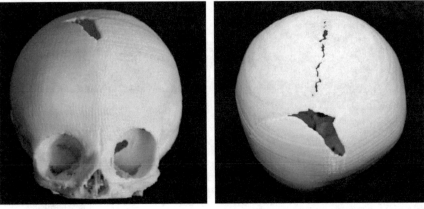

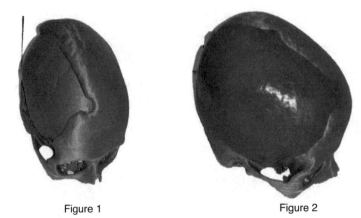

Figure 1   Figure 2

Customised 3D Printed model for fabrication of cranioplasty for a post traumatic
craniectomy patient (Figure 1).
The part in red is the cranioplasty waxup which can be later invested and converted into
PMMA cranioplasty (Figure 2).

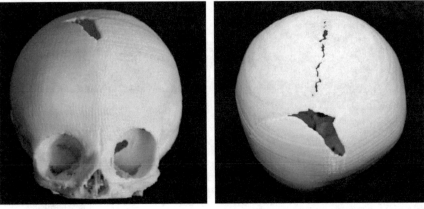

Figure 1   Figure 2

3D printed model of a 2 year old girl child with craniosynostosis (Figure 1).
Flattening of the forehead on the left side can be appreciated (Figure 2).
The model is used for planning the osteotomy.

Fig. 2.23 Customised 3D printed model for fabrication of cranioplasty

2.9   Conclusion

Digitalization is one of the most important aspects of current dentistry. If digitalization is implemented in clinical dentistry with proper knowledge, then it can bring
increased successful treatment outcomes with better care for patients. A detailed
knowledge and skills are required to achieve a fully digitalized workflow.

References

1. Srilatha A, Doshi D, Kulkarni S, Reddy MP, Bharathi V. Advanced diagnostic aids in dentalcaries—a review. J Global Oral Health. 2019;2(2):118–27.
2. Divya J, Deepak R, Medhavi S, et al. Contemporary diagnostic aids in endodontics. J Evol Med Dent Sci. 2014;3(6):1526–35.
3. Bennett TA. Emerging technologies for diagnosis of dental caries: the road so far. J Appl Phys. 2009;105
4. Yang J, Dutra V. Utility of radiology, laser fluorescence, and transillumination. Dent Cline North Am. 2005;49(4):739–52.
5. Ashley FP, Blinkhorn SA, Davies MR. Occlusal caries diagnosis: an in vitro histological validation of the electronic caries monitor (ECM) and other methods. J Dent. 1998;26:83–8.
6. Pretty AI. Caries detection and diagnosis: novel technologies. J Dent. 2006;34(10):727–39.
7. Lussi A, Imwinkelried S, Pitts N, Longbottom C, et al. Performance and reproducibility of a laser fluorescence system for detection of occlusal caries in vitro. Caries Res. 1999;33(4):261–6.
8. Novaes FT, Moriyama MC, De Benedetto MS, et al. Performance of fluorescence-based methods for detecting and quantifying smooth-surface caries lesions in primary teeth: an in vitro study. Int J Paediatr Dent. 2015;26:13.
9. Theocharopoulou A, Lagerweij MD, van Strijp AJ. Use of the ICDAS system and two fluorescence-based intraoral devices for examination of occlusal surfaces. Eur J Paediatr Dent. 2015;16(1):51–5.
10. Shivakumar KM, Prasad S, Chandu GN. International caries detection and assessment system: a new paradigm in detection of dental caries. J Conserv Dent. 2009;12(1):10–6.
11. Pretty AI. Caries detection and diagnosis. In: Limeback H, editor. Comprehensive preventive dentistry. Oxford: Wiley-Blackwell; 2013. p. 25–42.
12. Hall A, Girkin JM. A review of potential new diagnostic modalities for carious lesions. J Dent Res. 2004;83:89–94.
13. Bab I, Feuerstein O, Gazit D. Ultrasonic detector of proximal caries. Caries Res. 1997;31:322. (Abst)
14. Matalon S, Feuerstein O, Kaffe I. Diagnosis of approximal caries: bite-wing radiology versus the ultrasound caries detector. An in vitro study. Oral Surg Oral Med Oral Pathol Oral Radiol Endod. 2003;95:626–31.
15. Tagtekin DA, Öztürk F, Lagerweij O, Hayran O, et al. Thickness measurement of worn molar cusps by ultrasound. Caries Res. 2005;39:139–43.
16. Kimura Y, Wilder-Smith P, Matsumoto K. Lasers in endodontics: a review. Int Endod J. 2000;33:173–85.
17. Soo-ampon S, Vongsavan N, Soo-ampon M, Chuckpaiwong S, et al. The sources of laser Doppler blood-flow signals recorded from human teeth. Arch Oral Biol. 2003;48:353–60.
18. Gazelius, Lindh-Stromberg U, Pettersson H, Oberg PA. Laser Doppler technique—a future diagnostic tool for tooth pulp vitality. Int Endod J. 1993;26(1):8–9.
19. Eugene C, Paul AV. Dental pulp testing: a review. Int J Dent. 2009:1–12.
20. Roeykens H, Van Maele G, De Moor R, Martens L. Reliability of laser Doppler flowmetry in a 2-probe assessment of pulpal blood flow. Oral Surg Oral Med Oral Pathol Oral Radiol Endodont. 1990;87(6):742–8.
21. Ingolfsson AR, Tronstad L, Hersh EV, Riva CE. Effect of probe design on the suitability of laser Doppler flowmetry in vitality testing of human teeth. Endodont Dent Traumatol. 1993;9(2):65–70.
22. Ashraf EA, Donald YC. Dental pulp neurophysiology: part2. Current diagnostic tests to assess pulp vitality. JCDA. 2009;75(2):139–43.
23. Dakshita V, Ashish S. Pulse oximetry and laser Doppler flowmetry for diagnosing of pulp vitality. J Interdiscip Dent. 2011;1(1):14–21.
24. Sasano T, Nakajima I, Shoji N, et al. Possible application of transmitted laser light I for the assessment of human pulpal vitality. Endod Dent Traumatol. 1997;13(2):88–91.

25. Nissan R, Trope M, Zhang C-D, Chance B. Dual wavelength spectrophotometry as a diagnostic test of the pulp chamber contents. Oral Surg Oral Med Oral Pathol. 1992;74(4):508–14.
26. Nivesh R, Pradeep S. Recent diagnostic aids in endodontics—a review. IJPCR. 2016;8(8):1159–62.
27. Ramachandra SS, Dhoom M, et al. Periodontal probing systems: a review of available equipment. Res Gate. 2009;3(3):1–7.
28. Lynch JE, Hinders MK, McCombs GB. Clinical comparison of an ultrasonographic periodontal probe to manual and controlled force probing. Measurement. 2006;39:429–39.
29. Elashiry M, Meghil MM, et al. From manual probing to digital 3-D imaging to endoscopic capillaroscopy: recent advances in periodontal disease diagnosis. J Periodontal Res. 2019;54:1–9.
30. Jeffcoat MK. Diagnosing periodontal disease: new tools to solve an old problem. J Am Dent Assoc. 1991;122(1):54–9.
31. Kozlowski Z, Miklaszewska B, Konopka T, et al. Using halitometer to verify symptoms of halitosis. Adv Clin Exp Med. 2007;16(3):411–6.
32. Falcao DP, Miranda PC, Almeida TFG, et al. Assessment of the accuracy of portable monitors for halitosis evaluation in subjects without malodor complaint. Are they reliable for clinical practice? J Appl Oral Sci. 2017;25(5):559–65.
33. Zhou H, McCombs GB, Darby ML, et al. Sulphur by-product: the relationship between volatile Sulphur compounds and dental plaque-induced gingivitis. J Contemp Dent Pract. 2004;5(2):27–39.
34. McNamara TF, Alexander JF. M lee "the role of microorganisms in the production of oral malodor". Oral Surg OraMed Oral Pathol. 1972;34(1):41–8.
35. Kung RT, Ochs B, Goodson JM. Temperature as a periodontal diagnostic. J Clin Periodontol. 1990;17(8):557–63.
36. Kung RTV, Goodson JM. Diagnostic temperature probe. Accessed Oct 18, 2008.
37. Tanya P, Bozhkova. The T SCAN system in evaluating occlusal contacts. Folia Med. 2016;58(2):122–30.
38. Garg AK. Analyzing dental occlusion for implants: Tek Scan's T Scan III. Dent Implantol Updat. 2007;18(9):65–70. 28
39. Sultana MH, Yamada K, Hanada K. Changes in occlusal force and occlusal contact area after active orthodontic treatment: a pilot study using pressure-sensitive sheets. J Oral Rehabil. 2002;29(5):484–91.
40. Pyakural U, Long H, et al. Mechanism, accuracy and application of Tscan system in dentistry-review. JNDA. 2013;13(1):52–6.
41. Szentpetery A. Computer aided dynamic correction of digitized occlusal surfaces. J Gnathol. 1997;16:53–60.
42. Ruge S, Kordass B. 3D-VAS- initial results from computerized visualization of dynamic occlusion. Int J Comput Dent. 2008;11:9–16.
43. Kinuta S, Wakabayashi K, Sohmura T, Kojima T, et al. Measurement of masticatory movement by a new jaw tracking system using a home digital camcorder. Dent Mater J. 2005;24:661–6.
44. Minakuchi H, Clark GT, Haberman PB, Maekawa K, Kuboki T. Sensitivity and specificity of a miniature bruxism detection device. Oral Surg Oral Med Oral Pathol Oral Radiol Endodontol. 2005;99:440–1.
45. Vijaykumari B, Siddavaram SJ, et al. Joint vibration analysis a functional tool in diagnosis of temporomandibular disorders-a case report. Int J Contemp Med Surg Radiol. 2019;(2):B128–32.
46. Kondrat W, Sierpinska T, Radhke J. Assessment of the temporomandibular joint function in young adults without complaints from masticatory system. Int J Med Sci. 2018;15(2):161–9.
47. SUkhpal K, Riponjot S, Sandeep K. Digital revolution in orthodontic diagnosis. Ann Geriatr Educ Med Sci. 2017;2:38–40.
48. Graber TM. Orthodontics principles and practice. 3rd ed. Philadelphia, PA: W. B. Saunders; 1972.
49. Broadbent BH. A new X-ray technique and its application to orthodontia. Angle Orthod. 1931;1:45–66.

50. Alexandru O, Cosmin S, Emilia O et al. The digital decade in interdisciplinary orthodontics. ISSN:1792–5908.
51. Emilia T, Budi K, Carla AE 3D scanning, imaging, and printing in orthodontics. Issues in contemporary orthodontics, Farid Bourzgui, IntechOpen, 2015 doi: https://doi.org/10.5772/60010.
52. Vanessa P, Ljose G, Rosa C. Digital diagnosis records in orthodontics.An overview. Med Oral Patol Oral Cir Buccal. 2006;11:E88–93.
53. James M, Martin F. The cutting edge. J Clin Orthodont. 2003;37:101–3.
54. Kumar A, Ghafoor H. Rapid prototyping: a future in orthodontics. J Orthod Res. 2016;4(1):1–7.

Digital Oral Radiography

3

Carla Cabral dos Santos Accioly Lins,
Flávia Maria de Moraes Ramos-Perez,
Andrea dos Anjos Pontual, Maria Luiza dos Anjos Pontual,
and Eduarda Helena Leandro do Nascimento

3.1 Introduction

Since the discovery of X-rays and the first dental radiography, radiographic examination is essential for diagnosis. Until the mid-1980s, analog radiographic films were the only options for image receivers and played an important role in health services, clinics, and in teaching at dental schools. Besides the high radiation dose, there was a need for chemical processing to visualize the image, which is harmful to the environment.

Digital radiology was a revolution to dentistry and medicine. It was in 1987, in Geneva, that Francis Moyen demonstrated the first intraoral digital radiography system for dentistry. It was called radiovisiography. Since then, there were many technological advancements, which made it possible, that, nowadays, we have the best equipment available in the market [1]. The radiographic process waived the use of chemicals and started being digital, besides the advancement of the image manipulation resources, which greatly contributes to the diagnoses [1, 2].

The conventional radiographic examinations presented as two-dimensional images are widely used in dentistry, especially panoramic and intraoral radiographies (periapical and interproximal). Besides the innumerous advantages, such as high spatial resolution for the intraoral images and low radiation dose for both, some limitations are evident, such as the compression of three-dimensional

C. C. dos Santos Accioly Lins (✉)
Department of Anatomy, Center for Biological Sciences, Federal University of Pernambuco (UFPE), Recife, PE, Brazil

F. M. de Moraes Ramos-Perez · A. dos A. Pontual
M. L. dos Anjos Pontual
Oral Radiology Area, Department of Clinical and Preventive Dentistry, Federal University of Pernambuco (UFPE), Recife, PE, Brazil

E. H. L. do Nascimento
Department of Dentistry, Federal University of Sergipe (UFS), Aracaju, Brazil

© Springer Nature Switzerland AG 2021
P. Jain, M. Gupta (eds.), *Digitization in Dentistry*,
https://doi.org/10.1007/978-3-030-65169-5_3

anatomy, geometry distortion, and anatomical noise, which may impair the diagnosis. In cases where tridimensional assessment is required, patients will be referred for a computed tomography scan, CBCT being the most requested for dental and maxillofacial purposes.

This chapter will cover digital images features and acquisition, digital receivers, the pre- and post-processing phases of digital images, and the image manipulation tools. Additionally, many aspects of the CBCT will be described, emphasizing on the main indications of this examination and how to improve image quality for diagnosis.

3.2   Digital Radiograph

Intraoral radiographs are still considered the first-choice method for diagnosis, treatment, and patient follow-up, since they are efficient, low dose, and low cost. Digital radiographs have several advantages, such as image quality enhancements, nearly instantaneous availability of images, reduction of working time, the elimination of chemical processing, and easier image storage and communication [1, 2].

After exposure, the X-ray beam is attenuated by the tissues and reaches the image receiver, which receives analog information. This information is subsequently converted into numbers by a computerized process called analog to digital conversion [2]. This process takes place in two steps: sampling (a process that groups one voltage range) and quantification (a process that attributes a number to each range). Finally, the digital image is presented and stored in a computer.

Digital image is formed by a matrix that corresponds to a group of lines and columns of pixels (the smallest units of a digital image). Digital images are fundamentally composed of numbers that determine pixels' spatial distribution and the gray values attributed to them. The gray values vary according to the intensity of radiation absorbed during the digital receiver's exposure to the X-rays. Thereby, it is ensured that digital images are numerical and distinct [3].

Pixel matrix, pixel size, and bit depth determine important features of the digital image. Currently, the pixel size of radiographic images acquired through intraoral digital receptors is about 19–60 μm, thus providing a maximum spatial resolution that is no less than the usual radiographic film. Digital image acquisition software offers various bit depths, allowing image acquisition with 8, 10, 12, 14, or 16 bits generating images with respectively 256, 1024, 4096, 16,384, and 65,536 levels of gray. It is worth pointing out that the deeper the bit and the smaller the pixel, the bigger the contrast resolution and the spatial resolution, respectively. In theory, this allows better representation capacity of the different degrees of tissue attenuation, as well as the distinction of contiguous points in the image, resulting in better visualization of subtle differences [4]. Nevertheless, it is known that the human eye is only able to distinguish a limited amount of shades of gray.

3.3   Digital Image Acquisition

Digital image acquisition can be performed in three distinct ways: indirect acquisition by means of digitizing films, direct acquisition, using solid-state digital receivers and semi-direct acquisition using a phosphor plate system [1].

3.3.1   Indirect Digital Acquisition

On the indirect acquisition, the image is acquired through the usual method, using a conventional radiographic film and, after that, the information is captured and digitalized. The film's image capture and digitalization can be accomplished through a flatbed scanner with transparency adapted or digital cameras [1].This digital radiographic image acquisition method enables the use of the available digital tools to enhance the digital image in various software. However, a larger amount of working time is required for the digital image acquisition, thus adding one more step to the image acquisition.

3.3.2   Direct Digital Acquisition

In the direct digital radiographic acquisition, the radiographic film is replaced by a solid-state receiver, which can be charged coupled devices or complementary metal oxide semiconductors.

On the intraoral solid-state receivers, a thick, rectangular-shaped, rigid plastic casing protects a silicon chip and other components against deterioration and contamination. Most of these intraoral receivers are connected to the computer by a cable. The CCD receiver has a silicon matrix organized in the same way as the pixels. Above this matrix, there is a layer of scintillator material. Some manufacturers add an optic-fiber layer between the scintillator layer and the silicon chip to protect the matrix (pixels) from direct X-ray penetration and thus prolong the sensor life span. The CMOS-type sensors have a similar structure to the CCD type, consisting of a pixel array but differing from the aforementioned on the way charges are transferred and read [5].

There are intraoral direct digital systems that use wireless technology to transmit digital image information [1, 6]. These systems can use common radio-frequency waves [6] or bluetooth waves. On the systems that use bluetooth waves, the sensor is connected to a base station through a cable, and the data transmission from this station to the computer happens as waves. The base is magnetized, or the systems provide a holder to stow and fixate the equipment on any surface during image acquisition. The systems that use this technology usually have a receiver antenna in the form of a USB flash drive that must be inserted into the computer's USB port.

One of the systems that use bluetooth waves on data transmission (X-POD, MyRay, Imola, Italy) also allows image acquisition without a computer, since it has a base unit with a touch screen to control image acquisition, visualization, and managing. The images are saved and organized in folders for each patient, stored on the removable secure digital memory card. In this case, the images are stored in a memory card, and afterward synchronize the equipment with the computer software and use bluetooth waves or connect the base unit to the computer through a USB cable to transmit the radiographic images.

The CDR wireless system (Schick Technologies, Inc., Long Island City, NY, USA) was the first wireless solid-state digital system, and it uses a battery on the sensor's posterior surface (non-active side) and emits radio-frequency waves to a base station. This station captures the waves through a receiver antenna and transmits the information to a computer via an optic-fiber cable and a USB interface. The disadvantage of this system is the increased thickness of the sensor compared to other receivers [1, 6].

Extraoral direct digital sensor presents pixels on long, linear, and thin matrix. This matrix has few pixels widthwise and many pixels lengthwise. The long and narrow pixel matrix is aligned with the X-ray beam and, for the image acquisition, there is a scanning movement of the area to be exposed. When solid-state receivers are used, the extraoral radiography acquisition process takes a few seconds from the exposure to X-rays until the appearance of the image on the computer monitor [1].

The main advantage of solid-state digital systems is that the image appears almost instantly after the exposure of the receiver to X-rays. The smaller active area of image receivers and the reduced dynamic scale when compared to films and PSP plates are disadvantages of the intraoral solid-state receivers. Besides, the rigid and thicker plastic pack and the cable may bring discomfort to the patient and complicate the placement of the receiver.

3.3.3   Semi-Direct Digital Acquisition

In the semi-direct digital acquisition, the conventional radiographic film is replaced by the PSP plate. When exposed to X-rays, these plates absorb and store energy, forming a latent image. To visualize the image, the PSP plate must be processed after exposure by scanning the plate through each system's scanner (data reading) [3].

PSP plates are comprised of a polyester base with one of its surfaces covered by a europium-doped barium fluoride halide (active side). The combination of barium with chloride, iodine, or boron forms a crystalline gelatin. When those plates are exposed to X-rays, europium's valence electrons absorb energy and may jump to the conduction bands. These electrons might migrate to halide vacancies (F centers) and be captured in a latent state. While remaining in this state, the number of captured electrons is proportional to the exposure to X-rays, and it represents a latent image (invisible and nonpermanent).

During the scanning step, after adapting the plate on the system scanner, the scanner will perform the sweeping of the plate through a thin collimated laser beam that will stimulate the release the energy stored. The information is converted to electrical signals, subsequently converted into binary digits through an analog to digital converter, and the image is visualized. The time required for the plate reading step varies from some seconds to a few minutes depending on the digital system scan resolution, brand, and manufacturer. Usually, intraoral PSP scanners process and display images in a matter of seconds.

The spatial resolution of images acquired by PSP plates systems is determined by some factors, such as phosphor layer thickness and laser diameter. The thicker the plate and the bigger the laser diameter, the smaller the image resolution. Another important issue is the interval between exposure and scanning of the PSP plate. After exposure to X-rays, the plates must be scanned as swiftly as possible, since some studies have shown changes in pixel values and these changes may cause loss of quality and affect clinical image interpretation when too much time elapses between exposure and the scanning [7]. Furthermore, during plate manipulation for scanning, one must follow the manufacturer's recommendations regarding the ambient light since it can potentially alter image quality.

After the plate scanning process, some energy is still left on the plate, and thus some electrons remain as "energy traps" (residual image). To use the PSP plate for another radiographic acquisition, the residual image sign must be eliminated by the active side of the plate exposure to a bright light source [1]. This process is done within the scanner itself right after the scanning. Subsequently, the phosphor plates must be stored on a lightproof recipient. It is recommended that the intraoral plates be stored on polyvinyl envelopes to protect them from oral fluids. Extraoral phosphor plates are positioned in chassis without image intensifiers.

PSP plates are available in various sizes which are compatible with the many sizes of conventional radiographic films. There are PSP digital systems that have phosphor plates with sizes compatible with intraoral radiographic films (sizes 0, 1, 2, 3, and 4) and others that, in addition to these plates sizes, have plates with similar sizes to the extraoral radiographic films.

PSP digital system has a wide dynamic range that avoids retakes by under-exposed and over-exposed images [7]. Besides, the PSP plate is more acceptable to patients because it is a wireless receiver, has comparable flexibility to conventional films, and is thinner than a solid-state receiver [7]. On the other hand, image acquisition and visualization happens in a few seconds since more steps are needed to visualize the image. Besides, the PSP plates are easily damaged during handling in dental practice, which deteriorates image quality by the presence of image artifacts as scratches and stains and are sensitive to rubbing with some disinfectants [7]. It is a disadvantage as it represents the need for phosphor plate continual reposition. To reduce damage risk during handling, some intraoral systems have protective covers.

The intraoral digital receivers and the surfaces of head stabilizing and positioning apparatus of extraoral direct digital Xray machines must be protected by disposable surface barriers against cross-contamination. A two-layer barrier may be used to prevent contamination of the intraoral receivers [7]. Some manufacturers introduced an automated internal ultraviolet (UV) disinfection feature that according to them inactivates viruses and bacteria on the plate transport mechanism of intraoral PSP digital systems.

3.4   Digital Radiographic Processing

Digital radiographic systems have several tools that allow imaging adjustment, which generally aim to improve its quality and/or ease its assessment. These adjustments are called *radiographic processing* and can occur at two different moments: first at the digital reading and conversion of data by the computer immediately after the radiographic acquisition, but before the image display on the monitor, named *pre-processing*; and after the appearance of the image on the computer screen, also known as *post-processing*.

3.4.1   Pre-Processing of Digital Images

All the adjustments automatically made by the software owner of the digital systems before the image appears on the computer screen are classified as pre-processing. The occurrence and degree of adjustments to the images happen regardless of the professional's will and, in most systems, these adjustments cannot be disabled.

Among the main pre-processing adjustments, the replacement of defective pixel values in CCD systems and the automatic exposure compensation (AEC), present in most direct digital systems, can be mentioned. In the first case, the replacement of defective pixel values of CCD systems by the weighted average of the values of neighboring pixels is performed in order to homogenize the images and reduce noise. The AEC is a nonlinear enhancement of the image that identifies the lowest and highest pixel values and changes the grayscale to increase radiographic contrast. Thus, the AEC favors the production of images of high contrast even when there are variations in the exposure of the image receiver to the X-rays, possibly increasing the dynamic range of digital radiography (exposure range in which it is possible to obtain images clinically suitable) [8]. Furthermore, it was recently demonstrated that the presence of high-density materials in the imaged region, such as metallic restorations, endodontic materials, and dental implants, is able to alter the gray values of the whole image because of the presence of AEC, further increasing the contrast of the images [9]. However, little is known about the possible influence of this automatic correction on the diagnosis of different dental conditions.

One of the advantages of pre-processing integrated with digital systems is the improvement of image quality, often automatically correcting under- or overexposed images. On the other hand, the fact that this processing is hidden from the user often prevents such conditions to be perceived by the professional and corrected clinically.

3.4.2 Post-Processing of Digital Images

The post-processing of the images comprises the adjustments made manually and subjectively by the operator, after viewing the image on the computer monitor. Any operation that the professional performs to improve, restore, modify, or analyze the image is considered post-processing. Generally, such modifications can be undone in the software used during post-processing.

The main adjustments that can be made in digital radiography are related to the modification of the size of the pixels and changes in the histogram (distribution of gray values) of the image. Digital systems can have several image manipulations tools, and these can be accessed in the radiographic acquisition system software or in specific software for this purpose. Among the most commonly used tools, that we can mention are manipulation of brightness and contrast, zoom, linear and angular measurements. In addition, the inverted radiography and pseudocolor tools and the filters of relief, sharpness, and smoothing are also generally available in the post-processing software. The main modifications made to the image by each tool are described as follows.

Brightness and contrast: These are adjustments commonly made by profession-als. The brightness is related to the degree of darkening of the image. Increasing the brightness makes the image visibly clearer. On the other hand, the contrast refers to the visual difference between the densities of the structures X-rayed. Thus, increas-ing the contrast causes the difference between the gray tones of the image to increase. To increase the brightness of a radiograph, the software increases the gray values of the pixels evenly. To increase the contrast, the software must decrease the darker half of the gray values and increases the pixel values of the lighter half. The adjustment of the "histogram" tool allows simultaneous modification of the bright-ness and contrast of the images, controlled by the "gamma curve." Such modifica-tions must be used carefully, according to the professional's preference, so as not to mask areas of different densities (Fig. 3.1a–e).

Zoom: Zoom refers to the magnification of the image on the monitor and, together with the brightness and contrast, is one of the tools most used in the assessment of digital radiographs. The zoom facilitates the visualization of details in the image, but it must be used sparingly, since when enlarging the digital image, its pixels may become evident. The higher the spatial resolution of the image, the greater its power of magnification without loss of image quality.

Measurements: Linear and angular measurements are widely used in several spe-cialties in dentistry, and their precision has been proven by various studies. Examples of its applications involve the determination of the measurements of root canal sys-tems in endodontics, cephalometric measurements in orthodontics, and determining the height of the alveolar ridge in edentulous regions in implantology (Fig. 3.1f).

Sharpness and smoothing: These filters are intended, respectively, to enhance and soften the boundary between the structures. Both filters represent mathematical algorithms that reduce the blur or noise image, improving its quality. In this way, the radiograph becomes more attractive. However, the improvement in the diagnostic performance of images with filters is still controversial in the literature.

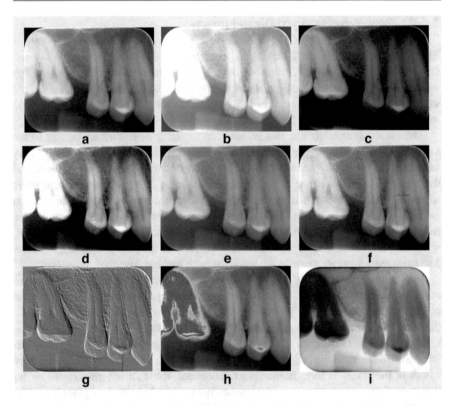

Fig. 3.1 Examples of post-processing of a digital image: original image (**a**) and enhanced images with brightness (**b**, **c**) and contrast (**d**, **e**) adjustments, linear measurements (**f**) and, high relief (**g**), pseudocolor (**h**), and radiographic inverted view (**i**)

High relief: The high relief, relief, or three-dimensional tool gives the appearance of relief to structures of greater density, highlighting the limits of structures of different degrees of attenuation to X-rays, such as enamel and dentin (Fig. 3.1g).

Pseudocolor: Consists in transforming gray tones to image color. This tool does not have clinical applicability, considering that it does not add any real factor that can improve the diagnosis. On the contrary, pseudocolor can modify the limits and the appearance of the real object (Fig. 3.1h).

Inverted radiography: The radiographic inverted view is based on the inversion of the gray values of the image pixels. With the use of this tool, radiolucent structures become radiopaque and vice versa on radiographs. However, this tool does not seem to bring benefits to the diagnosis in dentistry (Fig. 3.1i).

3.5   Digital Subtraction Radiography

In addition to these post-processing tools, in some software it is possible to perform a technique called *digital subtraction radiography*. It aims to compare two standardized radiographs from the same region, taken at different times. To do this, the software subtracts similar structures in the two images, that is, those that have not changed during the time interval, presenting them in an intermediate gray shade. In the areas of tissue loss and gain, respectively, a darker shade of gray and a lighter shade of gray are added to the image. Subtraction is indicated for the evaluation of tissue repair or healing, monitoring of patients with periodontal disease, among other indications. The main challenge for performing this technique, however, is the accurate standardization of the radiograph, since small changes in the image acquisition geometry can substantially interfere with the result of radiographic subtraction.

3.6   Cone Beam Computed Tomography (CBCT)

Cone beam CT (CBCT) is a three-dimensional imaging technique commonly used in dentistry. Initially, it was developed to use in angiography and, after that, based on the studies by Mozzo et al. [10] in 1998, a machine specifically designed for dental and maxillofacial evaluation was created. However, it was only in the mid-2000 that its use became more widespread. Since then, dental practitioners have been requesting CBCT for their patients. The criteria for referring patients to CBCT should be carefully selected because of its higher radiation dose compared to conventional radiographs, especially in cases of younger patients.

In all dental specialties, CBCT should be indicated only when it is believed that this examination will provide additional information that may alter the patient's diagnosis, treatment plan, or prognosis.

3.7   Clinical Applications of CBCT

3.7.1   Dental Implant Treatment Planning

Implant dental planning is one of the most common indications for CBCT, because this imaging modality offers cross-sectional and three-dimensional reconstructions, allowing preoperative evaluation of volume, architecture, and density of the residual alveolar ridge. The use of CBCT is indicated when clinical examination and two-dimensional radiography fail to identify local problems, topography, and relationship to important anatomic structures surrounding remaining alveolar bone, such as nasopalatine canal, maxillary sinus, nasal floor, mental foramen, submandibular fossa, and mandibular canal (Fig. 3.2).

CBCT is considered appropriate for diagnosis and treatment planning in the following cases: extensive bone augmentation procedures, sinus floor elevation procedures, computer-guided implant surgery, zygomatic implant placement, and osteogenic distraction [11]. Besides, before the elevation procedure and dental implant placement in the posterior maxilla, the evaluation of the maxillary sinus should consider the presence of pathology, evaluation of the Schneiderian membrane, and the presence and type of septa, since the presence of septa increases the risk for perforation of this membrane. In implant placement, CBCT allows proper

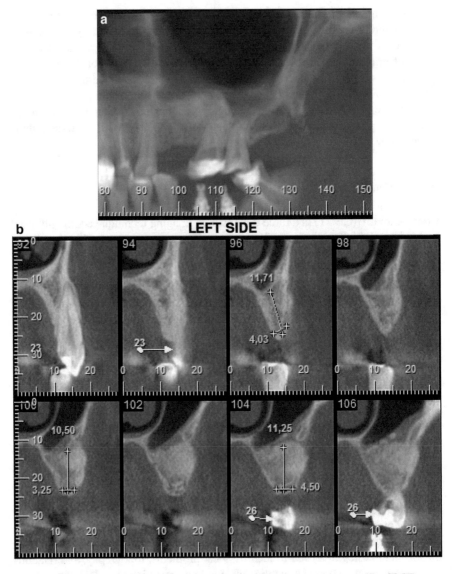

Fig. 3.2 Panoramic (a) and cross-sectional images (b) of a posterior maxilla CBCT scan. Measurements of alveolar bone height and width (cross-sectional image n. 96), and bone graft (cross-sectional n. 100, 102, and 104)

preoperative planning with a higher degree of prediction and agreement when compared to the surgical standard [12] and, additionally, the information obtained from this imaging modality can support the planning and improve the predictability of the prosthetic result [13].

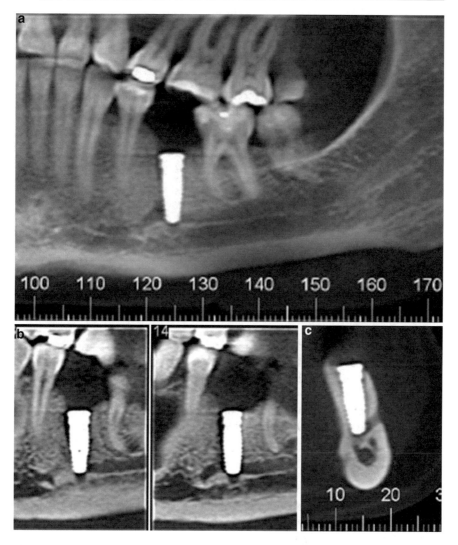

Fig. 3.3 Panoramic image shows an implant in mandibular premolars region (**a**). Sagittal (**b**) and coronal images (**c**) show an implant invading the mental foramen

Two-dimensional radiography techniques are adequate to follow-up the patients in the absence of symptoms. However, based on the clinical symptoms, CBCT may be helpful for the diagnosis and management of postoperative complications following implant placement, such as neurosensory disturbance, postoperative infections, injuries to adjacent teeth, and invasion of anatomic structures (e.g., maxillary sinus, mental foramen, and mandibular canal) (Figs. 3.3 and 3.4) [11].

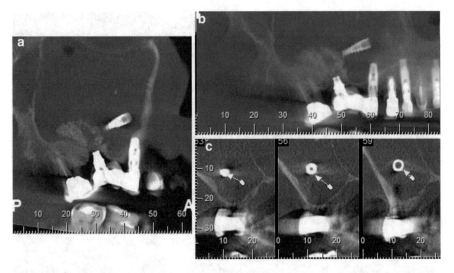

Fig. 3.4 Sagittal (**a**), panoramic (**b**), and cross-sectional (**c**) images show the implant displacement into maxillary sinus and the complete opacification of the maxillary sinus

3.7.2 Endodontics

CBCT should be preferred when periapical radiographs fail to provide enough information. It has been demonstrated that the evaluation of three-dimensional images positively influence endodontists in making decision. Due to the complexity of the root canal system and the need for images with a high level of detail, it is important to use smaller FOV and voxel to obtain high-quality images.

3.7.2.1 Canal Morphology

One of the reasons for endodontic therapy failures is the non-visualization of the canal complex anatomy. Despite this, CBCT is not indicated as the first choice technique to assess root canal anatomy. Three-dimensional images can be requested in cases of greater complexity, especially in multi-rooted teeth and in some cases of teeth with root canal anomalies.

3.7.2.2 Inflammatory Lesions

Periapical pathosis are common lesions in the jaws and, in most cases, are diagnosed during routine radiographic examination. Periapical radiography is the standard technique for diagnosis; however, the overlap of structures, anatomical noise, and distortion may impair the diagnosis. Additionally, the real size of the lesions can be underestimated. CBCT is important as a complementary method, in those cases when there are clinical signals and symptoms and the periapical radiography presented inconclusive findings.

In the presence of external root resorption, especially if these lesions are small and located in buccal or lingual surfaces, the diagnosis can be difficult with two-dimensional images. CBCT should be requested if a three-dimensional evaluation has an influence on treatment decision making and/or alter the prognosis.

3.7.2.3 Root Vertical Fractures

Periapical radiographs and their variations using the parallax technique are commonly used to evaluate teeth with suspected fracture. However, in some cases, in the absence of fragment displacement or if the central X-ray beam did not pass parallel to the fracture line, it will not be identified. To help with this task, dental practitioners may request high-resolution three-dimensional images, since they present high accuracy and may be useful to the diagnosis (Figs. 3.5 and 3.6). This diagnosis is challenging especially in the presence of teeth with high atomic dental materials (dental implants, metal restorations, metal posts, and gutta-percha and endodontics sealers), due to beam hardening artifacts formation, which may damage the image. In some cases, the presence of bone resorption adjacent to the fracture line may be helpful in its detection.

3.7.3 Maxillofacial Surgery

Among the applications of CBCT in surgery, the evaluation of paranasal sinuses, upper airway, craniofacial development changes, orthodontic (Fig. 3.7) and orthognathic planning and, mainly, the evaluation of impacted teeth can be mentioned (Figs. 3.8 and 3.9). Because the latter is the most common application in surgery, it is described in more detail below.

3.7.3.1 Impacted Teeth and Third Molars Evaluation

Impacted teeth are those that have complete root formation, are partially or completely covered by bone, but fail to erupt within the expected normal time. Several factors can contribute to dental impaction, such as skeletal and/or dental malocclusion (making the space available smaller than the space required for dental

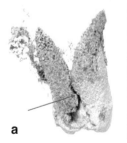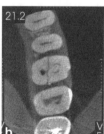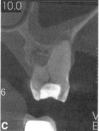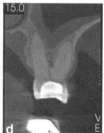

Fig. 3.5 CBCT in endodontics. (a) Three-dimensional, (b) axial, (c, d) cross-sectional images show a tooth fracture with crown and dental furcation involvement

Fig. 3.6 (**a**) Sagittal, (**b**) cross-sectional (**c**) axial and (**d**, **e**) three dimensional images show a tooth fracture involving both cown and roots

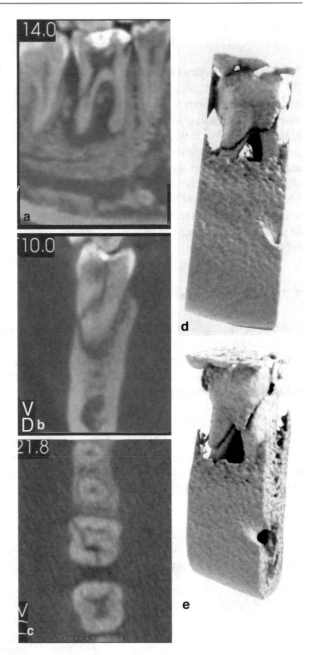

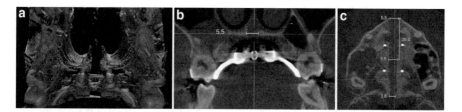

Fig. 3.7 Palatine disjunction. It is possible to assess treatment outcome after maxillary expansion using CBCT scans. (**a**) Three-dimensional, (**b**) coronal and (**c**) axial images

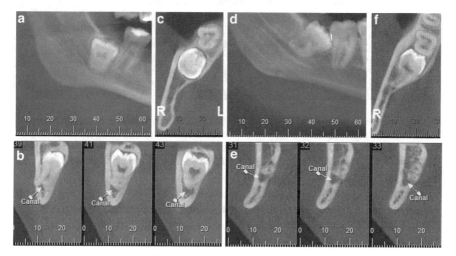

Fig. 3.8 Panoramic images show the angulation of impacted third molar (**a**—vertical and **d**—mesioangular). Cross-sectional images (**b**, **e**) demonstrate contact of third molars roots with inferior alveolar nerve (arrows). The axial images reveal the contact between third and second mandibular molars (**c**, **f**)

accommodation), developmental disorders (such as the presence of cleft palate), pathologies (which may directly involve the tooth in question or be adjacent to it, interfering with its eruption path), presence of supernumerary teeth, and ankylosis [14].

The teeth most frequently impacted are the third molars and canines. As consequences of dental impacts, external root resorption of adjacent teeth, intracoronary resorption of the involved tooth, malocclusion and development of pathologies

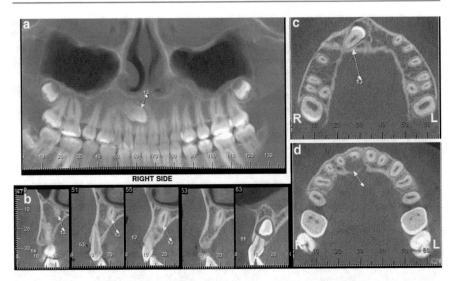

Fig. 3.9 (**a**) Panoramic, (**b**) cross-sectional, (**c**) and (**d**) axial images show a mesioangulated positioned impacted right maxillary canine with the root in contact with the floor of the nasal cavity and palatine cortical plate. The impacted tooth induced external root resorption of an adjacent tooth (maxillary central incisor-cross-sectional images n.61, 63, 65 and axial image **d**)

(inflammatory, cystic or tumor) can be mentioned. CBCT is especially important in the diagnosis of tooth resorption, as it also contributes significantly to the assessment of the degree of affected dental tissue. Besides, CBCT is important to assess the three-dimensional spatial location of the impacted tooth and its relationship with other adjacent teeth and anatomical structures, often improving surgical planning and predictability.

Impacted or not, the third molars are teeth that usually need to be removed, either because of the unfavorable anatomical position, lack of adequate space in the dental arch, association with infectious processes, or painful symptoms. For the assessment of third molars, CBCT should be indicated when a radiographic image shows specific signs of proximity between the tooth and the mandibular canal or the maxillary sinus. In addition to assessing the relationship of the tooth to these structures, attention should be paid to the presence of anatomical variations in the region, root morphology, relationship with the cortical bone, anatomical position, and possible associated pathologies. Although some studies have shown that CBCT does not change the prediction of neurosensory disturbances compared to panoramic radiography, recent studies indicate that the evaluation of CBCT changes the treatment plan for lower third molars, especially due to the diagnosis of external resorption of the second molar and the relationship between the tooth and the mandibular canal [15–17].

3.7.3.2 TMJ Bone Assessment

The morphology of the osseous joint components (mandibular condyle, glenoid fossa of the temporal bone, and articular eminence) and bone integrity are accurately visualized by three-dimensional images (Fig. 3.10). Consequently, CBCT is frequently requested to investigate bone temporomandibular joint (TMJ) alterations, such as intra-articular fractures (Fig. 3.11), osteoarthritis (Fig. 3.12), fibro-osseous ankylosis (Fig. 3.13), pathologies, hypoplasia [18], and outcome of orthognathic surgery in TMJ [19]. In addition, CBCT images also allow the assessment of joint space [19] and condylar mobility [20] (Fig. 3.14). This is important, once is associated with disk displacement, mainly in joints with reducible disk displacement [20].

For TMJ examinations, normally is used the one axial view of the examined condyles, then it is reconstructed sagittal (perpendicular to the long axis of the condyle) and coronal (parallel to the long axis of the condyle) of the joint. In addition,

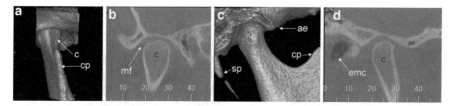

Fig. 3.10 CBCT imaging of TMJ. (**a**) Three-dimensional in frontal view; (**b**) Coronal (**c**) Three-dimensional in lateral view; (**d**) sagittal images: c (condyle), cp (coronoid process), mf (mandibular fossa), sp. (styloid process), ae (articular eminence), and eam (external acoustic meatus)

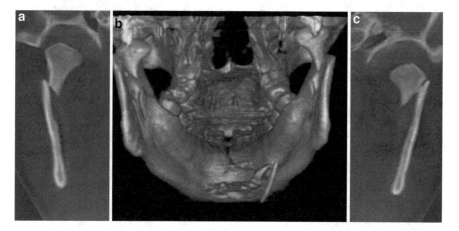

Fig. 3.11 (**a, c**) Coronal and (**b**) three-dimensional images show bilateral mandibular condylar neck fractures

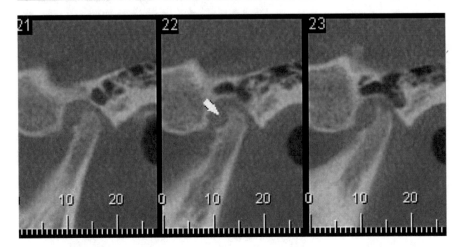

Fig. 3.12 Sagittal images show degenerative temporomandibular joint bone changes

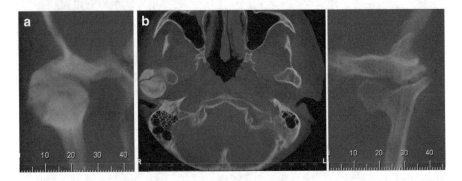

Fig. 3.13 (a, c) Coronal (b) Axial images presenting a fibro-osseous ankyloses

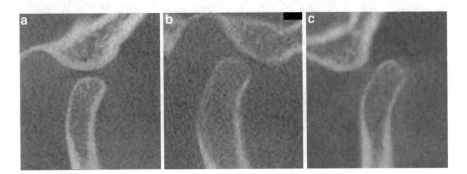

Fig. 3.14 Sagittal images are used to evaluate TMJ mobility. (a) Normomobility; (b) Hypomobility; and (c) Hypermobility

CBCT images of higher resolutions are preferred, with at least 0.2 mm of voxel to avoid that small alterations not be detected [21].

Based on imaginological evaluations, TMJ disorders affects 8% to 35% of the population, corresponding to the second most common reason for facial pain [22]. Osteoarthritis is the most frequent alteration of bone changes in TMJ, with the mandibular condyle being the most affected bone component [4]. It is more frequent in female patients and more probable that older patients have more expressive degenerative alterations than younger [22–24]. Several bone changes that characterize osteoarthritis: flattening, subcortical sclerosis, osteophyte, erosion and, subcortical cyst are presented in the Fig. 3.15.

The numerous advantages over this three-dimensional imaging modality explain why CBCT has been replacing Multi-detector Computed Tomography (MDCT) among dentists. CBCT presents a low radiation dose and a higher spatial resolution for hard tissues compared to MDCT. Additionally, CBCT machines are easy to operate, with faster scan time and low economic cost, besides allowing a comfortable positioning for the patients.

However, it is important to emphasize that effective dose varies according to the different CBCT units and their exposure parameters. For example, the higher the size of the field of view (FOV), number of basis images, and mAs, the greater the effective dose. These adjustments should be selected, keeping in mind their effects on image quality.

Despite the many advantages, some disadvantages should be considered such as the inability to assess soft tissue and the presence of artifacts. In CBCT machines, the gray values do not represent the real density of the tissues evaluated. These values are influenced by the FOV size, radiation scattering, artifacts, noise and reconstruction algorithms, different from those gray values (Hounsfield Units – HU) derived from MDCT, which are precise and reliable. This inability to represent the gray values leads to low contrast resolution images, especially for soft tissues.

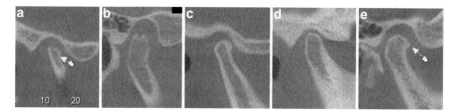

Fig. 3.15 Sagittal images with bone changes of degenerative joint disease in the condyle. (a) subcortical cyst; (b) erosion; (c) subcortical sclerosis; (d) flattening, and (e) osteophyte

3.7.4 Types of Artifacts

The artifacts are any type of distortion, which is not related to the scanned patient and can negatively influence the diagnosis. They may be classified according to the factor responsible for their origin into the following types/categories: beam hardening, photon starvation, partial volume effect, exomass, detector miscalibration, and patient motion.

Beam hardening and photon starvation artifacts are the most frequent because they are produced in the presence of high atomic number dental materials, usually present in the oral cavity, such as dental implants, metal restorations, gutta-percha and endodontics sealers, metal posts, among others. When the X-rays interact with the materials aforementioned, the incident beam is filtered, in the case of beam hardening, or completely absorbed, in the case of photon starvation. This results in the formation of hypodense (halo and dark bands) and/or hyperdense (white streaks) artifacts (Fig. 3.16). Their influence on image quality has been described extensively in the literature, mimicking root fractures, impairing viewing bone level around implants and simulating failures around restorations or metal posts. To reduce beam hardening and photon starvation effects and improve image quality, several methods have been recommended such as alteration/or combining of exposure parameters (i.e., high kVp, mAs, and degree of rotation) and the use of metal artifact reduction (MAR) algorithms. MAR tool is presented in some devices and its activation could be done before or after the acquisition. What is known is that the MAR tool only acts in the presence of artifacts generated by high-density materials present inside the FOV [25, 26].

The *partial volume* effect is related to the difference between the sizes of the evaluated structure and the voxel, which is defined as the smallest volume unit of the image. Thus, structures smaller than the voxel may be distorted or misrepresented in the image.

Exomass refers to any structure that is in the path of the X-ray beam but outside the field of view (FOV) of the exam (Fig. 3.17). Such structures, especially those with a high atomic number, can attenuate the beam to the point of negatively interfering with the signal reaching the image receiver and, consequently, decreasing the image quality. Interestingly, it is worth mentioning that MAR algorithms are not effective to correct CBCT artifacts arising from objects in exomass [27].

Detector miscalibration, on the other hand, is represented by flaws in the uniformity of data detection, which can be caused by altered or defective pixels in the image receiver or lack of maintenance of the CBCT device. Image errors are always projected in the same location as the receiver, causing loss of information in the affected area.

Motion artifacts are caused by the patient's movement during the CBCT scanning, which results in a change in the geometric positioning of the projected structures, often causing duplicity image at the limit of the structures and loss of image sharpness.

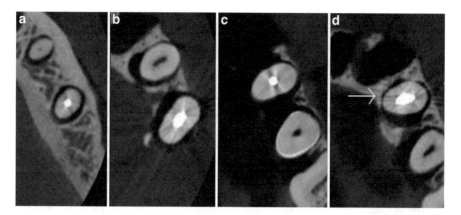

Fig. 3.16 Axial images of teeth restored with endodontic material filling. There is a more expressive artifact production of dark halo and bands in **a**, **c**, dark bands, and white streaks in **b** and **d**. In **d**, the arrow points to a dark band mimicking a root fracture

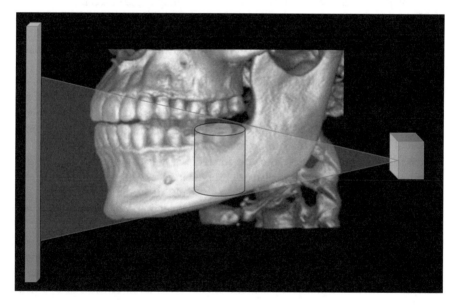

Fig. 3.17 Illustration of exomass. The cylinder represents a small FOV. Structures outside the FOV but in the path of the X-ray can negatively interfere in the image quality

Currently, several CBCT systems are commercially available, with different parameters of acquisition (type of exposure, degree of rotation, voltage, and tube current), FOV, and voxel size. All of them can directly influence the image quality. Thus, the choice of these parameters must consider the image quality for each specific diagnostic.

The first CBCT machines presented image intensifiers detectors, which were replaced to flat panel because of its features, such as distortion-free, higher dose efficiency, a wider dynamic range, and high spatial and contrast resolution [28]. Concerning the X-rays tube, the devices can present pulsed or continuous exposure. Several ones used pulsed exposure since they presented a better spatial resolution.

Some CBCT units allow acquisitions with partial/half (180°) instead of full (360°) rotation, which reduces the number of basis images and mAs, implying lower radiation dose for the patients. As a result, a loss of image quality can be observed. However, previous studies demonstrated good diagnostic images for implant planning [29], similar values of accuracy and sensitivity for root fracture detection [30], and good visualization of the anterior skull base and paranasal sinus [31].

The voltage or tube potential determines the energy of the X-rays. The higher the kVp, the higher the average energy photons, decreasing beam hardening artifacts formation. Besides that, a lower noise will also be observed, all of them contributing to improving the image quality. However, an increase in radiation dose for the patient will occur and this must be justifiable according to the criteria.

The product of the current tube (mA) with exposure time(s) is directly proportional to the dose. In some CBCT units, the current tube allows variation, while the voltage (kVp) is fixed. A combination of high kVp with low mAs should be considered to optimize CBCT images and maintain the radiation dose.

Based on the diagnostic task, the best scanning protocol should be chosen. As FOV size can vary from limited (4 × 4 cm) to large (up to 20 cm), exposure of the patient to a large volume for evaluating a small area is not justified due to the increase in effective dose for the patient. Besides that, larger FOVs lead to a decrease in spatial resolution, resulting in an image with more noise because there is an increase in scattered radiation after the interaction with the object. Nevertheless, impairment in image quality can also be observed in cases of smaller FOV sizes due to an indirect increase of the exomass that negatively affects the voxel values.

Smaller voxel sizes increase the accuracy in detecting longitudinal root fractures [32], external root resorption [33], and periodontal bone defects [34]. To assure the image quality, the size of the FOV, voxel and acquisition parameters will be selected, bearing in mind that doses should be kept "as low as reasonably achievable," following ALARA/ALADAIP principle. The last one has been introduced to refer to "as low as diagnostically achievable being indication-oriented and patient-specific" [35].

Concerns about the risks led the researchers to the development of guidelines, such as SEDENTEXCT [36] and DIMITRA [37], which focus on justification of patient exposure and dose optimization, later being specifically designed for pediatric dentistry.

The great value of CBCT images for dentistry is undoubted. Criteria for referring patients should be strictly selected, considering that the benefits must outweigh the risks. Professionals should attempt to choose the best image modality for each specific diagnostic task and consider low-dose protocols (mAs reduction, partial rotation, smaller FOVs, and larger voxel sizes), whenever is possible.

References

1. Van der Stelt PF. Better imaging: the advantages of digital radiography. J Am Dent Assoc. 2008;139(Suppl):7s–13s.
2. van der Stelt PF. Principles of digital imaging. Dent Clin N Am. 2000;44(2):237–48. v
3. van der Stelt PF. Filmless imaging: the uses of digital radiography in dental practice. J Am Dent Assoc. 2005;136(10):1379–87.
4. Heo MS, Choi DH, Benavides E, Huh KH, Yi WJ, Lee SS, et al. Effect of bit depth and kVp of digital radiography for detection of subtle differences. Oral Surg Oral Med Oral Pathol Oral Radiol Endod. 2009;108(2):278–83.
5. Sanderink GC, Miles DA. Intraoral detectors. CCD, CMOS, TFT, and other devices. Dent Clin N Am. 2000;44(2):249–55. v
6. Tsuchida R, Araki K, Endo A, Funahashi I, Okano T. Physical properties and ease of operation of a wireless intraoral x-ray sensor. Oral Surg Oral Med Oral Pathol Oral Radiol Endod. 2005;100(5):603–8.
7. Wenzel A, Moystad A. Work flow with digital intraoral radiography: a systematic review. Acta Odontol Scand. 2010;68(2):106–14.
8. Yoshiura K, Nakayama E, Shimizu M, Goto TK, Chikui T, Kawazu T, et al. Effects of the automatic exposure compensation on the proximal caries diagnosis. Dentomaxillofac Radiol. 2005;34(3):140–4.
9. Galvao NS, Nascimento EHL, Lima CAS, Freitas DQ, Haiter-Neto F, Oliveira ML. Can a high-density dental material affect the automatic exposure compensation of digital radiographic images? Dentomaxillofac Radiol. 2019;48(3):20180331.
10. Mozzo P, Procacci C, Tacconi A, Martini PT, Andreis IA. A new volumetric CT machine for dental imaging based on the cone-beam technique: preliminary results. Eur Radiol. 1998;8(9):1558–64.
11. Bornstein MM, Horner K, Jacobs R. Use of cone beam computed tomography in implant dentistry: current concepts, indications and limitations for clinical practice and research. Periodontol. 2017;73(1):51–72.
12. Guerrero ME, Noriega J, Jacobs R. Preoperative implant planning considering alveolar bone grafting needs and complication prediction using panoramic versus CBCT images. Imaging Sci Dent. 2014;44(3):213–20.
13. Harris D, Horner K, Gröndahl K, Jacobs R, Helmrot E, Benic GI, et al. E.a.O. guidelines for the use of diagnostic imaging in implant dentistry 2011. A consensus workshop organized by the European Association for Osseointegration at the Medical University of Warsaw. Clin Oral Implants Res. 2012;23(11):1243–53.
14. Scarfe WCA. Christos maxillofacial cone beam computed tomography: principles, techniques and clinical applications, vol. 2018. 1st ed: Springer; 2018. p. 1242.
15. Hermann L, Wenzel A, Schropp L, Matzen LH. Impact of CBCT on treatment decision related to surgical removal of impacted maxillary third molars: does CBCT change the surgical approach? Dentomaxillofac Radiol. 2019;48(8):20190209.
16. Matzen LH, Petersen LB, Schropp L, Wenzel A. Mandibular canal-related parameters interpreted in panoramic images and CBCT of mandibular third molars as risk factors to predict sensory disturbances of the inferior alveolar nerve. Int J Oral Maxillofac Surg. 2019;48(8):1094–101.
17. Matzen LH, Villefrance JS, Nørholt SE, Bak J, Wenzel A. Cone beam CT and treatment decision of mandibular third molars: removal vs. coronectomy-a 3-year audit. Dentomaxillofac Radiol. 2020;49(3):20190250.
18. Larheim TA, Abrahamsson AK, Kristensen M, Arvidsson LZ. Temporomandibular joint diagnostics using CBCT. Dentomaxillofac Radiol. 2015;44(1):20140235.
19. Guo Y, Qiao X, Yao S, Li T, Jiang N, Peng C. CBCT analysis of changes in dental occlusion and temporomandibular joints before and after MEAW Orthotherapy in patients with nonlow angle of skeletal class III. Biomed Res Int. 2020;2020:7238263.

20. Imanimoghaddam M, Madani AS, Mahdavi P, Bagherpour A, Darijani M, Ebrahimnejad H. Evaluation of condylar positions in patients with temporomandibular disorders: a cone-beam computed tomographic study. Imaging Sci Dent. 2016;46(2):127–31.
21. Patel A, Tee BC, Fields H, Jones E, Chaudhry J, Sun Z. Evaluation of cone- beam computed tomography in the diagnosis of simulated small osseous defects in the mandibular condyle. Am J Orthod Dentofacial Orthop. 2014;145(2):143–56.
22. Dumbuya A, Gomes AF, Marchini L, Zeng E, Comnick CL, Melo SLS. Bone changes in the temporomandibular joints of older adults: a cone-beam computed tomography study. Spec Care Dentist. 2020;40(1):84–9.
23. Walewski LA, Tolentino ES, Yamashita FC, Iwaki LCV, da Silva MC. Cone beam computed tomography study of osteoarthritic alterations in the osseous components of temporomandibular joints in asymptomatic patients according to skeletal pattern, gender, and age. Oral Surg Oral Med Oral Pathol Oral Radiol. 2019;128(1):70–7.
24. dos Anjos Pontual ML, Freire JS, Barbosa JM, Frazao MA, dos Anjos Pontual A. Evaluation of bone changes in the temporomandibular joint using cone beam CT. Dentomaxillofac Radiol. 2012;41(1):24–9.
25. Nascimento EHL, Fontenele RC, Santaella GM, Freitas DQ. Difference in the artefacts production and the performance of the metal artefact reduction (MAR) tool between the buccal and lingual cortical plates adjacent to zirconium dental implant. Dentomaxillofac Radiol. 2019;48(8):20190058.
26. Candemil AP, Salmon B, Freitas DQ, Haiter-Neto F, Oliveira ML. Distribution of metal artifacts arising from the exomass in small field-of-view cone beam computed tomography scans. Oral Surg Oral Med Oral Pathol Oral Radiol. 2020;130:116.
27. Candemil AP, Salmon B, Freitas DQ, Ambrosano GMB, Haiter-Neto F, Oliveira ML. Are metal artefact reduction algorithms effective to correct cone beam CT artefacts arising from the exomass? Dentomaxillofac Radiol. 2019;48(3):20180290.
28. Pauwels R, Araki K, Siewerdsen JH, Thongvigitmanee SS. Technical aspects of dental CBCT: state of the art. Dentomaxillofac Radiol. 2015;44(1):20140224.
29. Lofthag-Hansen S, Thilander-Klang A, Grondahl K. Evaluation of subjective image quality in relation to diagnostic task for cone beam computed tomography with different fields of view. Eur J Radiol. 2011;80(2):483–8.
30. Bechara B, McMahan CA, Noujeim M, Faddoul T, Moore WS, Teixeira FB, et al. Comparison of cone beam CT scans with enhanced photostimulated phosphor plate images in the detection of root fracture of endodontically treated teeth. Dentomaxillofac Radiol. 2013;42(7):20120404.
31. Guldner C, Ningo A, Voigt J, Diogo I, Heinrichs J, Weber R, et al. Potential of dosage reduction in cone-beam-computed tomography (CBCT) for radiological diagnostics of the paranasal sinuses. Eur Arch Otorhinolaryngol. 2013;270(4):1307–15.
32. Melo SL, Bortoluzzi EA, Abreu M Jr, Correa LR, Correa M. Diagnostic ability of a cone-beam computed tomography scan to assess longitudinal root fractures in prosthetically treated teeth. J Endod. 2010;36(11):1879–82.
33. Dalili Z, Taramsari M, Mousavi Mehr SZ, Salamat F. Diagnostic value of two modes of cone-beam computed tomography in evaluation of simulated external root resorption: an in vitro study. Imaging Sci Dent. 2012;42(1):19–24.
34. Icen M, Orhan K, Seker C, Geduk G, Cakmak Ozlu F, Cengiz MI. Comparison of CBCT with different voxel sizes and intraoral scanner for detection of periodontal defects: an in vitro study. Dentomaxillofac Radiol. 2020;49:20190197.
35. Kuhnisch J, Anttonen V, Duggal MS, Spyridonos ML, Rajasekharan S, Sobczak M, et al. Best clinical practice guidance for prescribing dental radiographs in children and adolescents: an EAPD policy document. Eur Arch Paediatr Dent. 2019;21:375.
36. Radiation protection no. 172: cone beam CT for dental and maxillofacial radiology (evidence-based guidelines), 2012.
37. Oenning AC, Jacobs R, Pauwels R, Stratis A, Hedesiu M, Salmon B. Cone- beam CT in pae-diatric dentistry: DIMITRA project position statement. Pediatr Radiol. 2018;48(3):308–16.

Digitalization in Endodontics

4

Saaid Al Shehadat and Priyanka Jain

4.1 Introduction

Digital technology is one of the most rapid and extensive evolution in dentistry. Remarkable developments of endodontic technology have been achieved in the last decades. The ultimate result in the digital transformation of endodontics has definitely improved the daily clinical practice of practitioner.

Endodontics is the only dental discipline where we cannot see what we are doing. It is based more on our clinical skills and tactile sensation. We must, therefore, rely on different technological methods to assure the predictability and prognosis of endodontic preparation and obturation.

Since the turn of the century, various advancements in endodontic technologies have allowed dentists to see what we could not see before. The technologies reviewed in this chapter include:

1. *Pulp testers* which help us correctly diagnose.
2. *Digital imaging* which helps us to read images more clearly and in more detail. Advances in radiographic techniques such as *CBCT* permits dentists to see what cannot be seen on a regular X-ray.
3. *Apex locators* which accurately identify the terminus for working length.
4. *Endodontic electric motors and nickel-titanium* (NiTi) endodontic shaping instruments which are credited for making mechanical cleaning and shaping more predictable, safer, efficient, and easier than ever before. This can be

S. Al Shehadat (✉)
College of Dental Medicine, University of Sharjah, Sharjah, UAE
e-mail: salshehadat@sharjah.ac.ae

P. Jain
Professor, Department of Endodontics, National University College of Dentistry, Manila, Philippines

© Springer Nature Switzerland AG 2021
P. Jain, M. Gupta (eds.), *Digitization in Dentistry*,
https://doi.org/10.1007/978-3-030-65169-5_4

attributed to changes in metallurgy. *Shaping* has been enhanced to produce smooth-tapered walled preparations.

5. Advances in the use of *Sonics and Ultrasonics* in endodontics for cleaning the complex root canal system.
6. *Carrier-based obturation techniques* which help dentists deliver a better and successful endodontic treatment and prognosis.
7. *Microscopes* which enable dentists to prepare a successful access cavity and facilitate the diagnosis of difficult cases through a combination of illumination and magnification.
8. 3D *guided endodontics and virtual reality which* offers interactive 3D visualizations of root canal systems, and makes it possible to practice virtual endodontics before ever treating a patient.

4.2 Digital Radiography

Radiography has always been a fundamental tool in endodontic practice [1, 2]. It is an essential component of all phases of root canal treatment (RCT) procedures from diagnosis to follow-up period [3–5]. Periapical radiographs provide useful diagnostic information including position of the tooth, size of pulp chamber, anatomy of roots, location and size of periradicular lesions, and the proximity of adjacent anatomical structures [6]. In addition, they are very useful during RCT procedures to determine the actual working length, monitor the progress of canal preparation, confirm the correct placement of master cones before obturation, and evaluate the quality of root canal filling. The conventional radiography that depended on the usage of X-ray films has been replaced by digital radiography.

The conventional X-ray films depend on chemicals for development and fixation. They have several disadvantages including the need for a light safe environment for storage, a relatively high radiation dose, more time for development and extra time to be digitized using a scanner with a transparency adaptor. In addition, they provide static images with no availability of post-image treatments except for modifying brightness. Digital radiography systems have become widely acceptable with continuous improvements and additions. When optimal exposure parameters and suitable processing of signals are used, optimal image quality of the digital radiograph is produced [7]. The diagnostic quality of digital intraoral X-ray was early reported to be comparable to the conventional X-ray films [8]. Moreover, digital X-ray systems depend on computer technology in the capture, process, display, treatment, and storage of digital images. Contrast enhancement of the digital radiograph is very useful for the diagnosis of many endodontic cases (Fig. 4.1).

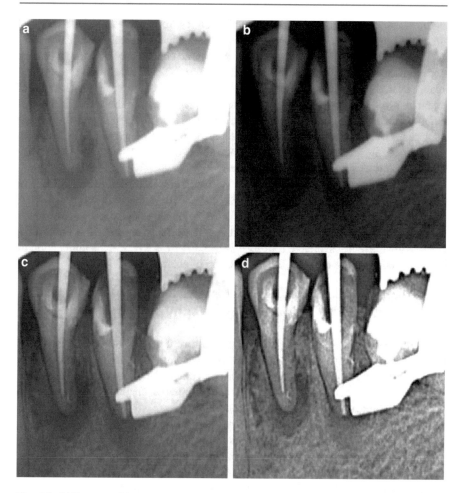

Fig. 4.1 Different useful treatments can be performed for the digital image including enhancement of brightness, sharpness, and contrast

4.3   Optical Coherence Tomography (OCT)

Optical coherence tomography (OCT) is a noninvasive and nonhazardous method of imaging, it depends on the analyzing the scattered reflections of light close to the infrared region, to determine the microstructural details of the oral biological tissue. OCT is comparable to ultrasound as the general principle of using reflections to create the images is the same for both but the methods for detecting these reflections are different. Dental OCT has the potential to detect and diagnose early stages of demineralization, remineralization, recurrent caries, restorative failures, root canal anatomy/calcification, periodontal disease, and precancerous lesions in real time.

In endodontics, OCT has been used to determine enamel cracks, coronal cracks, and vertical root fractures, along with the fracture's location along the root. The main advantage of using OCT in endodontics is that it does not require a dry root canal and in fact gives a microscopic detailed image through the surrounding root canal circumferential from dentin to cementum. This further helps in preventing root canal over preparation and possible perforation of canal walls. In addition, OCT imaging can also reveal transportation of the canals and accessory canals, if any.

There are different types of OCT such as endoscopic OCT, polarization-sensitive OCT, Doppler OCT, and high-resolution OCT. We believe that endoscopic OCT has the potential to be used in endodontics if suitable tips are developed [9]. However, all the studies with OCT imaging in dentistry have been in vitro, and no clinical devices are currently available for this purpose. Figure 4.2 shows the application of optical coherence tomography in the detection of enamel cracks [10].

4.4   Cone Beam Computed Tomography (CBCT)

The true innovation in radiographic imaging in recent years has been the advent of CBCT. This technology allows imaging and observation of the tooth and its surrounding structures in the coronal, sagittal, and axial planes, and has many advantages which have already been discussed in the previous chapter. This section will discuss its applications in the field of endodontics.

New generations of CBCT machines are currently able to provide high-resolution images using smaller submillimeter voxel sizes, more dynamic multiplane imaging navigation, and data correction applying imaging filters. Currently, the CBCT is considered as an effective tool for diagnosis and treatment planning with great facilities to manipulate brightness and contrast and change slice thicknesses [11].

The benefits of a CBCT imaging should outweigh any potential risks. Imaging with CBCT should only be considered in cases where conventional imaging does not provide sufficient information to allow proper diagnosis and management of the problem. The ALARA principle that is, "as low as reasonably achievable" should be always maintained to avoid unnecessary radiation exposure of the patient. CBCT systems can be further classified into limited and full CBCT. The limited CBCT, known also as dental or regional, has a field of view (FOV) ranging in diameter between 40 and 100 mm, whereas the full CBCT, also known as ortho or facial CBCT has a FOV that ranges between 100 and 200 mm.

The American Association of Endodontists (AAE) has stated that limited CBCT systems are considered better for endodontic applications [10]. CBCT machines can be further classified based on the scan position. The majority of CBCT machines are seated position. Few of them are supine or upright position machines.

CBCT is very valuable in diagnosis of endodontic and non-endodontic origin pathosis, canal morphology, external and internal resorption, invasive cervical

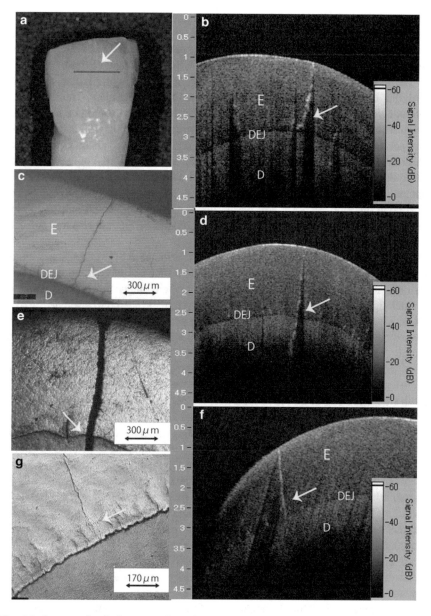

Fig. 4.2 Images of a distinct enamel crack. (a) A visual examination of enamel crack. (b) A swept-source (SS)-OCT image along the red line in (a). The crack extended to the DEJ. (c) A CLSM image corresponding to the cross-sectioned enamel crack along the red line in (a). The crack ended up to the DEJ. (d) A SS-OCT image of a sample determined as a deep enamel crack trans-illumination. The crack was seen extending beyond the DEJ. (e) A Confocal Scanning Laser Microscopy (CLSM) image corresponding to the cross-sectioned enamel crack in (d). The crack penetrated deep into the dentin. (f) A SS-OCT image of a sample determined as a superficial enamel crack with trans-illumination. The crack had extended into the DEJ. (g) A CLSM image corresponding to the cross-sectioned enamel crack in (f). The crack had not extended into the DEJ (E: enamel; D: dentine; DEJ: dentin–enamel junction) [10] (*Reproduced with permission from Journal of Endodontics, Elsevier Publishing*)

resorption, root fractures, and presurgical endodontics planning. However, compared to intraoral film, CBCT has high levels of scatter and noise, higher contrast resolution but inferior spatial resolution. The spatial resolution is even higher than that with medical-grade CT scan. The cost of CBCT is also much more [12, 13].

For all these reasons, CBCT should not be considered as a preliminary diagnostic tool, that is, the usage of CBCT is not indicated for every patient. There is no sufficient evidence that CBCT is needed for routine dental and should be restricted to cases where benefits outweigh the potential risks. CBCT imaging can be used in preoperative phase as it provides better visualization of canal anatomy, canal morphology, periodontal ligament, bone abnormalities, and internal and external root resorption. It is recommended to detect apical periodontitis occult, evaluate developmental anomalies, and provide more information in cases of cysts, fractures, cortical bone invasion, adjacent soft tissue invasion, traumatic dental injuries, and all difficult cases where special attention and more information are required for diagnosis [14–16].

In a systemic review conducted by *Aminoshariae* et al., [17] CBCT has almost double odds to locate a lesion compared to the traditional radiograph for the same lesion. This is quite important for clinical cases where diagnosis or decision making is challenging. *Rosen* et al. [18] conducted a systematic search to evaluate the diagnostic efficacy of CBCT in endodontics using an efficacy model. It was found that the expected ultimate benefit of CBCT to the endodontic patient is not clear and mainly limited to its diagnostic accuracy efficacies. Therefore, one should be cautious and follow rational approach when considering CBCT for endodontic patients.

In another meta-analysis study to determine the diagnostic accuracy of CBCT for tooth fracture, *Long* et al. [19] found that the pooled prevalence of tooth fractures was 91% for cases of clinically suspected and radiographically undetected tooth fractures using periapical radiographs. The CBCT appeared to have a high diagnostic accuracy for tooth fractures and was highly recommended to be used in clinical settings. The authors were very confident with the results of positive test, but they recommended to be careful when interpreting the negative test results, especially for endodontically treated teeth. However, this meta-analysis has some limitations including following small sample sizes in some researches, the lack of applying reference standard test for all patients in some researches, and the lack of data for horizontal and oblique tooth fractures for some subgroups.

In 2015, the AAE committee in conjunction with members of the American Academy of Oral and Maxillofacial Radiography (AAOMR) delivered a position statement for the use of CBCT in endodontics (Table 4.1).

In summary, CBCT might become the first choice to manage and assess endodontic cases, especially if lower radiation doses and better resolution become available. There is still a need for clinical trials to provide evidence of increased efficacy possible for endodontic applications of CBCT. Furthermore, adequate training to use CBCT software and interpret CBCT images is needed to all CBCT practitioners. Examples of benefits of CBCT imaging in endodontics can be seen in Fig. 4.3.

Table 4.1 Recommendations of the joint position statement

Diagnosis	*Recommendation 1* Intraoral radiographs should be considered the imaging modality of choice in the evaluation of the endodontic patient *Recommendation 2* Limited FOV CBCT should be considered the imaging modality of choice for diagnosis in patients who present with contradictory or nonspecific clinical signs and symptoms associated with untreated or previously endodontically treated teeth
Initial treatment	
Preoperative	*Recommendation 3* Limited FOV CBCT should be considered the imaging modality of choice for initial treatment of teeth with the potential for extra canals and suspected complex morphology, such as mandibular anterior teeth, and maxillary and mandibular premolars and molars, and dental anomalies
Intraoperative	*Recommendation 4* If a preoperative CBCT has not been taken, limited FOV CBCT should be considered as the imaging modality of choice for intra-appointment identification and localization of calcified canals
Postoperative	*Recommendation 5* Intraoral radiographs should be considered the imaging modality of choice for immediate postoperative imaging
Re-treatment	
Nonsurgical	*Recommendation 6* Limited FOV CBCT should be considered the imaging modality of choice if clinical examination and 2D intraoral radiography are inconclusive in the detection of vertical root fracture. *Recommendation 7* Limited FOV CBCT should be the imaging modality of choice when evaluating the nonhealing of previous endodontic treatment to help determine the need for further treatment, such as nonsurgical, surgical, or extraction. *Recommendation 8* Limited FOV CBCT should be the imaging modality of choice for nonsurgical retreatment to assess endodontic treatment complications, such as overextended root canal obturation material, separated endodontic instruments, and localization of perforations
Surgical	*Recommendation 9* Limited FOV CBCT should be considered as the imaging modality of choice for presurgical treatment planning to localize root apex/apices and to evaluate the proximity to adjacent anatomical structures

4.5   Ultrasound (US) Imaging

US combined with color power Doppler (real-time imaging) is another noninvasive imaging technology that does not utilize ionizing radiation. Real-time ultrasound imaging, also called real-time echotomography or echography, has been the widely used diagnostic technique in many fields of medicine. The imaging system in echographic examination is based on the reflection of US waves called "echos" and its application to endodontics has shown success.

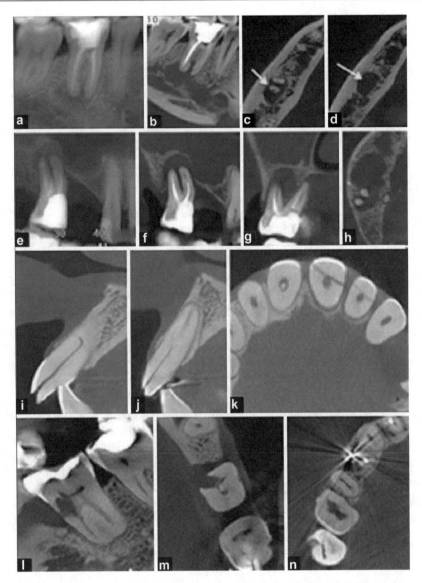

Fig. 4.3 (**a**) apical periodontitis is observed at the apices of a left first mandibular molar on a panoramic X-ray. (**b**) The CBCT scan of the same tooth shows that there is no root filling in the mesiobuccal canal with extensive apical periodontitis (sagittal plane). (**c, d**) the axial plane shows that there is no root filling in both the mesial canals with extensive apical periodontitis. (**e**) A panoramic X-ray view for the right second maxillary molar suggests the presence of apical periodontitis near the maxillary sinus. (**f**) A sagittal plane view of a CBCT scan of the same tooth confirms the presence of the apical periodontitis close to the maxillary sinus. (**g, h**) The frontal and axial planes (respectively) confirm the intimate contact with the maxillary sinus. (**i, j**) The sagittal plane of a CBCT scan reveals vertical root fracture of the left maxillary central and lateral incisors (respectively). (**k**) The same teeth with the vertical fractures in the axial plane. (**l, m**) A cervical radicular resorption can be observed on the sagittal and axial planes (respectively) of a CBCT scan of the left first mandibular molar. (**n**) artifacts in mesiobuccal root canal on a CBCT scan of an upper right first premolar because of the presence of an intra-canal post [20]

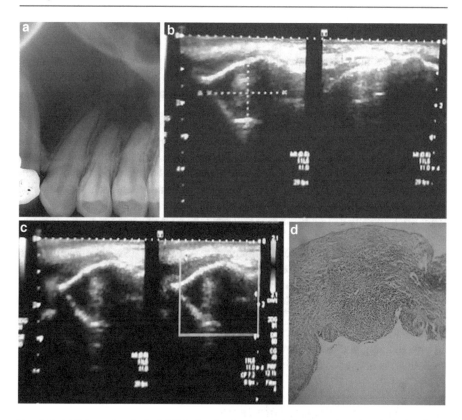

Fig. 4.4 (a) Intraoral periapical IOPA showing large well-defined, corticated periapical radiolucency associated with maxillary left canine, first and second premolar suggestive of periapical cyst. (b) Ultrasound image shows surface of thinned buccal cortical plate of bone as hyperechoic border and the deep surface of the periapical lesion, and the anechoic area in between the two due to fluid contents suggestive of periapical cyst. (c) No evidence of vascularization in the wall on color Doppler examination also suggestive of periapical cyst. (d) Histopathological section of lesion confirming the diagnosis of periapical cyst [23]

US was found to be a reliable diagnostic technique in the differential diagnosis of periapical lesions (granulomas versus cysts). Drawbacks include its use only in the anterior region where there is little or no overlying cortical bone, since sound waves are blocked by bone. In addition, the interpretation of US images is usually limited to radiologists who have extensive training.

Recent studies have shown US imaging use in monitoring the healing of periapical lesions following endodontic treatment, thereby stating that that ultrasound can detect healing earlier than radiography [20–22]. However, they are still not widely used as the differential diagnosis of granuloma and cyst is not considered important in treatment planning. Figure 4.4 describes the application of ultrasound in endodontics.

4.6   Magnetic Resonance Imaging (MRI)

MRI is also a noninvasive imaging technology which uses radio waves instead of ionizing radiation, and so does not have health hazards and is safe to use. The concept behind its use is a strong magnetic field that leads to excitation of the hydrogen atoms within tissues.

MRI may be used for the investigation of pulpal and periapical conditions, along with their extent and the anatomic implications. However, it has several drawbacks. These include poor resolution compared with conventional radiographs, longer scanning times compared to CT, increased costs, and limited access only in dedicated radiology units. Different hard tissues such as enamel and dentine cannot be differentiated from each other or from metallic objects as they all appear radiolucent. MRI imaging cannot be used in patients with a pacemaker due to the presence of a strong magnetic field.

A recent modification in MRI imaging, SWIFT-MRI (Sweep Imaging with Fourier Transform), shows promising use in endodontics as it offers simultaneous three-dimensional hard- and soft-tissue imaging of teeth (Fig. 4.5) [24].

Other advancements in endodontic imaging such as *Tuned aperture computed tomography (TACT), Micro-CT, and Spiral computed tomography (SCT)* are not discussed as they are not still widely used in practice. Micro-CT is not used for in vivo imaging due to the high radiation dose required. TACT (an alternative CT technique) is not yet commercially available for dental applications.

4.7   Electrical/Digital Pulp Testers

The determination of the status of dental pulp tissue is essential for the correct diagnosis in dental clinic. Currently, there is no single reliable technique that can diagnose all pulp conditions. However, carful analyzing of the chief complaint, dental history, clinical examination, radiographs, and other investigations usually lead to the diagnosis of the underlying diseases.

Histological examination of sections of pulp tissue specimen is considered the most accurate way of evaluating the pulp status as it allows to assess the presence and extent of inflammation or the presence of tissue necrosis. However, it is impractical and not feasible in dental practice, and thus clinicians have to use other investigations including pulp test devices to assess the dental pulp status during diagnosis. For long time, all pulp tests suffered from shortcoming related to accuracy, reliability, and reproducibility. The application of the suitable pulp test is important as not all pulp testing are appropriate for all clinical situations.

It is quite important to differentiate between vitality test and sensibility test. The pulp vitality test includes an assessment of the pulp's blood supply. The pulp sensibility tests asses the pulp sensory response, that is, the ability of the pulp to respond to a stimuli. The positive response of the pulp to a stimulus indicates the presence of innervation, and clinicians assume that the pulp has a viable blood circulation.

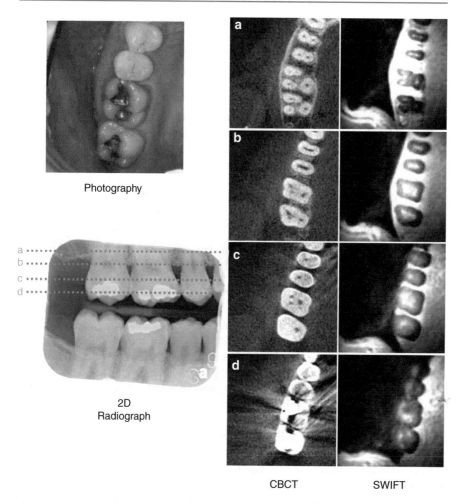

Fig. 4.5 In vivo images of the right posterior teeth. The photograph depicts the maxillary teeth that are also imaged with a traditional 2D radiograph used to detect interproximal caries. The dotted lines, represented by **a**, **b**, **c**, and **d**, correlate with the cross-sectional CBCT and SWIFT images at those levels, from more superior closer to the root tip moving inferiorly to the crown of the teeth. Note the lack of image distortion associated with the occlusal amalgam restorations in the SWIFT sections compared to the CBCT sections. (SWIFT: selected slices with FOV diameter 110 mm and isotropic voxel size 430 μm) [24] (*Reproduced with Permission from Journal of Endodontics, Elsevier Publishing*)

Thus, the pulp is either healthy or inflamed. The negative pulp response to a stimulus may suggest the necrosis of pulp tissues. However, one should be careful for the limitation of the sensibility tests and the possibility of false, positive or negative, responses.

Electric pulp testing (EPT) is one of the sensibility tests. EPT technology is based on the production of impulses of negative polarity that is able to reduce the voltages required to stimulate nerve response in the pulp and periodontium tissue [25].

The electrical stimuli can cause an ionic change across the neural membrane, and this induces an action potential with a rapid hopping action at the nodes of Ranvier in myelinated nerves [26]. There were two modes EPTs: bipolar and monopolar. Both of them can be subdivided into wire or wireless devices [27, 28]. The most common types are wireless, battery-operated EPTs.

Bipolar devices were common till the mid-1950s. They involved using two electrodes, one is placed on the tooth buccal surface and the other on the palatal/lingual surface. The electrical current passes from one electrode to the other through the crown. In monopolar EPT, only one electrode is applied to the tooth surface. The circuit should be completed by placing the metal clip on the patient's lip. Touching the probe handle by the patient's hand can also complete the circuit [29–31]. To test the pulp status, the current intensity is increased gradually. In cases of vital pulp tissue, the patient starts feeling a "tingling" sensation once the voltage reaches the level of pain threshold [32]. The threshold is reached when sufficient number of nerve terminals are activated [28, 33]. Pain threshold level varies between teeth as well as patients. It is affected by patient's age, tooth surface conduction, pain perception, and other factors [34].

Early animal study on dogs showed that EPT may interfere with a pacemaker resulting in risk of precipitating cardiac arrhythmia [35]. Based on this study, a recommendation not to use EPT in patient with pacemaker was established. However, more recent in vitro and human studies have shown that with the new generations of pacemakers that have better shielding, there is no interference from EPT or any other electrical dental devices on pacemakers [36, 37].

EPTs have the limitation of being unreliable in many cases. For example, they may produce false results in healthy immature teeth [26]. This is because it may take up to 5 years after tooth eruption for the myelinated fibers to reach the pulp-dentine border at the plexus of Rashkow. Patients undergoing orthodontic treatment may also show false EPT results because of disturbance of sensory elements due to the orthodontic treatment [38]. Similarly, recently traumatized teeth may show false results for the same reason [39]. Pulp canal calcification is another situation of false EPT reading. In such a case, the sensory response threshold is increased. This might be due to complete blockage of sensory response. Patients of hyperthyroidism may require higher intensity of electrical current compared to normal patients to elicit an EPT response [26]. Loss of pulp sensibility to EPT may also be observed in case of pulp hyperemia [40]. On the opposite, the breakdown products from necrotic pulp tissues may cause EPT stimulation leading to false positive responses [41]. False positive response in necrotic teeth was also reported to be caused by current passing through periodontal or gingival tissues [42].

4.7.1 Clinical Considerations

The EPT device is technique-sensitive with multiple limitations [43]. To avoid false reading, an EPT requires an appropriate application method, adequate stimulus, and careful interpretation [44]. The correct method includes first the good isolation of the tooth and the tight placement of the probe tip on the tooth surface. The occlusal two-thirds of the labial surface is recommended as it allows more consistent results [45]. However, it was reported that placing the electrode at the incisal edge of anterior teeth triggers a response with the least amount of electrical current [46]. For permanent molars, the highest concentration of neural elements is observed in the pulp horns, and the lower is in the cervical region of the pulp [47]. Thus, the optimum site for EPT electrode placement was reported to be at the tip of the mesiobuccal cusp [25].

It is highly recommended to use a conducting medium between the probe tip and the tooth surface to improve the electrical conductivity [48]. It is also important to confirm that the target tooth does not contact with the adjacent teeth, as this may cause inaccurate response as observed when two adjacent teeth have proximal metallic restorations. The same can be said for patients wearing orthodontic bands [42, 49].

4.8   Apex Locators

The procedures of RCT (i.e., cleaning, shaping, and root filling) should be confined within the root canal system. Working length (WL) determination is an essential step in the RCT. WL is usually defined as "the distance between a coronal reference point and the apical limit of preparation" [50]. Many dental schools consider the dentinoce-mental junction (DCJ) as ideal point to end the preparation (Fig. 4.6) [51]. However, the DCJ is a histological point that cannot be located clinically. However, the apical constriction (AC) is almost at the level of the DCJ and are usually located at about 1 mm far from the root apex [50]. For many clinicians, the AC is considered the end of the root canal, and any instrumentation or filling beyond this point is considered as over-instrumentation/overfilling. Other clinicians consider the anatomical apex as the end of root canal and over-instrumentation/overfilling starts only beyond this level.

Traditionally, the WL has been determined by taking PA radiographs when a file is inserted to a previous estimated length of the canal. However, the development of new electronic devices known as electronic apex locators has proven to determine WL more accurate, precise, and predictable [52, 53]. Apex locator is defined as an electronic

Fig. 4.6 Anatomical and histological structures of the apex described by Kuttler. 1. Apical constriction 2. Foramen. 3. Dentino-cemental junction. 4. Radiographic apex. 5. Anatomical apex (*Reproduced with permission from Elsevier Publishing*) [51]

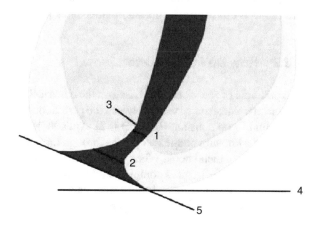

endodontic device used to determine the length of the root canal space by determining the position of the AC. The AC has found to have an electric resistance of 6.5 kilo ohms (kΩ), and this specific characteristic was behind the development of apex locators.

4.8.1 Development of Electronic Apex Locators

Electronic apex locators have been in practice for more than 40 years. The apical constriction of the root has a specific resistance to electric current. This resistance can be measured using a pair of electrodes. The electrodes in apex locator are the endodontic file and the lip clip. These devices are able to detect the point where file becomes in contact with the periodontal tissue [54, 55]. The first generations of apex locators were unreliable and suffered from a lot of errors. The presence of fluids in the root canal led to errors. However, the new generations are more accurate, more reliable, and become basic devices used in endodontic treatment.

The first electronic method to determine WL was developed by Sunada (1962), who constructed a simple device that can be used clinically to determine the root canal length [54]. The device depended on the constancy of the electrical resistance between the mucosa and periodontium which is about 6.5 kΩ. This value was found to be constant at any part of periodontium regardless of the patient's age, tooth type, and root shape. A great evolution was achieved in 1970 by Inoue who reported the use of Sono Explorer. Later, based on Inoue researches, an oscillator loop was used to calibrate and measure frequency at periodontal pockets depth of each tooth. The third generation of apex locators was launched in the late 1980s when a multiple channel impedance ratio-based device was used by Kobayashi to measure the impedance of two different frequencies simultaneously [54].

The ability of apex locators to determine the moment when a file becomes in contact with periodontal tissue extends their benefits. They are very useful to detect perforations in roots or pulp chambers, horizontal fractures, internal and external resorptions. They are also helpful in RCT of immature teeth that have incomplete root formation. Some apex locators can be used to detect the sensibility of the teeth. Others are combined with electronic handpiece (e.g., Root Zx II) and are able to determine WL precisely as the stand-alone units [56].

4.8.2 How Do Apex Locators Work?

The principle of apex locator is based on the electrical resistance of different tissues. The electrical resistance value between the periodontal ligament and the oral mucosa was found to be constant (6.5 kΩ) [57]. Apex locators produce a direct electrical current of a known voltage that passes through the endodontic file and being recaptured back by a metal hook. When the tip of the file reaches the periodontal ligament ($R = 6.5$ kΩ), the circuit is complete and the apex locator beeps and displays a "0" value on its screen. Some devices may show other signals like flashing light or pointer on screen display, digital readout or a Buzzer sound.

4.8.3   Generations of Apex Locators

The *first* generation of apex locators, the "Resistance-Based Apex Locator" was designed to measure the resistance of the electrical current considering that the resistance of periodontal ligament equals that of oral mucous membrane. The device should be used in a dry canal and K-file can be used with it. However, many shortcomings were reported for these devices. Accuracy is reduced in a wet canal, that is, the presence of remaining pulp tissue, excessive hemorrhage, or inflammatory exudate in the root canal system. False reading may also be encountered in case of obstructed canals, carious teeth, and presence of defective restorations, metallic restorations, and case of perforations [54, 58]. The devices used a direct electrical current that may cause the feeling of electric shock sensation by the patient. Furthermore, compared with WL determined by radiographs, these devices were found to be unreliable as many of the readings were significantly longer or shorter than the real WL [55]. Some examples of apex locators from the first generation: The Root Canal Meter (Onuki Medical Co., Japan), (Fig. 4.7a), Meter S II (Onuki Medical Co., Japan), the Dentometer (Dahin Electro medicine, Denmark), and the Endo Radar (Electronica Liarre, Italy).

The *second* generation was known as impedance-type apex locators because the devices here depended on the principle of impedance. Impedance principle suggests

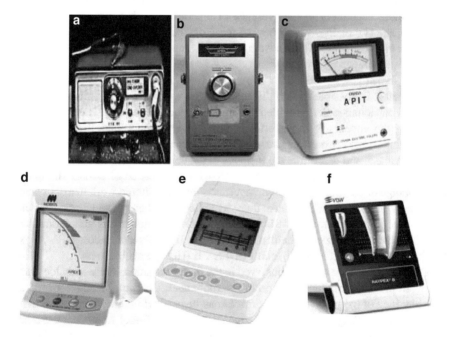

Fig. 4.7 Different models of apex locators; (**a**): Root Canal Meter (First generation); (**b**) Sono-Explorer (second generation); (**c**) Endex apit locator (third generation); (**d**) Root ZX II (Fourth generation); (**e**) Endometer-Magic Finder EMF-100 (Fifth generation); (**f**) Raypex® 6 Apex Locator (sixth generation)

the presence of electrical impedance across the canal wall of the tooth. This imped-ance increases gradually and reaches its greater value at the apical part before being dropped dramatically at the cemento-dentinal junction. The devices in this genera-tion used alternating electrical current which allowed the design of an electronic system. However, similar problems of incorrect readings were observed. To obtain accurate reading, the root canal should be free of electroconductive materials [59]. Other disadvantage of the devices were that they required calibration before using, complicated calculations after using, and no digital readout was present. In addition, there was a need to use special coated probes with these devices instead of endodon-tic instrument. The coated probes have the problem to be difficult place in narrow canals, and they lose their benefit after autoclaving [53, 58]. Sono-Explorer M-III (Hayashi Dental Supply, Japan) and Analytic/Endo (Orange, USA) (Fig. 4.7b) are some examples of devices from this generation.

The *third* generation is also known as frequency-dependent apex locators. In this generation, the devices use multiple frequencies to determine how far the instru-ment is from the end of the canal. The device here depended on the fact that differ-ent sites of the root canal show different impedances between low and high frequencies (400 Hz to 8 kHz). The lowest value is at the coronal part. As the file progress deeper into the canal, difference in impedances increases and reaches the highest value at CDJ. The devices contain more microprocessors that can do the required algorithm calculation. Unlike the previous generations, the devices can operate more accurately in the presence of electrolyte such as saline or sodium hypochlorite. The main disadvantage of these devices is that they need to be cali-brated for each canal [53, 58]. An example of this generation is Apit or Endex/Apit-Endex (Osada, Japan) (Fig. 4.7c).

In the *fourth* generation (Ratio Type Apex Locators), the devices depended on the fact that it is possible to find difference in the combination of values of resis-tance and capacitance that provide the same value of impedance. Thus, instead of measuring the impedance as performed in the previous generation, the locators of this generation measure the resistance and capacitance separately, compare them with a database, and determine the distance to the apical foramen of the root canal. The accuracy of the devices becomes better with less chance of errors. The main disadvantage of the fourth-generation devices is that they should work in a dry canal or partially dried canal which make them inapplicable in heavy exudate cases or in the presence of bleeding [55, 58]. Some of the devices under this generation are RootZX® (Morita, France), Elements Diagnostic Unit (SybronEndo), AFA Apex Finder, ROOT ZX II (Fig. 4.7d), and PROPEX II (Henry Schein Dental).

A great improvement can be observed in the **fifth** generation where apex locators can work precisely in any condition of the root canal: dry, wet, bleeding, or filled with any type of irrigants [59]. The devices can be used without the need for previ-ous calibration. They use multiple frequencies instead of dual frequencies. Some examples of electronic apex locators from this generation are currently available in the market: Raypex 5®, VDW, Allemagne, Apex Pointer+® (Micro-Mega, France), Propex II® (Dentsply Maillefer, France), Novapex® (VDW, Munich), and Endometr e-Magic Finder (S-Denti Co., Ltd) (Fig. 4.7e).

The *sixth* generation, also known as adaptive apex locators, continue using multifrequency system. They can operate with good accuracy in dry and wet conditions, even with the presence of blood or exudates [60]. It can continuously adapt to the humidity degree in the root canal [55]. Furthermore, the devices are able to produce different kinds of sound to indicate the progress of the file in the root canal. Raypex® 6 Apex Locator (VDW) and ProPex Pixi (Dentsply, USA) are examples of this generation (Fig. 4.7f).

4.8.4   Clinical Tips to Avoid False Reading

To ensure accuracy and reproducibility and avoid false reading, the following precautions should be considered:

- The tooth should be isolated probably, and metallic parts of restoration should be removed or avoided.
- Delay using apex locators till the initial preparation of the coronal part of the root canal (crown-down technique) to increase the accuracy of the devices [54, 58]. This is highly recommended in case of curved roots.
- Minimize the presence of remaining intact vital pulp tissue, inflammatory exudates as they can cause false reading [53, 58].
- The root canal should be damp with a minimal amount of irrigant. For example, the Root ZX was found more accurate in the presence of sodium hypochlorite [61].
- The pulp chamber should be free of irrigant.
- Ensure good contact between the device hook and lip. Be sure the mucous membrane is damp.
- Select a suitable size of the instrument (file) to be used with the apex locator. The diameter of the tip of the instrument should fit that of the canal. The tip should not float in the canal; it should come in contact with the canal walls at the estimated WL.
- Connect the selected file to the device, place it in the canal, and move it apically in a slow watch winding motion.
- Some recommend stopping when the locator displays "0" reading. However, from our clinical experience, we recommend moving the file 0.5–1 mm apically to confirm having (red/out of apex) reading. This helps to avoid false reading caused by remaining vital pulp tissue at the apical part.
- Repeat the measurement at least three times.
- Confirm the determined WL by digital or conventional P.A. X-ray.
- Consider that calcified/very narrow canals and accumulation of dentine debris can affect the work of apex locators negatively.
- If the determined length always differs from that estimated on the X-ray, the device should be turned off and restarted again.
- If the device showed repeated wrong readings, the batteries should be checked and may be re-changed.

4.9   Sonics and Ultrasonic

Ultrasonic in dentistry was first introduced by Richman [62] in 1957. Its main use in dentistry is for scaling and root planning of teeth and in root canal therapy [58]. The term *endosonics (Ultrasonics in endodontics)* was first coined by Martin and Cunningham [63, 64] and was defined as the ultrasonic and synergistic system of root canal instrumentation and disinfection.

In endodontics, ultrasonic devices can be used either in instrumentation or passive ultrasonic irrigation (PUI). However, due to their aggressive nature, and difficulty in controlling dentin removal, they are no longer used for instrumentation [65–67].

Advantages of using ultrasonic in endodontics include access preparation and refinement of root canals, removal of intra-canal obstructions such as broken instruments and posts, root-end cavity preparation and refinement, placement of retrograde filling materials, ultrasonic condensation of gutta-percha, passive irrigation (sonic or ultrasonic), and needle activation during sonic or ultrasonic irrigation (active irrigation).

Ultrasonic and, more recently, sonic irrigation is a technology that relies on vibrating the irrigating needle itself, thus enhancing the flushing and increased permeation of the root canal system by the irrigating solution.

4.9.1   Types of Sonic Devices

Rispi-Sonic file and EndoActivator	These devices facilitate penetration of the irrigant, and improve mechanical cleansing, compared to needle irrigation [68]
Vibringe	This uses traditional syringe–needle delivery, in addition to the sonic vibration, thus showing better results than traditional syringe irrigation in the apical part of the canal [69]

Activation of irrigants is attributed to cavitation and acoustic streaming phenomena, created by the ultrasonic devices. Cavitation occurs when ultrasound generates bubbles to create a pressure-vacuum effect. This effect is minimal and restricted to the area of the device tip. Acoustic streaming is steady, unidirectional circulation of fluid in the vicinity of a small vibrating object [70].

Sonic devices generate significant back-and-forth movement of the device tip, which is effective in disinfecting canals [71]. Sonic technology has flexible, noncutting, polymer tips that maintain the anatomical integrity of the final preparation [67, 72, 73]. On the contrary, ultrasonic insert tip that contacts dentin will cut dentin and generate its own smear layer, as they are manufactured from metal alloys.

A sonically driven polymer tip will continue to move even while constrained as opposed to an ultrasonic vibrating tip [74]. A loss of tip movement may compromise the exchange of irrigant.

The introduction of ultrasonic technology has significantly enhanced the treatment outcome and prognosis root-end surgeries [75]. Most relevant clinical advantage is the improved access to the root end area. Availability of different sizes of retro-tips with different angulations leads to a smaller osteotomy for surgical access [76]. Careful monitoring of the intensity of ultrasonic energy is required so as to avoid fracture of the tips in the apical surgical site.

4.9.2 Note on Active and Passive Root Canal Irrigation

Passive irrigation is conducted by slowly dispensing the root canal irrigating solution through different gauged needles [77]. Needle should be loose in the canal, and smaller gauge needles should be chosen in order to achieve deeper and effective penetration. Care should be taken not to push irrigants beyond the apical foramen.

In order to allow the irrigant to reflux and move the debris coronally, the needle should be loose in the canal. To achieve deeper and more effective placement, smaller gauged needles should be chosen. Passive irrigation has limitations because the static reservoir of irrigant restricts the penetration, circulation, and cleansing potential of the irrigation solution of a root canal system. On the other hand, active irrigation initiates dynamics and flow within the fluid and thus improves root canal disinfection. During cleaning and shaping, fluid activation facilitates enhanced fluid penetration through all aspects of the root canal system and improves cleaning and disinfection of the canal [78].

4.10 Digital Delivery of Local Anesthetics

It is very important to control the pain and anxiety during an endodontic procedure. In the last two decades, a variety of different injecting devices without the use of a needle have been developed.

Electronic dental anesthesia (EDA), introduced by Shealy in 1967, involves the use of the principle of transcutaneous electrical nerve stimulation (TENS) to help control chronic pain. EDA is highly successful in periodontal procedures but is mainly unsuccessful in surgical and endodontic procedures [79].

Iontophoresis was first introduced in 1993. Although Gangarosa described the use of iontophoresis for the basic applications in dentistry [80] such as treatment of hypersensitive dentine, treatment of oral ulcers, and herpes labialis lesions and topical anesthesia, there is not enough evidence and recent studies regarding the application of iontophoresis in dentistry.

Computer-controlled local anesthetic delivery (CCLAD) is a new concept to deliver dental anesthesia, and was first introduced in the mid-1990s. Computer technology is used to control the rate of the flow of the anesthetic solution through a needle [81]. A constant volume of anesthetic solution is delivered at a preset pressure, thus making the delivery less painful and more controlled. This gives the advantage of better tactile sensitivity to the clinician. Disadvantages include higher cost and speed of injection at the slowest pump rate. Since the time frame of whole 4 min is required to completely express a local anesthetic cartridge, it may cause impatience and stress among some patients [81]. Another disadvantage is the fact that this method does not eliminate the use of a needle.

The *Wand*™ (Milestone Scientific, Inc., Livingston, NJ, USA), a CCLAD device, was introduced in 1997. It does not use a traditional syringe and has three main components, namely, base unit, foot pedal, and disposable headpiece assembly. Due to the greater control over the syringe and the fixed flow rates of the LA drug, the Wand is considered effective in reducing pain, particularly in painful injection sites such as palatal infiltration, periodontal ligament, or intraosseous injections and incisive blocks. The lack of a traditional syringe makes it useful to reduce apprehension in children. Three rate-mode injections are available: slow (0.005 ml/s), fast (0.03 ml/s), and turbo (0.06 ml/s).

In 2006, Milestone Scientific introduced a new device called the *Single Tooth Anesthesia (STA)*. STA incorporates dynamic pressure-sensing (DPS) technology that provides a constant monitoring of the exit pressure of the local anesthetic solution during the drug's administration. DPS also helps to determine the pressure at the needle tip in order to identify the ideal needle placement for PDL injections. With STA system, a greater volume of LA solution can be administered since the amount and pressure is calculated by the system instead of operator, and thus provides increased comfort and less tissue damage than traditional syringe to the patient. STA has three rate modes of injection, namely, STA mode: single, slow rate of injection; normal mode, and turbo mode: faster rate of injection—0.06 ml/s.

The *Comfort Control Syringe* is a new device that differs from the other CCLAD systems in that there is no foot pedal. The injection and aspiration can be controlled directly from the syringe, making it easier to use. But the drawback is that the syringe is bulky and more difficult to use than the other computer-controlled devices. A comparison between the traditional dental syringe and the Comfort Control Syringe revealed no meaningful differences in ease of administration, injection pain and efficacy, and patient acceptability [82].

4.11 Automated Instrumentation Systems (Endodontic Electric Motors)

Automated instrumentation systems are devices developed to improve speed efficiency of the endodontic process. They allow the use of mechanically driven instruments [83]. The history of automated preparation devices goes back to 1871 where the first clockwise foot engine drill came in use. Straight handpieces were well known in the 1880s. They were permanently attached to a flexible foot-engine cable and converted to angle handpieces by connecting an additional attachment to the front end [84]. In 1960, the nickel-titanium (NiTi) alloy was developed by William Bueller (Maryland, USA). The benefits of NiTi alloy to fabricate endodontic rotary files was soon recognized. A new generation of low torque control motors (known as endodontic motors) has been developed to improve root canal preparation using NiTi instruments. By time, endodontic motors have been improved in terms of controlling torque and kinematics that become adjustable in different directions.

Endodontic motors usually contain a central unit that controls the whole device, a micro motor, and a contra angle handpiece where rotary files can be adapted. Some motors have a pedal that allows to proceed the different functions using foot. Endodontic motors take into consideration the low torque at failure values of the NiTi rotary files and can provide as low torque as 1 N/cm^2 which is considered very safe for root canal preparation [85]. Some systems are provided with programmable settings and automatic reverse functions. Others are integrated with apex locators. Dental companies that produce files recommend using their own endodontic motors. However, the current endodontic motors are considered completely independent of the file system, and thus, any endodontic motor can be used with any file system if it provides the suitable function. The new generation of motors has been widely improved by adding many valuable features including the touchscreen, small size, lightweight, autoclavable devices, and the ability to produce both high and low speed with less noise and vibration (i.e., StarETorque, DentalEZ).

4.11.1 Conventional Endodontic Motors

Automated instrumentation systems have been designed to prepare root canals properly with less risk of file deformation or separation [85, 86]. File life span can be prolonged by reducing the maximum stress on their surfaces using specific values of torque and speed [87]. A balance between speed and torque is the key for the proper cutting efficiency [88].

The high torque makes the rotary instrument very active but increases the possibility of instrument lock, deformation, and separation. Vice versa, low torque is safer and causes lower cyclic fatigue in NiTi rotary instruments [89, 90]. However, low torque reduces the cutting efficiency and makes it difficult for the instrument to progress in the canal. The operator may push the instrument apically to compensate the weak progress, which in turn increases the possibility of instrument lock, deformation, and separation. Each rotary file has its ideal right torque. The right torque is usually low for the smaller diameter or less tapered files. The right torque should be set carefully just below the limit of the file elasticity [90]. Similar to high torque, the greater speed increases the cutting efficiency, but it has the disadvantages of increasing the possibility of instrument separation, changing the canal anatomy especially in curved parts, losing the control and the tactile sensation. Conventional endodontic motors provide a wide variety of speeds range from 150 rpm to 4000 rpm. The operator has to be careful when selecting the speed and torque. The recommendation of the manufacture of the rotary system is usually followed. However, it is believed that these recommendations would not be optimal in all clinical situations. Thus, new generations of endodontic motors with additional smart tasks have been developed.

4.11.2 New Endodontic Motors

Three mode motions can be available in some recent endodontic motors. These are continuous, reciprocating, and noncontinuous motions (known as optimum torque reverse mode or OTR). In the continuous mode, when the torque levels applied on the file is equal to the torque values set on the motor, the rotation will be stopped, or the rotating will be reversed. Thus, file deformation/separation would be avoided.

The first reciprocating system used was Giromatic (MicroMega), which was introduced in 1964. Giromatic, and other early reciprocating systems like Endo-Gripper (Moyco Union Broach, Montgomeryville, PA, USA), Intra-Endo 3 LD (KaVo, Biberach, Germany), and Dynatrak (Dentsply DeTrey, Konstanz, Germany), have used equal angles of 90° clockwise (CW) and counterclockwise (CCW) motion [91]. The performance of this reciprocating motion was found to be beyond the hand files. Thus, new equal 30° angles of CW and CCW rotation was dependent in other handpieces such as the M4 (SybronEndo, Orange, A, USA), Endo-Eze (Ultradent Products Inc., South Jordan, UT, USA), and Endo-Express SafeSider (Essential Dental Systems, South Hackensack, NJ, USA) systems.

Over time, many disadvantages of the equal reciprocating motion were reported. Compared to the continuous motion, equal reciprocating motion is less efficient in cutting, limited in debris removal out of the canal, and requires more inward pressure to progress in the canal. Thus, asymmetric reciprocating motion was developed with new generations of NiTi rotary files. Currently, the Wave One motor (Dentsply Maillefer, Switzerland) provides asymmetric motion of 150°CCW and 30°CW. The VDW Silver Reciproc motor (VDW, Munich, Germany) provides asymmetric motion of 170°CCW and 50°CW. In both motors, three reciprocating cycles complete one complete reverse rotation. This allows the rotary file gradually advance into the canal with less apical pressure. New motors with adjustable reciprocating angle are currently available. These motors provide adjustment range between 20° and 240° with possible 10° interval (Ai-Motor, Woodpecker, China).

Optimum torque reverse (OTR) function is another function that was added to a new generation of endodontic motor (DentaPort ZX OTR) (Fig. 4.8). The main purpose of this module is to prevent file jamming inside the root canal. The system is able to switch automatically from the regular filing to the OTR action depending on the shape and condition of the file in the canal. Thus, filing efficiency is not

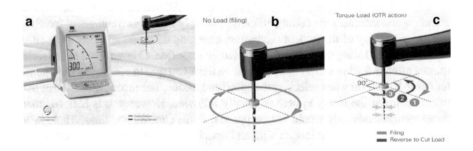

Fig. 4.8 Example of a new generation of Endodontic motor with OTR mode. (a) DentaPort ZX OTR. Morita. (b) When load is less than torque setting. Filing is performed normally. (c) When load exceeds torque setting, file reverses for 90° then goes forward 180°; this is repeated as necessary (*Adapted from Tri Auto ZX Manual, Morita*)

reduced greatly and the file can be used at maximum torque (usually 3.5 Ncm) in the coronal part of the canal for pre-flaring. Files with positive rank angles (cutting action in forward rotation) are recommended with the OTR function. If the contrary electrode is attached to the corner of the patient's mouth, the apex locator is activated, and the file tip can be monitored during shaping the canal. This allows the preparation of the root canal without damaging the apex.

4.12 Obturation

The use of heat to condence the gutta-percha mass was described first by Herbert Schilder in 1967 to better fill the intricacies of the root canal system. Studies have shown that different obturation techniques, whether or not they utilize heat, do not seem to affect the prognosis [92]. However, recent analysis of healing of periapical lesions following endodontic treatment with CBCT showed that the density of root filling is a predictor of healing [93].

Down pack technologies is one of the technologies utilized to aid in the efficiency and improved density of the root canal filling *material*. Heating devices like Touch and N Heat and System B (SybronEndo) have been available for more than a decade. These devices eliminate the need for a flaming torch used in Schilder's technique and decrease the incidence of burnt lips. They allow the operator to perform vertical compaction of gutta-percha by using autoclavable tips of various sizes. These electrical devices have the advantage of delivering a precise amount of heat for a long period of time. The temperature at the tip of the heat carrier can be monitored at the integrated screen (Fig. 4.9). Recent wireless devices such as DownPak (EI, Hu-Friedy, Chicago, IL) or the Endotec II (Medidenta International Inc.; Woodside, NY) are battery operated and allow convenience during the technique. The DownPak utilizes heat and vibration for vertical and lateral condensation. This minimizes the need for high temperatures during obturation. However, regardless of the system/device used, the potential for significant overfilling of the canal remains.

The Obtura 3 (Obtura), Calamus (Tulsa, Dentsply), Ultrafil 3D (Hygienic-Coltene-Whaledent, Akron, OH), or Elements Obturation unit (SybronEndo) are the most commonly used devices for *thermoplasticized gutta-percha*. The effective technique necessitates that this be done incrementally, with vertical compaction performed between the increments, to assure better compaction of gutta-percha. Many companies have introduced integrated devices that contain handpieces for down pack and backfill (flow) techniques (Calamus Dual, Dentsply Tulsa Dent Specialties; Elements obturation Unit, Kerr).

Carrier-based techniques is another heat-based obturation technique. It consist of a carrier coated in with GP. Traditionally, the carriers were made from stainless steel and titanium (Successfil, Hygienic-Coltene-Whaledent) but are now manufactured from plastic (Thermafil, Dentsply-Tulsa Dental; SimpliFill, Discus Dental, Culver City, CA) or cross-linked GP (Gutta Core, Dentsply Maillefer, Ballaigues, Switzerland). In all these techniques, a carrier coated with gutta-percha that is

Fig. 4.9 Gutta-percha root canal obturator SYSTEM B, Sybron Endo, USA. The temperature at the tip of the heat carrier can be monitored at the integrated screen

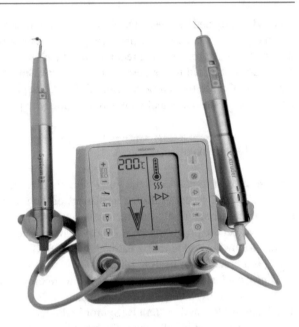

slightly larger in size than the sizing instrument is placed in an oven until the gutta-percha is sufficiently soft and inserted to the working length. The oven offers a stable heat source with more control and uniformity for plasticizing the gutta-percha. These carrier-based systems are popular because of the simplicity and ease of use. However, they are usually more difficult to remove for post preparation or during retreatment than other root canal obturation methods.

Each of these techniques has its share of benefits and limitations. Variables such as the complexity of the root canal anatomy, the type of sealer used, the residual microbial irritants in the canal, the promptness and effectiveness of restoration etc. should be taken into consideration when choosing an obturation technique.

4.13 Surgical Operating Microscope (SOM)

RCT involves many procedures that can be described as "blind"! These procedures are usually performed using tactile sensation as nothing can be seen beyond the canal orifice. The only way to see inside the root canal was, for long time, by taking radiograph.

The surgical operating microscope (SOM) was first introduced to otolaryngology in the 1950s, followed by neurosurgery in the 1960s. Using SOM in endodontics was suggested in the early 1990s. In 1999, Gary Carr introduced an operative microscope that had Galilean optics where parallel optics that allowed the user to focus at infinity eyestrain [94]. The device was ergonomic, provided five magnifications (3.5× to 30×), and had some documentation accessories. Since then, different generations of microscopes with more improvements were introduced in markets. Currently, there are many brands, multiple models, and different generations and properties.

4.13.1 Components of SOM

Regardless of the brand and the generation, SOM contains four main components (Fig. 4.10a): 1, body of microscope; 2, light source housing; 3, supporting structures; and 4, documentation components. The body of SOM (Fig. 4.10b) is the main part. It contains eyepieces, binoculars, magnification changer, focusing knob, objective lens, and beam splitter.

4.13.1.1 Eyepieces
These are magnification glasses (Fig. 4.10b) with different ranges of powers that may reach to 20×. They have adjustable diopter settings (from −5 to +5) that is used to adjust for object accommodation, that is, the ability to focus the lens of the eyes. This is especially important when assistant scope or documentation equipment are used. At the end of each eyepiece, there is a rubber cup that can be turned down to suit clinicians who wear glasses. The distance between the two eyepieces can be modified by specific key (interpupillary distance key), so that both left and right field of the view become one when looking through the eyepieces [95].

There are three types of eyepieces based on the quality and the properties of optical aberration correction: Huygens (H), wide field (WF), and Plössl (PL). The H

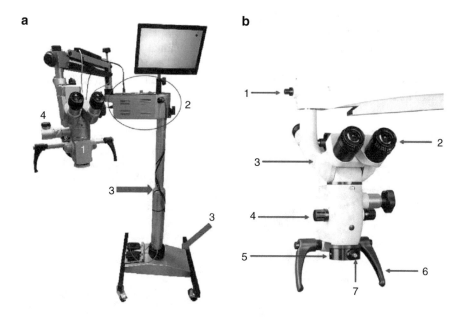

Fig. 4.10 (**a**) The main parts of SOM. 1, body of microscope; 2, light source housing; 3, supporting structure; 4, documentation components. (**b**) The components of the body. 1, brightness control knob; 2, eyepieces; 3, binoculars; 4, magnification changer (MC); 5, objective lens; 6, handgrip; 7, fine focusing knob (*Adopted from* http://www.zumazmedical.com/product/)

eyepieces are simple and cheap but have less quality in terms of vision compared with the others. The WF eyepieces provide good vision in all the field. The PL eyepieces are considered the most sophisticated and high quality with good correction of the optical aberrations [95].

4.13.1.2 Binoculars
The binocular (Fig. 4.10b) contains the eyepieces and allow for the adjustment of the interpupillary distance. The main role of the binocular is to project the intermediate image into the focal plane of the eyepieces so that the two divergent circles of light combine to effect a single focus. They can be modified manually or by a small knob. Once the interpupillary distance and the diopter setting have been determined, they should not be changed unless the microscope will be operated by another person. There are three types of binoculars: straight, inclined, and inclinable tubes (Fig. 4.11). The tubes in the straight binoculars are parallel to the head of the microscope. Such design is not suitable for dental work and usually used in otology. The inclined tubes are oriented at constant 45° whereas the angulation of the inclinable tubes are adjustable through a range of angles. The inclined tubes provide more comfortable working position and are more suitable for dental works. Some recent SOMs have an additional ergonomic tool known as "Carr extender," which allows more ergonomic position to the operator by bringing the binoculars away from the microscope and closer to the operator [95].

4.13.1.3 Magnification Changer (MC)
The MC is located within the head of the microscope and consists of lenses with different magnification factors. The MC might be manual with a 3, 5, or 6 steps; or automatic (power zoom changer). The automatic MC consists of a series of lenses that move back and forth on a focusing ring to provide different magnification factors. The main advantage of power zoom changer is to avoid the momentary visual

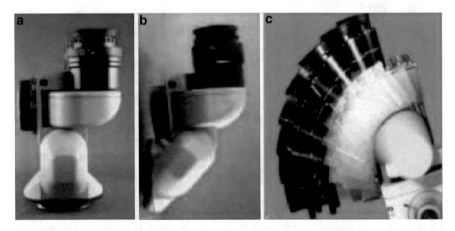

Fig. 4.11 Binoculars are available in three different kind of tubes: (a) straight tube; (b) inclined tube; and (c) inclinable tube [94]

disruption that occurs with manual step changers when the clinician changes the magnification. However, it has the following disadvantages when compared to the manual MC:

- Number of lenses is much higher.
- Moving from the minimum to the maximum magnification is slow.
- A greater absorption of light.
- Much more expensive.

4.13.1.4   Objective Lens

This is a biconvex lens that contains multiple layers of an antireflective coating on both surfaces. These layers reduce return light loss from normally 2% per lens surface to only 0.5% per lens surface. The focal length (which is the distance between the focal point of the objective lens and the central of the lens (Fig. 4.12) determines the working distance (which is the microscope and the surgical field). The longer the focal length the shorter the working distance, the greater the magnification and the narrower the field of view. The range of focal length varies usually from 100 mm to 400 mm. For endodontic work, a 200 mm focal length is considered suitable as it allows approximately 20 cm (8 inches) of working distance.

4.13.2 Total Magnification (TM)

The total magnification (TM) depends on four different factors. They are focal length of binocular (FLB), focal length of objective lens (FLOL), eyepiece power (EP), and magnification factor of the changer (MF). TM can be calculated using the following formula:

$$TM = \left(FLB / FLOL \right) \times EP \times MF$$

The total magnification for the SOM ranges from 2.5× to 32 ×.

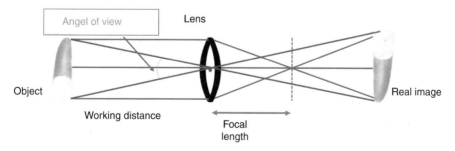

Fig. 4.12 The relation between the focal length, the distance length, and the angle of view. The longer the focal distance, the greater the magnification, the narrower field of view, and the shorter working length

4.13.3 Light Source Housing

The light sources in SOM might be one of three common systems: halogen, Xenon, or light emitted diode (LED). The halogen light has intensity of about 100 watts. It shows lower color temperature (yellowish) and does not provide enough illumination for good quality documentation. Recently, a new generation of Fiber Optic Halogen Light Source, which is comparable to the Xenon light has been introduced. The Xenon light provides natural look and is better for documentation. It has intensity of about 180 watts, which is suitable for the Endodontic work. In addition, the life of lamp is much more than that of the halogen light (e.g., it can reach to 500 h in OMPI microscopes). Similar to the Xenon light, the LED provides white light with little lower intensity and much better lifetime compared to Xenon (lifetime for LED might reach 70,000 h in Zumax OMS2350). One should note that light intensity decreases either when magnification is increased or when working distance is increased. For example, if the working distance is doubled, the intensity of light at the object is reduced to a quarter.

4.13.4 Supporting Structure

This is the structure that carries the other SOM parts. The type of the supporting structure determines the mount type of the SOM, that is, floor, ceiling, wall, or table mount. The supporting structure contains a "Counterbalanced Adjustable Connection Arms" that allow for easily maneuver of the head of microscope, and stop when the operators want during the work. In the recent SOMs, all maneuvers can be achieved using one hand and a little force. A balancing system is usually needed to be added to the supporting structure if additional documented accessories (like camera) is planned to be attached to the SOM. This will increase the safety of the SOM and prevent undesirable movement of the SOM body.

4.13.5 Documentation Components

These are additional accessories that help for documentation of the cases. Some microscopes do not allow the insertion of any accessories, but others do. Assistant scope eyepieces, SLR camera, CCD camera, video camera, and monitor are some examples of these accessories.

4.13.6 Advantages and Disadvantages of SOM

SOM provides magnification and intense illumination. This definitely improves the performance in endodontics and provides many advantages as it helps to [95–101]:

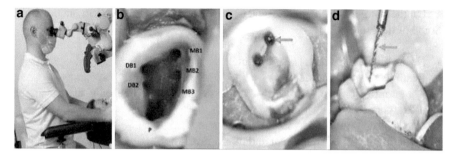

Fig. 4.13 (a) Ergonomic position is achieved when using SOM [95]. (b) SOM helps finding extra and hidden canals in upper first molar [101]. (c, d) management and retrieval of instruments separated in root canals should be always done using SOM

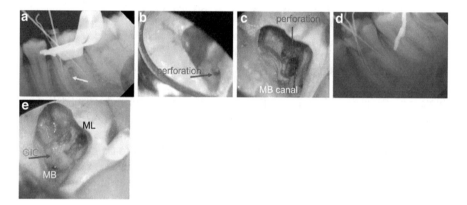

Fig. 4.14 (a) a perforation during searching for MB canal in lower first molar with calcified pulp chamber. (b) the perforation was located under SOM; MB orifice cannot be seen due to presence of tertiary dentin. (c) the orifice of MB canal was found using ultrasonic tip. (d) P.A. X-ray to confirm finding MB canal. (e) sealing the perforation with GIC under SOM to avoid wrong insertion of the material in the MB canal

- Improve ergonomics for the clinician (Fig. 4.13a).
- Improve diagnostic power.
- Prepare optimal access cavity.
- Preserve more tooth structure.
- Find hidden and accessory canals (Fig. 4.13b).
- Negotiate calcified canals.
- Locate and retrieve separated instruments (Fig. 4.13c, d).
- Locate and seal perforations (Fig. 4.14).
- Recognize and locate tooth fracture.
- Remove old root filling in context of retreatment.
- Place retro-filling material.
- Identify resected root-end cracks.
- Reduce surgical trauma.
- Reduce postoperative pain.

On the other hand, there are some disadvantages of using SOM in endodontics. Some of them are:

- Needs high skills and a lot of training.
- Restricts the working field.
- Less control on the instrument as operator is able to see only the tip of the instrument.
- Needs more time and longer session.
- High initial cost of equipment and micro-instruments.

4.14 How to Use Dental Microscope

The preparation of dental microscope should involve patient positioning, operator positioning, and microscope positioning.

4.14.1 Patient Positioning

In general, the patient should be at flat position for lower teeth and at Trendelenburg position (head slightly lowered to the pelvis) for upper teeth (Fig. 4.15). The chair should be raised to get sufficient space for operators' legs below and microscope above. The head of the patient should be then adjusted slightly to right or left according to the working field. In case of poor visibility, the patient's head is moved 10–20° back (Fig. 4.16). Table 4.2 summarizes the position of the patient in different situations.

4.14.2 Operator Positioning

Any ergonomic position that allows for good view and sufficient illumination of the surgical field is acceptable. For right-handed dentists, sitting position is between 7 and 12 o'clock [102]. 11–12 o'clock positions are the most common

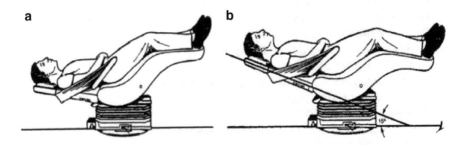

Fig. 4.15 (**a**) Patient position for upper teeth (Trendelenburg position). (**b**) Patient position for upper teeth (flat position) (*Adapted from Ergonomics in Dentistry by Hams Hamed*)

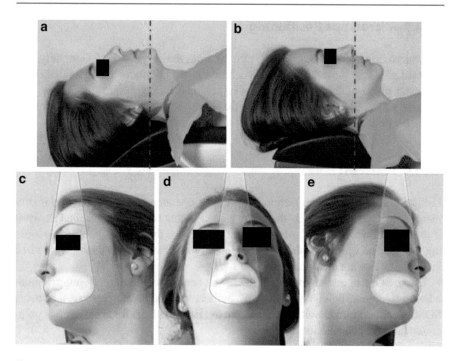

Fig. 4.16 (**a**) Mandibular occlusal plane should be vertical when treating lower teeth. (**b**) Maxillary occlusal; plane should be vertical when treating upper teeth. (**c, d, e**) The head of the patient should be placed right, straight, or lift of left according to the working field [95]

Table 4.2 Position of the patient

Maxillary	Anteriors	Patient looking ahead, occlusal plane 45° to the floor
	Premolars	Facing slightly to the other side
	Molars	Lying on his/her other side
Mandibular	Anteriors	Patient looking straight ahead
	Right posteriors	Facing slightly to the left
	Left posteriors	Lying on the right side with the head turned up

for all sides and all teeth. Some prefer the 11–12 o'clock positions for upper teeth and 8–9 o'clock for lower teeth. For endodontics work, indirect view is always considered. Operator position is selected with consideration to the patient position and microscope position. The operator should adjust the seating position so that the back is perpendicular to the floor, the knees are 90° to the hips, and the forearms are 90° to upper arms. Feet are placed flat on the floor. The eyepieces are inclined so that the head and neck are comfortably sustained. These recommendations are maintained regardless of the arch or quadrants being worked on.

4.14.3 Microscope Positioning

The microscope should be 200–250 mm far from the surgical field. Generally, it is directed at 90° to floor. To improve visibility, it can be modified and angled down the axial plane of the roots when necessary. The interpupillary distance is then adjusted followed by adjustment of the fine focus positioning to get the better view of the surgical site.

4.14.4 Assistant Role

Using SOM requires good training from both operator and assistant. The instruments, materials, and devices should be placed so that they can be reached easily. It is recommended to use endodontic cart nearby. Since the dentist should keep looking through the eyepieces, the assistant should be trained how to hand the required instruments and materials properly.

Using SOM in endodontics provides great benefits and definitely improve endodontic treatment outcome. Therefore, authors of this chapter believe that using SOM in endodontics should be considered as "must" at least for access cavity preparation and root canals' location.

4.15   3D Guided Endodontics

The concept of "minimally invasive endodontics" should be considered during access cavity preparation. The destructive or unnecessary removal of tooth tissue should always be avoided [103]. To preserve more dental tissue, new conservative (contracted) access cavity, and ultraconservative (ninja) access cavity were introduced [104]. However, in some clinical scenarios, the conservative access cavity preparation becomes a challenge. For example, in case of teeth with calcified coronal pulp chamber (pulp stone) or sclerosed canals, the calcific deposits might cover the orifices of root canals or block the canal spaces. Endodontic treatment for such teeth is considered one of the most challenging tasks in dentistry. Locating and preparation the calcified canals may result in unnecessary removal of dentin with the risk of perforating or fracturing the root [105]. This might occur even with the possibility of presence of a remaining narrow soft tissue in the root canal [106]. The prognosis in such teeth may be considerably impaired due to excessive loss of tooth material [107]. The use of surgical operative microscope (SOM) is highly recommended.

More recently, a new "guided endodontics" solution was introduced as a novel approach to manage teeth with calcified pulp canals and apical pathology [108]. The concept of this new approach depends on using data from computed tomography to generate a computer-aided guide that serves in accurate access cavity preparation. As a matter of fact, this approach was developed first in dental implantology to guide the surgeon for accurate placement of implants. The optimum position of the implant can be determined previously using CBCT analysis and then applied on to the patient using different static and dynamic guidance techniques [109].

4.16   Static Guidance (3D Printed Surgical Guidance)

In the static guidance, a guided surgical stent is designed by means of a computer-aided design (CAD) software based on a CBCT scan and printed using a 3D printer. The stent contains metal sleeves within an acrylic base that guide the drills during surgical procedure. "Static" refers to the fact that the implant is placed as predetermined using the surgical stent without the ability to modify or change the position.

One of the major disadvantages of the static guidance systems that restricted their use is that they require big space to accommodate for the guide. This makes them difficult to be used for posterior teeth or in patient with limited mouth opening. The other disadvantages include the difficulty to modify the planned dimensions and/or angulations after fabrication, irrigations to cool bone during preparation is limited, consuming time as it requires laboratory works, and expensive considering the cost of the pre-CBCT prosthetic plan and the surgical stent [109, 110].

Moving this technology to endodontics to manage teeth with calcified pulp tissue was just a matter of time. For clinicians, the concept of 3D guided endodontics presented a promising valuable technique for a higher predictable endodontic outcome with less invasive and lower risk of iatrogenic damage. In 2016, Buchgreitz et al. and Zehnder et al. confirmed the accuracy of using a static drill guide for access cavity preparations in ex vivo researches [111]. However, two more restrictions should be considered to use static guidance in endodontic work. First, the endodontic patient commonly comes to dental clinic with acute pain that requires immediate interference and cannot wait the time required to plan and prepare for the static guidance procedures. Second, each root canal should have its own drill guide. This means the need to have multiple drill guides for multiple-canal teeth like posterior teeth with more expense [112].

The virtual optimal access cavity can be planned using a computer software, preoperative CBCT scan, and (CAD/CAM) technology. Based on this plan, a template is fabricated using a 3D printer. The template will be very helpful to guide for a minimally invasive drill into the calcified root canal system [113]. Access cavity preparation was performed by two operators. Postoperative CBCT scan was superimposed on the virtual planning. The deviation of planned and prepared cavities was measured in three dimensions and used to evaluate the accuracy. The results showed that the printed templates used for "guided endodontics" enabled the operators to access all root canals up to the apical third of root with low deviation of planned and prepared access cavities (Fig. 4.17) [111].

The same team has applied the static guided endodontics technique to treat a tooth with pulp canal calcification endodontically (Fig. 4.18) [108].

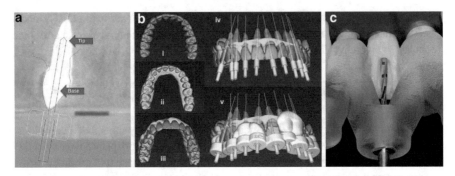

Fig. 4.17 (a) The virtual bur is superimposed with the tooth to create straight line access to the apical third of the root canal. The base of the bur (red arrow) and the tip of the bur (blue arrow) can be seen. (b) The matching between CBCT and teeth scans, (i) CBCT scan, (ii) teeth scan, (iii) matched scans, (iv) virtual Bur in the matched scan, (v) designed template (sleeves and burs). (c) Clinical application, the bur was guided through the sleeve to the apical third of the root canal (*Reproduced with permission from John Wiley & Sons*) [111]

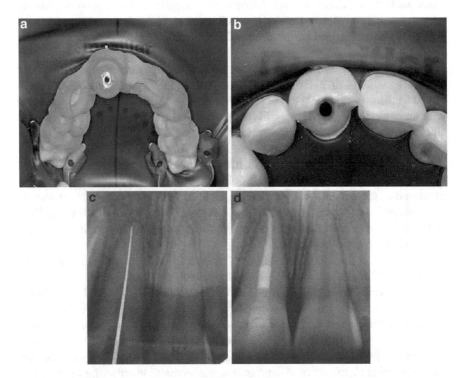

Fig. 4.18 (a) Template positioned on the maxillary teeth to check its correct and reproducible fitting. (b) View of the endodontic access cavity after root canal location. Control radiograph with silver cone in the root canal. (c) Successful instrumentation of the calcified root canal (d) Postoperative radiographic examination. (*Reproduced with permission from John Wiley & Sons*) [108]

4.17   Dynamic Guidance (Live 3D Navigation)

Dynamic guidance was initially introduced for cranio-maxillofacial surgery (115) and improved later to determine the ideal position of dental implants [113]. The dynamic guidance system contains optical technologies that allow direct views of the surgical site and provides real-time visualization. This technology is very similar to systems of global positioning or satellite navigation. The Trace Registration method is known as "trace and place" or TAP technique. With this technique, the CBCT scan is uploaded and registered by selecting three to six accessible radiographic landmarks (points) on the screen. Next, the selected points are traced in the patient's mouth. The advantages of TAP technique include the reduction of patient exposure to radiation; first, because the possibility to use a small volume CBCT, and second because it eliminates the need for a second CBCT that is usually needed with metallic fiducial-markers placed on the jaw via a thermoplastic stent. In addition, TAP technique will save time, minimize the cost of the procedure, and reduce the chance of errors caused by possible dislocation of the stent during scanning [112]. Some of the current available systems are Navident (ClaroNav), (Fig. 4.19), RoboDent (RoboDent), Image Guided Implantology (Image Navigation), and X-Guide (X-Nav Technologies).

In 2016, Dr. Charles Maupin used this technology for the first time in endodontics for access cavity preparation in calcified teeth. It was obvious that dynamic guidance solves most of the problems that static drill guides have in endodontic application. For endodontic application, the locations of the root canals should be determined using computer software and preoperative CBCT data. The dynamic guidance systems that involves motion-tracking system with optical cameras is then used to provide a real-time dynamic plus visual feedback to intraoperatively guide canal preparation. The preplanned information is transferred to the real-life clinical case, and the exact position of the handpiece is tracked continuously during canal preparation.

Buchannan & Maupin reported three cases using a Dynamic Guidance System, the X-Guide (X-Nav Technologies, LLC, Lansdale, PA) [114]. Two scanning drums were used as reference points; one was secured to the patient's jaw prior to CT scanning, and the other was secured to a latch-grip handpiece attachment. Two overhead cameras connected to computer processor were used to trace the reference points allowing to generate an avatar of the target tooth on the computer screen. This enabled the operator to observe drilling into tooth in real time. The technique was less invasive and very effective in locating canals in the calcified teeth.

Nahimas [112] demonstrated the accuracy of the Dynamic Guidance System when compared to traditional techniques in preparing access cavity in a clinical case (Fig. 4.20–4.28). They were able to use the navigation software and the dynamic guidance to locate much calcified canals through much smaller access cavities preserving more tooth structure by using the Dynamic Dental Navigation System, Navident.

Fig. 4.19 Navident unit
used for dynamic
navigation (ClaroNav,
Toronto, Canada)

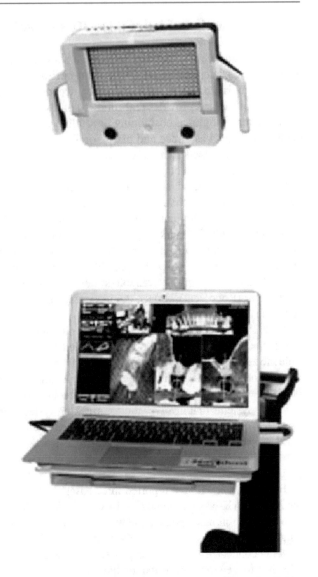

Another advantage of the dynamic guidance systems is that they afford flexibility
and possibility to modify the treatment plan at any time during the procedure [110].
The dynamic guidance systems are more applicable for posterior teeth or with
patient with limited mouth opening as they do not require long drills or burs. They
require no laboratory work and thus no waiting time. They also increase operative
safety and reduce technical errors. In endodontic work, Zehnde et al., (2016)
reported 0.21 mm as the mean of absolute difference in mesial/distal direction, 0.2
the mean for buccal/oral aspect, and 0.16 mm for the mean of apical/coronal deviation with a maximum error of 0.76 mm in all directions [111].

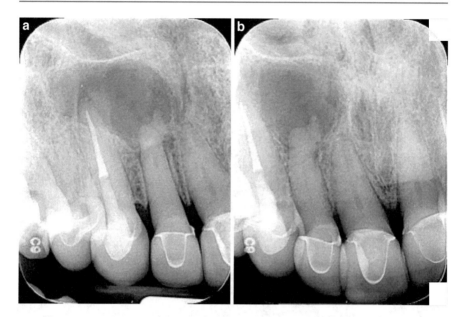

Fig. 4.20 *(Courtesy Oral health and Dr. Nahmias)* [112]. (**a, b**) Periapical radiographs of teeth 12 and 13. Please note that the radiolucency appears to be affecting both teeth. The canal appears to be calcified on tooth # 12 in addition to the ceramic crown's orientation is not parallel to the inclination of the root making the access and localization of the canal very difficult. 3D guided Endodontics procedures is indicated

In 2017, Buchanan and his team evaluated the accuracy of Dynamically Guided Access (DGA) when used for access cavity preparation in teeth with calcified pulp tissues using X-Nav system (X-Nav Technologies, LLC, Lansdale, PA). The study was performed in 3D printed jaws (TrueJawTM by Dental Engineering Laboratories, Santa Barbara, CA) where teeth were designed with eliminate pulp chambers to simulate teeth with calcified pulp tissues. Each canal was accessed through its own 1 mm opening in the occlusal surface (Fig. 4.29). The results showed remarkable accuracy as all canals were easily instrumented using size 15 files through the limited occlusal opening [114]. These results are sufficient enough to apply the dynamic technique in clinical practice to manage calcified teeth, and a series of successful cases were published next year [114]. The advantages of accessing calcified canals through a very small access (1 mm wide access) or through crowns were met in these cases. The authors of this chapter suggest a possible application for removing fiber posts from root canals.

Although the concept of guided endodontics has been established and used in several cases, there are a number of considerations for this technology to make it applicable and reliable in the daily practice. First, the technology is expensive considering the cost of the software, equipment, CBCT, and other running costs. However, it could

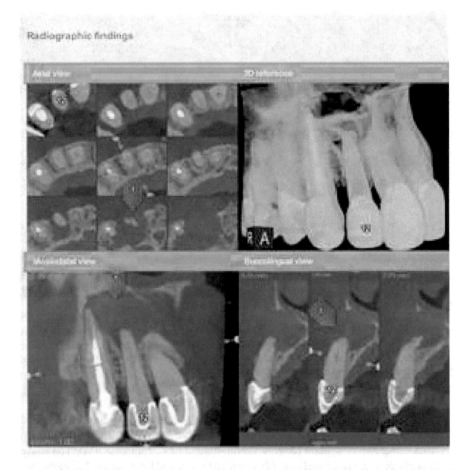

Fig. 4.21 The CBCT report (by Canaray, Mississauga, Canada) indicates that a large area of infection is associated with tooth 1.2. It concludes that 1.3 does not appear to be the source of the infection and that root canal treatment or extraction is indicated for 1.2

be argued that the successful application of this technology results in successful RCT and allows the tooth to retain and save the cost of replacement that might be needed later in case of extraction. Second, the current dynamic navigation systems are designed for implant surgery where the drill tag fits a slow-speed contra-angle handpiece. However, access cavity preparation is better performed by high-speed hand pieces that can penetrate enamel and dentine more efficiently and effectively. Besides, the current implant-design software allows only for straight line preparation. This would not be suitable for calcified canals where the obliteration is not in a straight line to the canal entrance or if it is in the middle or apical third of the root canal. In some cases, a buccal (facial) access cavity might be required to access the patent part of the

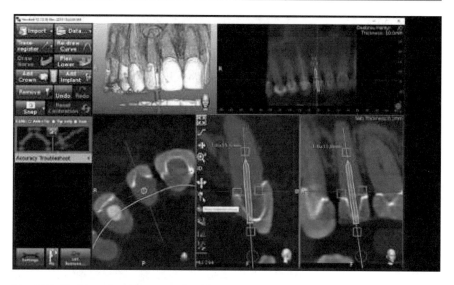

Fig. 4.22 Navident planning screen. Used for planning the endodontic access cavity (appears in yellow) through the calcified pulp chamber directly into the radiographically visible coronal entrance to the canal. The operator adjusts the yellow "implant" image, which will be used for the guidance (diameter, length, position, and direction) until they are satisfied that this is the best path to take. Axial, coronal, and sagittal views are aligned to set up the correct path for the bur to follow

Fig. 4.23 CBCT image determining that approximately 14 mm is calcified before the canal location

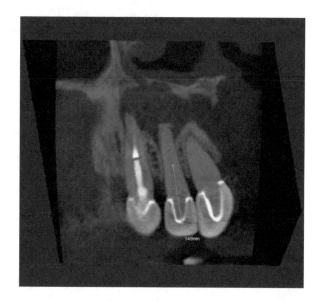

Fig. 4.24 IOPA confirming the visibility of the cabal at around 14 mm into the tooth, same as on the CBCT

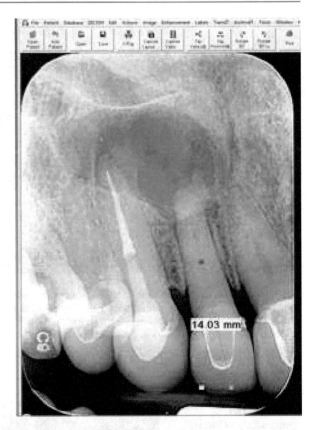

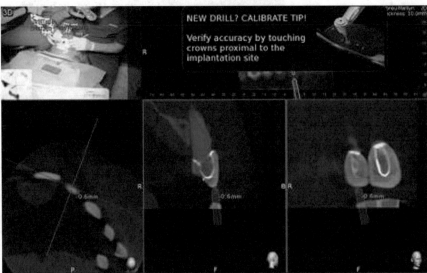

Fig. 4.25 "Accuracy Check"—After calibrating the drill-tip and just prior to drilling, the operator is prompted to perform a "sanity check" step, where the system's accuracy is verified. This is done by touching with the drill-tip on distinct rigid landmarks (such as teeth cusps) in the treated jaw, and comparing the physical drill's location to its on-screen position representation (in light blue). This check can be repeated at any time during the procedure

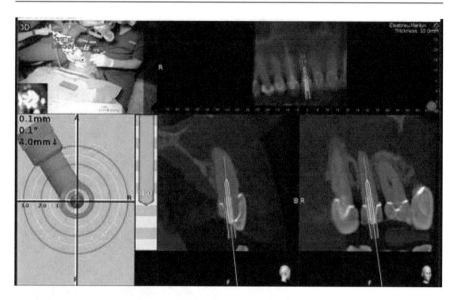

Fig. 4.26 "Accuracy Check"—After calibrating the drill-tip and just prior to drilling, the operator is prompted to perform a "sanity check" step, where the system's accuracy is verified. This is done by touching with the drill-tip on distinct rigid landmarks (such as teeth cusps) in the treated jaw, and comparing the physical drill's location to its on-screen position representation (in light blue). This check can be repeated at any time during the procedure

Fig. 4.27 The actual view the operator follows during active dynamic navigation. The operator aligns the head of the hand piece and the tip of the bur into the center circle ("Bulls eye"). The main center circle has a diameter of 1.0 mm. Each Orange circle is separated by 1 mm orange intervals. The green bar on the right shows the distance (in mm) left to drill to the pointed tip of the planned trajectory (in yellow). Here we are 4 mm away from the predetermined target

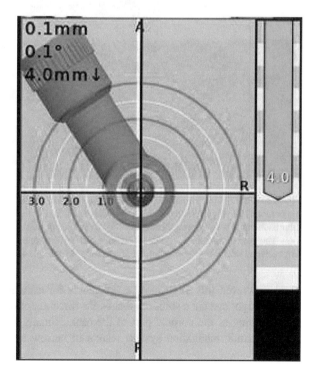

Fig. 4.28 Postoperative
X-ray of the case
completed

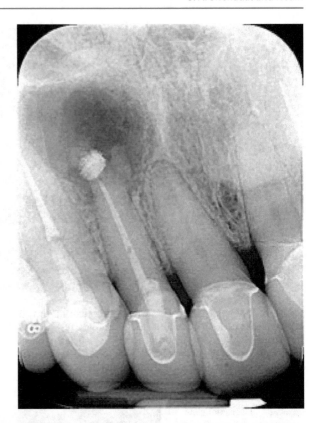

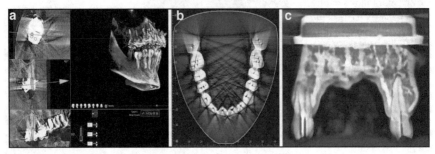

Fig. 4.29 (a) Computer treatment plan is shown after access paths have been plotted in a calcified upper molar. The highlighted path is for the MB canal. (b) Occlusal CBCT view of TrueJaw replica after each canal was entered through its own dynamically guided access path. (c) Sagittal CBCT view showing dynamically guided access paths cut on opposite sides of the TrueJaw arch *(Reproduced with Permission from Dr. Stephen Buchanan)* [114]

canal. However, this might not be acceptable for esthetic reasons. A two stages of drilling might present a solution, that is, the direction of drilling is modified after initial accessing of the coronal part of the canal. Finally, the access cavities prepared using dynamic navigation system results in narrow and parallel walls that might

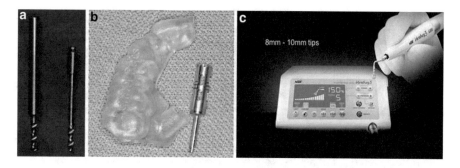

Fig. 4.30 (**a**) A commercially available twist bur with a diameter of 1.2 mm (left) and the same bur modified to be used through the guide sleeve (right) *(Reproduced with permission from John Wiley & Sons)* [115]. (**b**) Three-dimensional–printed surgical guides with custom fit trephine bur *(Reproduced with permission from Elsevier Publishing)* [116]. (**c**) Piezotomes with a chisel [117]

hamper the following RCT procedures including cleaning, shaping, and obturation of the root canal system. Thus, further investigation is needed to overcome the challenges and make the dynamic guided applicable in everyday clinical practice.

For instruments used to prepare the tooth tissues, longneck drills and endodontic ultrasonic tips were routinely used to manage calcified canals under microscope. For guided endodontic procedures, Buchanan used micro-burs designed for minimally invasive access procedures (Guided Access burs by SS White) [114], Zehnde et al. (2016) used a diamond bur to penetrate enamel and then used a specific bur (drill) through the dentine to gain access to the root canal [111]. Buchgreitz et al. (2016) used a high-speed bur to penetrate enamel and/or filling and a modified twist bur with a diameter of 1.2 mm to drill into the calcified root (Fig. 4.30a) [115]. For static guided surgical endodontics, Giacomino et al. (2018) used trephine burs (Fig. 4.30b) [116], and Mohame et al. (2018) [117] used piezotome chisel to elevate the cortical bone and Lindeman burs to perform root resection (Fig. 4.30c), but it is not clear if these types of burs can be calibrated for dynamic guidance procedures.

4.18   3D Guided Surgical Endodontics

Both static and dynamic guidance have applications in Endodontic Microsurgery (EMS). Giacomino et al. (2018) have developed a technique known as "Targeted Endodontic Microsurgery" (Targeted EMS) where trephine burs can be used within a stent for root-end resection; osteotomy; and biopsy in single step (Fig. 4.30b) [108]. Not far from this design, Mohamed et al., (2018) introduced the "Computer Guided Cortical Window Approach" where a cortical bone window (bone lid) is elevated to access the apical region using a piezotome chisel [109]. The dynamic guidance enabled an undergraduate student to proceed surgical endodontic treatment of a lesion in an upper lateral incisor precisely using Navident dynamic navigation system (ClaroNav, Toronto, Ontario, Canada) [118].

Guided EMS allows precise localization of the root and precise cutting and removal of the periapical pathological tissue (Fig. 4.31). It is a minimally invasive

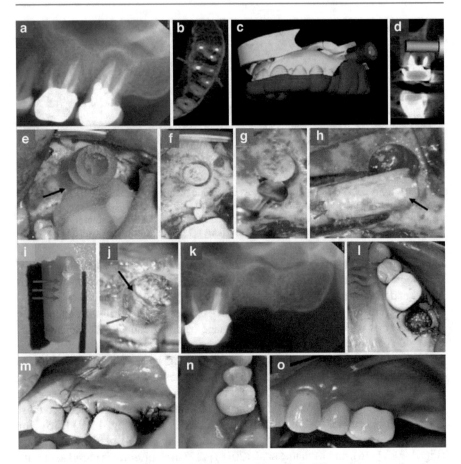

Fig. 4.31 The palatal root of tooth #17. (**a**) Preoperative periapical X-ray shows two sinus tracts (black arrows). (**b**) The gutta-percha cone tracing the distal sinus tract to palatal root of tooth #17. (**c**) 3D surgical guide (3DSG) was fabricated on the digital cast. Note the trephine port that was designed for contralateral occlusal clearance. (**d**) A coronal view of CBCT shows the planned trephine path. (**e**) The trephine path avoids the GPA traced in yellow from the greater palatine foramen running anteriorly. (**f**) 3DSG with custom fit trephine. (**g**) To produce bleeding points, 3DSG with trephine is inserted in port. (**h**) Bleeding points and subsequent incision for mucosal window. (**i**) Mucosal window after trephine osteotomy with core in place. (**j**) Core specimen with palatal cortical bone (black arrow), resected root end, and soft tissue (blue arrows). (**k**) Immediate postoperative radiograph. (**l**) Immediate postoperative image with replanted palatal mucosa. (**m**) One week postoperative. (**n**) Four weeks postoperative. (**o**) Three months postoperative with healed palatal tissue and sinus tracts (*Reproduced with permission from Elsevier Publishing*) [116]. (**Disclaimer**—*"Targeted Endodontic Microsurgery U.S. patent Application No. 16/396,185 was filed April 26, 2018. All rights, title, and interest have been assigned to the Government of the United States. One or more embodiments of the inventions described in these patent applications are described in this textbook chapter. The views expressed are those of the author's and do not reflect the official views or policy of the United States Department of Defense or the Uniformed Services University of the Health Sciences"*)

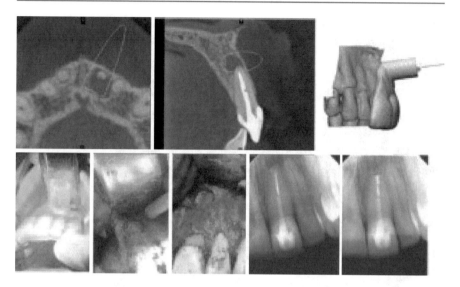

Fig. 4.32 3D printed guides are being used in surgical endodontics. Tooth 21 with a 10-month recall. Hollow cylindrical trephine burs traditionally used to remove implants combined with a 3D-printed surgical guide for osteotomy and root-end resection of tooth #9 (*Reproduced with permission from AAE, Courtesy Dr. Ray*) [119]. (**Disclaimer**—*"Targeted Endodontic Microsurgery U.S. patent Application No. 16/396,185 was filed April 26, 2018. All rights, title, and interest have been assigned to the Government of the United States. One or more embodiments of the inventions described in these patent applications are described in this textbook chapter. The views expressed are those of the author's and do not reflect the official views or policy of the United States Department of Defense or the Uniformed Services University of the Health Sciences"*)

and safe approach that preserves bone structure and reduces the risk of iatrogenic damage to adjacent anatomic structures. Thus, the postoperative patient discomfort is less, and the healing is faster. Figures 4.32 and 4.33 show another clinical application for the use of a static guide in endodontic surgery [119].

4.19   See Footnote

"Targeted Endodontic Microsurgery U.S. patent Application No. 16/396,185 was filed April 26, 2018. All rights, title, and interest have been assigned to the Government of the United States.

One or more embodiments of the inventions described in these patent applications are described in this textbook chapter. The views expressed are those of the author's and do not reflect the official views or policy of the United States Department of Defense or the Uniformed Services University of the Health Sciences."

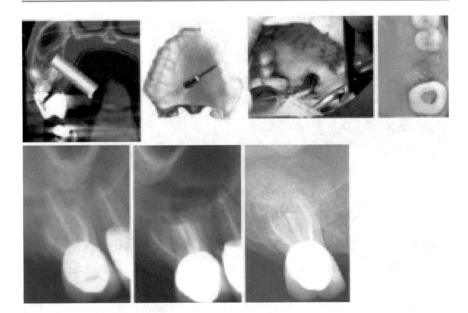

Fig. 4.33 Tooth 17 with 18-month recall. Similar procedure applied for a flapless palatal approach to the palatal root of tooth #2 and called the procedure Targeted Endodontic Microsurgery (TEMS) (*Reproduced with permission from AAE, Courtesy Dr. Ray*) [119]. **Disclaimer**—*"Targeted Endodontic Microsurgery U.S. patent Application No. 16/396,185 was filed April 26, 2018. All rights, title, and interest have been assigned to the Government of the United States. One or more embodiments of the inventions described in these patent applications are described in this textbook chapter. The views expressed are those of the author's and do not reflect the official views or policy of the United States Department of Defense or the Uniformed Services University of the Health Sciences".* See Sect. 4.19

4.20   The Assistive Augmented Reality (AR) Technology

Song et al. (2018) have introduced a new assistive augmented reality (AR) technology on the head-mounted see-through display (HMD). This system can assist the operator to prepare optimal access cavity and avoid preparation mishaps. It contains a warning and correction system that is designed to provide visual and audio guides during the preparation procedure. The position of the tool is oriented all the time, and clinician can avoid a wrong or risky tool pose. In addition, the dentist can review the radiograph during the work without the need to look at separate monitor. The dentist can display the radiographs on the HMD when needed or hidden them not to cause distraction. This feature can be easily controlled by voice orders only. This makes the application intuitive and easy to use without the need to use the operator's hands. One of the advantages of this application is that it can be deployed on the Microsoft HoloLens as HMD or on a PC that has an external display. The primary results of laboratory study show that this system is able to provide useful information to the operator to correct wrong poses of the instrument during access cavity procedure and help to make decisions in shorter time [120]. However, the system should be improved to be applicable on the real size human teeth and submitted for more clinical researches.

4.21 Conclusion

Advancements in digital technology continue to improve the techniques used in endodontic diagnosis and treatment. With proper use and training, the application of these new technologies will reduce patient treatment time and pain, and improve the overall outcome of endodontic treatment.

References

1. Naoum HJ, Chandler NP, RM L. Conventional versus storage phosphor-plate digital images to visualize the root canal system contrasted with a radiopaque medium. J Endod. 2003;29(5):349–52.
2. Wenzel A, Gröndahl HJ. Direct digital radiography in the dental office. Int Dent J. 1995;45(1):27–34.
3. Deepak B, Subash T, Narmatha V, Anamika T, Snehil T, Nandini DJ. Imaging techniques in endodontics: an overview. J Clin Imaging Sci. 2012;2
4. Gröndahl HG, Huumonen S. Radiographic manifestations of periapical inflammatory lesions: how new radiological techniques may improve endodontic diagnosis and treatment planning. Endod Topics. 2004;8(1):55–67.
5. Patel S, Dawood A, Whaites E, Pitt Ford TJ. New dimensions in endodontic imaging: part 1. Conventional and alternative radiographic systems. Int Endod J. 2009;42(6):447–62.
6. Sonoda M, Takano M, Miyahara J, Kato HJR. Computed radiography utilizing scanning laser stimulated luminescence. Radiology. 1983;148(3):833–8.
7. Tyndall DA, Ludlow JB, Platin E, Nair MJOS. A comparison of Kodak Ektaspeed plus film and the Siemens Sidexis digital imaging system for caries detection using receiver operating characteristic analysis. Oral Med Oral Pathol Oral Radiol Endod. 1998;85(1):113–8.
8. Van Der Stelt PF. Filmless imaging: the uses of digital radiography in dental practice. 2005;136(10):1379–87.
9. Walther J. Optical coherence tomography in the oral cavity. Technical University of Dresden. SPIE Photonics West 2018, San Francisco.
10. Imai K, Shimada Y, Sadr A, Sumi Y, Tagami J. Noninvasive cross-sectional visualization of enamel cracks by optical coherence tomography *in vitro*. J Endod. 2012;38:1269–74.
11. Bueno MR, Estrela C, Azevedo BC, Diogenes AJ. Development of a new cone-beam computed tomography software for endodontic diagnosis. Braz Dent J. 2018;29(6):517–29.
12. Patel S, Dawood A, Ford TP, Whaites EJ. The potential applications of cone beam computed tomography in the management of endodontic problems. Int Endod J. 2007;40(10):818–30.
13. Nair MK, Nair UP. Digital and advanced imaging in endodontics: a review. J Endod. 2007;33(1):1–6.
14. Cotton TP, Geisler TM, Holden DT, Schwartz SA, Schindler WG. Endodontic applications of cone-beam volumetric tomography. J Endod. 2007;33(9):1121–32.
15. Bueno MR, Estrela C, De Figueiredo JAP, Azevedo BCJ. Map-reading strategy to diagnose root perforations near metallic intracanal posts by using cone beam computed tomography. J Endod. 2011;37(1):85–90.

16. Venskutonis T, Plotino G, Juodzbalys G, Mickevičienė LJ. The importance of cone-beam computed tomography in the management of endodontic problems: a review of the literature. J Endod. 2014;40(12):1895–901.
17. Aminoshariae A, Kulild JC, AJ S. Cone-beam computed tomography compared with intraoral radiographic lesions in endodontic outcome studies: a systematic review. J Endod. 2018;44(11):1626–31.
18. Rosen E, Taschieri S, Del Fabbro M, Beitlitum I, Tsesis IJ. The diagnostic efficacy of cone-beam computed tomography in endodontics: a systematic review and analysis by a hierarchical model of efficacy. J Endod. 2015;41(7):1008–14.
19. Long H, Zhou Y, Ye N, Liao L, Jian F, Wang Y, et al. Diagnostic accuracy of CBCT for tooth fractures: a meta-analysis. J Dent. 2014;42(3):240–8.
20. Mamede-Neto I, Bandeca MC, Tonetto MR, Nogueira AL, Borba AM, Pereira TM, et al. The role of the cone-beam computed tomography as an incremental tool in endodontic diagnoses. J Int Oral Health. 2016;8(10):978.
21. Rajendran N, Sundaresan B. Efficacy of ultrasound and color power Doppler as a monitoring tool in the healing of endodontic periapical lesions. J Endod. 2007;33:181–6.
22. Maity I, Kumari A, Shukla AK, Usha H, Naveen D. Monitoring of healing by ultrasound with color power doppler after root canal treatment of maxillary anterior teeth with periapical lesions. J Conserv Dent. 2011;14:252–7.
23. Khambete N, Kumar R. Ultrasound in differential diagnosis of periapical radiolucencies: a radiohistopathological study. J Conserv Dent. 2015;18:39–43.
24. Idiyatullin D, Corum C, Moeller S, Prasad HS, Garwood M, Nixdorf DR. Dental magnetic resonance imaging: making the invisible visible. J Endod. 2011;37:745–52.
25. Lin J, Chandler N, Purton D, Monteith BJ. Appropriate electrode placement site for electric pulp testing first molar teeth. J Endod. 2007;33(11):1296–8.
26. Bender I. Reversible and irreversible painful pulpitides: diagnosis and treatment. J Aust Soc Endod. 2000;26(1):10–4.
27. Ehrmann EJADJ. Pulp testers and pulp testing with particular reference to the use of dry ice. Aust Dent J. 1977;22(4):272–9.
28. Närhi M, Virtanen A, Kuhta J, Huopaniemi T. Electrical stimulation of teeth with a pulp tester in the cat. Eur J Oral Sci. 1979;87(1):32–8.
29. Penna K, Sadoff R. Simplified approach to use of electrical pulp tester. N Y State Dent J. 1995;61(1):30–1.
30. Kolbinson DA, Teplitsky PE. Electric pulp testing with examination gloves. Oral Surg Oral Med Oral Pathol. 1988;65(1):122–6.
31. Guerra JA, Skribner J, Lin LM. Electric pulp tester and apex locator barrier technique. J Endod. 1993;19(10):532–4.
32. Kleier D, Sexton J, RJJodr A. Electronic and clinical comparison of pulp testers. J Dent Res. 1982;61(12):1413–5.
33. Johnsen DJ. Innervation of teeth: qualitative, quantitative, and developmental assessment. J Dent Res. 1985;64:555–63.
34. Mumford J. Thermal and electrical stimulation of teeth in the diagnosis of pulpal and periapical disease: SAGE Publications; 1967.
35. Woolley LH, Woodworth J, Dobbs JLJT. A preliminary evaluation of the effects of electrical pulp testers on dogs with artificial pacemakers. J Am Dent Assoc. 1974;89(5):1099–101.
36. Miller CS, Leonelli FM, Latham EJOS. Selective interference with pacemaker activity by electrical dental devices. Oral Med Oral Pathol Oral Radiol Endod. 1998;85(1):33–6.
37. Wilson BL, Broberg C, Baumgartner JC, Harris C, JJJoe K. Safety of electronic apex locators and pulp testers in patients with implanted cardiac pacemakers or cardioverter/defibrillators. J Endod. J Endod. 2006;32(9):847–52.
38. Sailus J, Trowbridge H, Greco M, Emling R, editors. Sensitivity of teeth subjected to orthodontic forces. Journal of dental Research; 1987.: Amer Assoc Dental Research 1619 Duke ST, Alexandria, VA 22314.

39. Waikakul A, Kasetsuwan J, Punwutikorn JJOS. Response of autotransplanted teeth to electric pulp testing. Oral Med Oral Pathol Oral Radiol Endod. 2002;94(2):249–55.
40. Pileggi R, Dumsha T, Myslinksi NJDT. The reliability of electrical pulp test after concussion injury. Dental Traumatol. 1996;12(1):16–9.
41. Peters DD, Baumgartner JC, LJ L. Adult pulpal diagnosis. I. Evaluation of the positive and negative responses to cold and electrical pulp tests. J Endod. 1994;20(10):506–11.
42. Rowe A, Ford TP. The assessment of pulpal vitality. Int Endod J. 1990;23(2):77–83.
43. Millard HJ. Electric pulp testers. Council on dental materials and devices. J Am Dental Assoc. 1973;86(4):872–3.
44. Lin J, Chandler N. Electric pulp testing: a review. Int Endod J. 2008;41(5):365–74.
45. Jacobson JJOS. Probe placement during electric pulp-testing procedures. Oral Med Oral Pathol. 1984;58(2):242–7.
46. Bender I, Landau MA, Fonsecca S, Trowbridge HO. The optimum placement-site of the electrode in electric pulp testing of the 12 anterior teeth. 1989;118(3):305–10.
47. Lilja JJAOS. Sensory differences between crown and root dentin in human teeth. Acta Odontol Scand. 1980;38(5):285–91.
48. Cooley RL, Robison SFJOS. Variables associated with electric pulp testing. Oral Surg Oral Med Oral Pathol. 1980;50(1):66–73.
49. Myers JW. Demonstration of a possible source of error with an electric pulp tester. J Endod. 1998;24(3):199–201.
50. Simon S, Machtou P, Adams N, Tomson P, Lumley PJD. Apical limit and working length in endodontics. 2009;36(3):146–53.
51. Franco V, Tosco E. The endodontic line: a clinical approach. Societa'Italiana di Endodonzi. 2013;27(1):2–12.
52. Nekoofar M, Ghandi M, Hayes S, Dummer P. The fundamental operating principles of electronic root canal length measurement devices. Int Endod J. 2006;39(8):595–609.
53. Ebrahim AK, Wadachi R, Suda HJ. Electronic apex locators—a review. J Med Dent Sci. 2007;54(3):125–36.
54. Khadse A, Shenoi P, Kokane V, Khode R, Sonarkar S. Endodontics. Electronic apex locators—an overview. Ind J Conserv Endod. 2017;2(2):35–40.
55. Sonal Soi SM, Vinayak V, Kaur P. Electronic apex locators. J Dent Sci Oral Rehabil. 2013:24–7.
56. Steffen H, Splieth C, KJIej B. Comparison of measurements obtained with hand files or the canal leader attached to electronic apex locators: an in vitro study. Int Endod J. 1999;32(2):103–7.
57. Sunada IJ. New method for measuring the length of the root canal. J Dent Res. 1962;41(2):375–87.
58. Gordon M, Chandler N. Electronic apex locators. Int Endod J. 2004;37(7):425–37.
59. Fouad AF, Krell KV. An in vitro comparison of five root canal length measuring instruments. J Endod. 1989;15(12):573–7.
60. Dimitrov S, Roshkev DJ. Sixth generation adaptive apex locator. J Endod. 2009;15(2009):75–8.
61. Tınaz AC, Sevimli LS, Görgül G, Türköz EG. The effects of sodium hypochloride concentrations on the accuracy of an apex locating device. Int Dent J. 2002;28(3):160–2.
62. Stock CJR. Current status of the use of ultrasound in endodontics. Int Dent J. 1991;41:175–82.
63. Martin H, Cunningham W. Endosonic endodontics: the ultrasonic synergistic system. Int Dent J. 1984;34:198–203.
64. Martin H, Cunningham W. Endosonics: the ultrasonic synergistic system of endodontics. Endod Dent Traumatol. 1985;1:201–6.
65. Mohammadi Z, Abbott PV. The properties and applications of chlorhexidine in endodontics. Int Endod J. 2009;42(4):288–302.
66. Van der Sluis L, Versluis M, Wu M, Wesselink P. Passive ultrasonic irrigation of the root canal: a review of the literature. Int Endod J. 2007;40(6):415–26.
67. Klyn SL, Kirkpatrick TC, Rutledge RE. In vitro comparisons of debris removal of the EndoActivator TM system, the F file TM, ultrasonic irrigation, and NaOCl irrigation alone after handrotary instrumentation in human mandibular molars. J Endod. 2010;36(8):1367–71.

68. Mozo S, Llena C, Forner L. Review of ultrasonic irrigation in endodontics: increasing action of irrigating solutions. Med Oral Patol Oral Cir Bucal. 2012;17(3):e512–6.
69. Pitt WG. Removal of oral biofilm by sonic phenomena. Am J Dent. 2005;18:345–52.
70. Ruddle CJ. Endodontic disinfection: tsunami irrigation. Endod Prac. 2008;11(1):7–15.
71. Neuhaus KW, Liebi M, Stauffacher S, Eick S, Lussi A. Antibacterial efficacy of a new sonic irrigation device for root canal disinfection. J Endod. 2016;42(12):1799–803.
72. Lumley PJ, Walmsley AD, Laird WR. Streaming patterns produced around endosonic files. Int Endod J. 1991;24(6):290–7.
73. Townsend C, Maki J. An in vitro comparison of new irrigation and agitation techniques to ultrasonic agitation in removing bacteria from a simulated root canal. J Endod. 2009;35:1040–3.
74. Rodig T, Bozkurt M, Konietschke F, Hülsmann M. Comparison of the vibringe system with syringe and passive ultrasonic irrigation in removing debris from simulated root canal irregularities. J Endod. 2010;36:1410–3.
75. Sumi Y, Hattori H, Hayashi K, Ueda M. Ultrasonic root-end preparation: clinical and radiographic evaluation of results. J Oral Maxillofac Surg. 1996;54:590–3.
76. Mehlhaff DS, Marshall JG, Baumgartner JC. Comparison of ultrasonic and highspeed- bur root-end preparations using bilaterally matched teeth. J Endod. 1997;23:448–52.
77. Ahangari Z, Samiee M, Yolmeh MA, Eslami G. Antimicrobial activity of three root canal irrigants on enterococcus faecalis: an in vitro study. Iran Endod J. 2008;3(2):33–7.
78. Gulabivala K, Ng YL, Gilbertson M, Eames I. The fluid mechanics of root canal irrigation. Physiol Meas. 2010;31(12):R49–84.
79. Clark MS, Silverstone LM, Lindenmuth J, Hicks MJ, Averbach RE, Kleier DJ, et al. An evaluation of the clinical analgesia/anesthesia efficacy on acute pain using the high frequency neural modulator in various dental settings. Oral Surg Oral Med Oral Pathol. 1987;63:501–5.
80. Gangarosa LP, Park NH, Fong BC, Scott DF, Hill JM. Conductivity of drugs used for iontophoresis. J Pharm Sci. 1978;67:1439–43.
81. Tharian EB, Tandon S. Iontophoresis. A novel drug administration for extraction of deciduous teeth. A clinical evaluation. Indian J Dent Res. 1994;5:97–100.
82. Hochman MN. Single-tooth anesthesia: pressure sensing technology provides innovative advancement in the field of dental local anesthesia. Compend Contin Educ Dent. 2007;28:186–93.
83. Revathi M, Rao C, Lakshminarayanan LJE. Revolution in endodontic instruments—a review. J Endodont. 2001;13:43–50.
84. Sanghvi Z, Mistry KJ. Design features of rotary instruments in endodontics. J Ahmedabad Dent Coll Hosp. 2011;2(1):6–11.
85. Yared G, Bou Dagher F, Machtou PJIEJ. Failure of ProFile instruments used with high and low torque motors. Int Endod J. 2001;34(6):471–5.
86. Pessoa OF, Silva JM, Gavini G. Cyclic fatigue resistance of rotary NiTi instruments after simulated clinical use in curved root canals. Braz Den J. 2013;24(2):117–20.
87. Kawakami DAS, Candeiro GTM, Akisue E, Caldeira CL, Gavini GJB. Effect of different torques in cyclic fatigue resistance of K3 rotary instruments. Braz J Oral Sci. 2015;14(2):122–5.
88. Yared G. In vitro study of the torsional properties of new and used ProFile nickel titanium rotary files. J Endod. 2004;30(6):410–2.
89. Gambarini G. Cyclic fatigue of nickel-titanium rotary instruments after clinical use with low- and high-torque endodontic motors. J Endod. 2001;27(12):772–4.
90. Berutti E, Negro AR, Lendini M, Pasqualini D. Influence of manual preflaring and torque on the failure rate of ProTaper rotary instruments. J Endod. 2004;30(4):228–30.
91. Prichard J, editor Rotation or reciprocation: a contemporary look at NiTi instruments? Br Dent J; 2012.: Nature Publishing Group.
92. Ng YL, Mann V, Rahbaran S, Lewsey J, Gulabivala K. Outcome of primary root canal treatment: systematic review of the literature—part 2. Influence of clinical factors. Int Endod J. 2008;41:6–31.
93. Liang YH, Li G, Wesselink PR, Wu MK. Endodontic outcome predictors identified with periapical radiographs and cone-beam computed tomography scans. J Endod. 2011;37:326–31.
94. Carr GB, Murgel CAJDC. The use of the operating microscope in endodontics. Dent Clin. 2010;54(2):191–214.

95. Microscopic dentistry a practical guide, Ziess.
96. Kim SJ. Principles of endodontic microsurgery. Dent Clin North Am. 1997;41(3):481–97.
97. Görduysus MÖ, Görduysus M, Friedman S. Operating microscope improves negotiation of second mesiobuccal canals in maxillary molars. J Endod. 2001;27(11):683–6.
98. Buhrley LJ, Barrows MJ, BeGole EA, Wenckus CS. Effect of magnification on locating the MB2 canal in maxillary molars. J Endod. 2002;28(4):324–7.
99. Yoshioka T, Kobayashi C, Suda H. Detection rate of root canal orifices with a microscope. J Endod. 2002;28(6):452–3.
100. Selden HS. The role of a dental operating microscope in improved nonsurgical treatment of "calcified" canals. Oral Surg Oral Med Oral Pathol. 1989;68(1):93–8.
101. Al-Habboubi TM, Al-Wasi KA. Maxillary first molars with six canals confirmed with the aid of cone-beam computed tomography. 2016;6(3):136.
102. Sarakinakis M. Dental assisting notes- dental assistants chair-side pocket guide: F. A. Davis; 2015.
103. Elsevier. E S. Preparation of the root canal system. Harty's endodontics in clinical practice. Edinburgh: Churchill Livingstone: Elsevier; 2017. p. 113–28.
104. Clark D, Khademi JJDC. Modern molar endodontic access and directed dentin conservation. Dent Clin. 2010;54(2):249–73.
105. Selden HS. The role of a dental operating microscope in improved nonsurgical treatment of "calcified" canals. Oral Surg Oral Med Oral Pathol. 1989;68(1):93–8.
106. Amir FA, Gutmann JL, Witherspoon E. Calcific metamorphosis: a challenge in endodontic diagnosis and treatment. Quintessence Int. 2001;32(6)
107. Cvek M, Granath L, Lundberg MJAOS. Failures and healing in endodontically treated non-vital anterior teeth with posttraumatically reduced pulpal lumen. Acta Odontol Scand. 1982;40(4):223–8.
108. Krastl G, Zehnder MS, Connert T, Weiger R, Kühl S. Guided endodontics: a novel treatment approach for teeth with pulp canal calcification and apical pathology. Dent Traumatol. 2016;32(3):240–6. https://doi.org/10.1111/edt.12235.
109. D'haese J, Ackhurst J, Wismeijer D, De Bruyn H, Tahmaseb AJP. Current state of the art of computer-guided implant surgery. Periodontol 2000. 2017;73(1):121–33.
110. Block MS, Emery RW, Cullum DR, Sheikh AJ. Implant placement is more accurate using dynamic navigation. J Oral Maxillofac Surg. 2017;75(7):1377–86.
111. Zehnder MS, Connert T, Weiger R, Krastl G, Kühl S. Guided endodontics: accuracy of a novel method for guided access cavity preparation and root canal location. Int Endod J. 2016;49(10):966–72. https://doi.org/10.1111/iej.12544.
112. Nahmias Y. Dynamic endodontic navigation: a case report.
113. Block MS, Emery RW. Static or dynamic navigation for implant placement—choosing the method of guidance. J Oral Maxillofac Surg. 2016;74(2):269–77.
114. Buchanan LS. Dynamic CT-Guided Endodontic Access Procedures. Dent Edu Lab; 2018.
115. Buchgreitz J, Buchgreitz M, Mortensen D, Bjørndal L. Guided access cavity preparation using cone-beam computed tomography and optical surface scans–an ex vivo study. Int Endod J. 2016;49(8):790–5.
116. Giacomino C, Ray J, Wealleans J. Targeted endodontic microsurgery: a novel approach to anatomically challenging scenarios using 3-dimensional-printed guides and trephine burs-a report of 3 cases. J Endod. 2018;44:671–7.
117. Mohamed N, Nahmias Y, Serota KJOH. The cortical window: part two computer guided endodontic surgery (CGES). OralHealthGroup. 2018.
118. Gambarini G, Galli M, Stefanelli LV, Di Nardo D, Morese A, Seracchiani M, et al. Endodontic microsurgery using dynamic navigation system: a case report. J Endod. 2019;45(11):1397–402. e6
119. Ray J. Targeted endodontic microsurgery- narrowing the gap between novice and adept. Endodontic surgery. American Association of Endodontists 2019.
120. Song T, Yang C, Dianat O, Azimi EJHTL. Endodontic guided treatment using augmented reality on a head-mounted display system. Healthc Technol Lett. 2018;5(5):201–7.

Digitization and Dental Lasers

5

Donald J. Coluzzi, Zahra Al Timimi,
and Mohammed Saleem

5.1   Introduction

Lasers have gained immense use due to the optimization of the wavelength for human tissue interactions. Initially, dental lasers were primarily used for soft tissue surgical procedures, such as excisions and incisions. Instruments then evolved for use on both hard and soft oral structures [1, 2]. Photobiomodulation (PBM) is now universally used as a substitute for low-level laser therapy, has been shown to have a positive effect on living tissues, and as such have been used as a noninvasive alternative in the treatment of various pathological conditions [3, 4].

The biomedical and therapeutic application of the photonic energy is based on the light-tissue interactions leading to laser absorption by cellular components such as mitochondria cytochromes and endogenous chromospheres, which give rise to phenomena such as fluorescence, chemical reactions, and thermal effects [5].

PBM is NOT a thermal interaction in the sense of significantly raising the tissue temperature. These laser therapies often involve red blood cells due to the high optical absorbance of hemoglobin; thus, have proved to be the "most versatile" [6, 7]. The red blood cells are also found in many organs in high concentration. Therefore, the damaging effect of these irradiations occurs at the cell level since hemoglobin is located in red blood cells [8]. The damage is thermal and is related to mechanical stress, vapor bubbles, and overheating because of irradiation [9]. These

D. J. Coluzzi (✉)
Department of Preventive and Restorative Dental Sciences, University of California San Francisco School of Dentistry, San Francisco, CA, USA

Z. Al Timimi
Department of Laser Physics, College of Science for Women, Babylon University, Babylon, Iraq

M. Saleem
Private Practice, Arar, Saudi Arabia

© Springer Nature Switzerland AG 2021   141
P. Jain, M. Gupta (eds.), *Digitization in Dentistry*,
https://doi.org/10.1007/978-3-030-65169-5_5

physiological phenomena stimulate other processes in the cell such as enzyme inactivation, alteration of metabolic rate, and coagulation among other structural changes in the cell [10].

Important effects of low-energy laser light have been highlighted in the scientific works of literature, which are tissue regeneration, reduction of inflammation, pain relief, and immune system enhancement [11]. The low-energy intensity lasers have in recent years being used in the noninvasive treatment of musculoskeletal and cutaneous complications and have also gained increased use in wound healing, nerve repair, and pain management, among other clinical applications. In diabetic conditions where wound healing is compromised, low-energy intensity lasers have shown beneficial effects of healing impaired wounds [12, 13].

Laser used in clinical dentistry has spanned over 30 years. Prior to that, carbon dioxide lasers (CO_2, wavelength 10.6 μm) were used in general medical surgeries and subsequently were applied to the soft tissue surgical procedures within the mouth [14]. Neodymium YAG (1.064 μm) was the first dental laser which was launched in 1989, and from there the next 10 years witnessed the emergence of different major wavelengths Er:YAG and Er,Cr:YSGG and diode semiconductor-based technology [15, 16].

5.2   Laser and its Components

LASER is an acronym for **L**ight **A**mplification by **S**timulated **E**mission of **R**adiation, which is based on theories and principles first put forth by Einstein in the early 1900s. The first actual laser system was introduced by Maiman in 1960 [17].

Laser energy is a man-made product and consists of photons of a single wavelength. The process of lasing occurs when an excited atom is stimulated to remit a photon before it occurs spontaneously; spontaneous emission of light results in unorganized light waves similar to light emitted by a light bulb [18]. **Stimulated emission** of photons generates a very coherent, collimated, monochromatic ray of light that is found nowhere else in nature. As that light is so concentrated and focused, it can have a decided effect on target tissue at a much lower energy level than natural light. The effect of laser energy on target tissue is dependent on its wavelength, which is determined by the lasing medium inside the laser device [19].

Laser irradiation is a type of electromagnetic radiation which exhibits the properties of a wave, and discrete energy packages referred to as photons. The short wavelengths such as high-energy ionizing irradiation cause the ionization of molecules in an indiscriminate manner with the far-infrared heating biological tissues [20, 21].

Materials, which can be used for stimulation to produce lasers, include ruby, dyes, crystals of common and rare earth minerals, semiconductors, and mixtures of gases [20]. Each will produce a laser of different wavelength. Lasers can be further categorized into four groups:

- Gas discharge lasers.
- Semiconductor diode lasers.

- Optically pumped laser.
- The final group that consists of X-ray lasers, combustion lasers, chemical lasers, and gas dynamic lasers.

Gas discharge lasers include the common type: helium neon lasers, carbon dioxide lasers, noble gas lasers. Semiconductor lasers include the high-power diode laser. The optically pumped laser uses photons of light to pump directly the lasing medium to higher energy levels [22, 23]. Lasers have their basic components, which are the power source, which provide energy, lasing medium (which is the active medium and can be solid or gas), and reflecting mirrors (two or more in number that forms an optical cavity or a resonator) with production of light of particular wavelength, which defines the type of laser as shown in Fig. 5.1.

The optical cavity contains the active medium and reflective surfaces. Initial energy is provided by an excitation source. Photons within the active medium are reflected, amplified, and then collimated. Those are emitted into a lens assembly, which then produces the useful laser beam [24].

In a diode laser, the semiconductor medium is a wafer that contains layers of positively and negatively charged compounds, bounded by reflective coating. Several of these wafers are grouped together to produce a useful laser beam [25, 26].

Laser radiation is specific wave generated and is a highly focused directional beam as opposed to the visible light which is mainly white light and nondirectional and nonfocused. Commercially available dental laser instruments all have emission

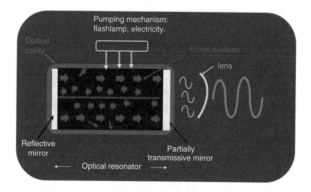

Fig. 5.1 A representational graphic of the basic components of a dental laser. The optical cavity contains the active medium and reflective surfaces. Initial energy is provided by an excitation source. Photons within the active medium are reflected, amplified, and then collimated. Those are emitted into a lens assembly, which then produces the useful laser beam. In a diode laser, the semiconductor medium is a wafer that contains layers of positively and negatively charged compounds, bounded by reflective coating. Several of these wafers are ganged together to produce a useful laser beam

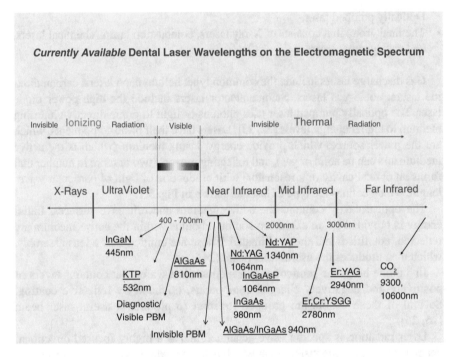

Fig. 5.2 Approximate absorption curves of the currently available dental laser wavelengths. The curves represent hemoglobin, melanin, water, and tooth enamel (carbonated hydroxyapatite.) Above the light green line, there is absorption, and below it is transmission of the photonic energy

wavelengths in the range of 488 nm to 10,600 nm [27, 28]. All are of nonionizing radiation and span the visible, near, mid, and far-infrared portions of the electromagnetic spectrum as shown in Fig. 5.2.

5.3 Laser Delivery Systems and Laser Emission Modes

Laser energy can be delivered to the surgical site by various means that are accurate and precise. These include the fiber-optic system, hollow fiber, articulated arm delivery system, and handpieces [29, 30]. See Figs. 5.3 and 5.4 below.

Lasers in the visible (445 and 532 nm) and near-infrared (from 810 nm to 1064 nm) range use fiber-optic strands by means of a handpiece with straight and precise tips that deliver the laser energy to the target tissue. This type of delivery system can degrade with time but is lightweight with a good tactile sensation and is easy to use and sterilize. Some newer models have more rugged fibers [31].

Erbium and CO_2 devices are lasers with more rigid glass fibers, semiflexible hollow waveguides, or articulated arms. However, there is a loss of energy over time with lack of control due to internal reflection, with these systems [5]. For

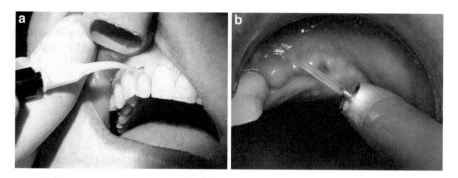

Fig. 5.3 (a) A small diameter glass fiber is paired with a disposable tip, used in contact with the target tissue. (b) A fiber optically delivered laser with a handpiece and a reusable tip, employed slightly of contact with the target tissue

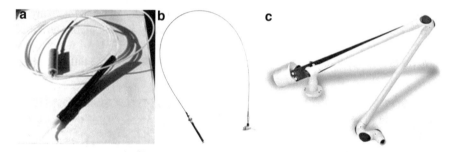

Fig. 5.4 (a) An optic fiber. (b) A hollow waveguide. (c) An articulated arm assembly. Usually, with an optic fiber, the laser beam is emitted with a contact tip; conversely with a hollow waveguide or an articulated arm, the beam is delivered without a tip in a non-contact mode

hard tissue procedures, a water spray is used for cooling, and that can be switched off for soft tissue surgery. In addition, lasers with articulated arm delivery systems utilize a progression of verbalized mirrors (generally 7) associated one to each other, prompting transmission of vitality [32, 33].

Two basic emission modes are used for dental lasers, based on their excitation source:

1. Continuous wave mode where the laser energy/beam is transmitted continuously as long as the laser is activated. Carbon dioxide, argon, and diode lasers operate in this manner. Variations in this mode include the "gated emissions" where there is a periodic alteration of the laser energy being on or off (similar to blinking), thereby preventing laser light transmission. This design helps minimize some of the undesirable residual thermal damage associated with continuous wave devices. It is very important to pay attention to this effect during laser use in order to protect damage to the surrounding tissues. Some of the recent models of "gated" lasers feature pulse durations in the microsecond range.

2. Free-running pulse lasers only operate in a unique pulsed mode, never continuously, where emission is in very short pulses in the microsecond range followed by a long time when the laser is off. Nd:YAG and Er:YAG as well as Er,Cr:YSGG devices operate as free-running pulsed lasers.

5.4　Types of Tissue Interactions

When laser light is exposed to the tissue, it can reflect, scatter, be absorbed, or be transmitted to the surrounding tissues. Different wavelengths have different absorption coefficients, and this property accounts for their variable effect on human tissue as shown in Fig. 5.5. The curves represent hemoglobin, melanin, water, and tooth enamel (carbonated hydroxyapatite.) Above the light green line, there is absorption, and below it is transmission of the photonic energy [34, 35].

The hydroxyapatite crystals of teeth and bone absorb carbon dioxide, and the erbium family's photons. The visible and near-infrared wavelengths have virtually no interaction with either enamel or water. The erbium family is very highly absorbed in water, while carbon dioxide is about 10 times less absorbed [21]. All wavelengths have different depths of penetration through soft tissue because of the different water

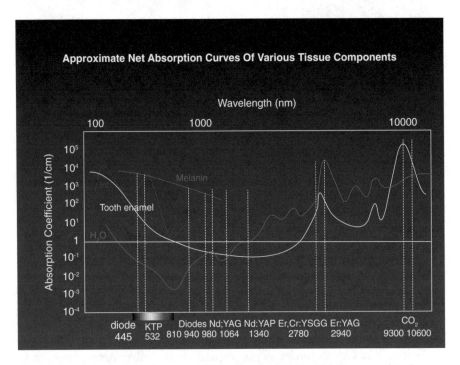

Fig. 5.5 Approximate absorption curves of the currently available dental laser wavelengths

absorption characteristics. Diode lasers can reach deeper into the tissue approximately several thousand layers, whereas the erbium lasers are absorbed on the surface [33, 36].

Lasers can have various effects on the target tissue. One effect is photothermal: simply stated, light is converted to heat. When the tissue absorbs the photonic energy used during surgical procedure, it elevates the temperature. When a temperature of 100 °C is reached, vaporization of the water within the tissue occurs. This process is called ablation. At temperatures between 60 and 100 °C, denaturization of the proteins starts occurring, without dehydrated and then burned, resulting in an undesirable effect called carbonization or vaporization [37, 38].

Nonsurgical, low-level power laser applications include photo-bio modulation (PBM), diagnostics, photo-activated antibacterial processes, laser tooth whitening, and laser scanning of tooth cavity preparations [39]. Another effect is photochemical effects such as curing of the composite resin [40]. Lastly, some lasers can also produce tissue fluorescence, which is used as a diagnostic method for caries detection [41, 42].

5.5   Lasers in Dentistry

The use of LASER technology in the dental industry is a subject of continuous researches and advancements. In Fig. 5.6, a systematic review on how the laser interacts with the dental tissue is shown.

Table 5.1 lists the currently available dental lasers whose emission is on the *visible spectrum.*

The currently available dental lasers whose emission is in the *invisible spectrum* is listed in Table 5.2.

5.6   Lasers Generally Practiced in Dentistry

5.6.1   Carbon Dioxide Laser

CO_2 laser's photonic energy has a very high affinity for water; it causes rapid soft tissue removal and hemostasis. The penetration of depth is relatively shallow. A newly available model of CO_2 with ultrashort pulse duration can be used for hard and soft dental tissue.

5.6.2   Neodymium Yttrium Aluminum Garnet Lasers

Absorption of this wavelength is high in pigmented tissue; therefore, it is sufficient for cutting and coagulating dental soft tissues, with high-grade hemostasis. Other uses include nonsurgical periodontal therapy.

Fig. 5.6 How the laser works on the tooth

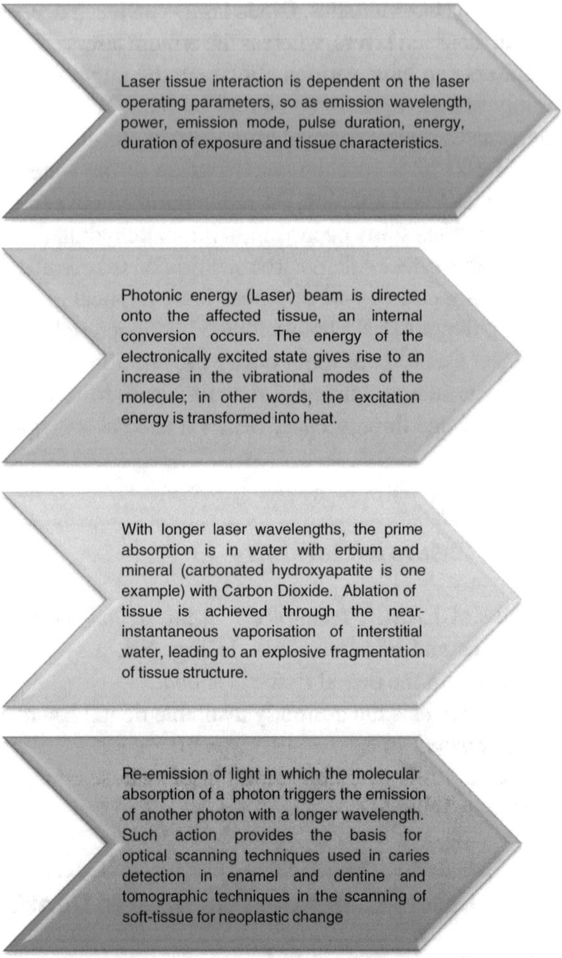

Laser tissue interaction is dependent on the laser operating parameters, so as emission wavelength, power, emission mode, pulse duration, energy, duration of exposure and tissue characteristics.

Photonic energy (Laser) beam is directed onto the affected tissue, an internal conversion occurs. The energy of the electronically excited state gives rise to an increase in the vibrational modes of the molecule; in other words, the excitation energy is transformed into heat.

With longer laser wavelengths, the prime absorption is in water with erbium and mineral (carbonated hydroxyapatite is one example) with Carbon Dioxide. Ablation of tissue is achieved through the near-instantaneous vaporisation of interstitial water, leading to an explosive fragmentation of tissue structure.

Re-emission of light in which the molecular absorption of a photon triggers the emission of another photon with a longer wavelength. Such action provides the basis for optical scanning techniques used in caries detection in enamel and dentine and tomographic techniques in the scanning of soft-tissue for neoplastic change

Table 5.1 lists the currently available dental lasers whose emission is on the **visible spectrum.** Column 1 lists the generic name of the laser and the color of light emitted; column 2 describes the typical uses of that laser; column 3 lists the elements of the active medium; column 5 lists the emission wavelength; and column 5 shows abbreviations for the emission modes

Generic name of laser	Typical uses	Active medium	Emission wavelength	Emission mode
Semiconductor diode, visible blue	Soft tissue procedures, tooth whitening	Indium gallium nitride	445 nm	CW, GP
KTP solid state visible green	Soft tissue procedures, tooth whitening	Neodymium-doped yttrium aluminum garnet (**Nd:YAG**) and potassium titanyl phosphate (**KTP**)	532 nm	CW, GP
Low-level lasers, visible red semiconductor, or gas lasers	Photobiomodulation therapy (PBM), photodynamic therapy (PDT), or carious lesion detection.	Variations of gallium arsenide or indium gallium arsenide phosphorus diodes Helium neon gas	600–670 nm 632 nm	CW, GP

CW continuous wave, *GP* acquired or gated pulse

Table 5.2 This table lists the currently available dental lasers whose emission is on the **invisible spectrum**. Column 1 lists the generic name of the laser; Column 2 describes the typical uses of that laser; Column 3 lists the elements of the active medium; Column 4 lists the emission wavelength or range of wavelengths; and Column 5 shows abbreviations for the emission modes

Generic name of laser	Typical uses	Active medium	Emission wavelength (nm)	Emission mode
Low-level diode lasers, near infrared	Photobiomodulation therapy (PBM), photodynamic therapy (PDT)	Variations of aluminum gallium arsenide diodes	800–900	CW, GP
Semiconductor diode, near-infrared	Soft tissue procedures	Aluminum gallium arsenide	800–830	CW, GP
Semiconductor diode, near-infrared	Soft tissue procedures	Aluminum/indium gallium arsenide	940	CW, GP
Semiconductor diode, near-infrared	Soft tissue procedures	Indium gallium arsenide	980	CW, GP
Semiconductor diode, near-infrared	Soft tissue procedures	Indium gallium arsenide, phosphorus	1064	CW, GP
Solid state, near-infrared	Soft tissue procedures	Neodymium-doped yttrium aluminum garnet (**Nd:YAG**)	1064	FRP
Solid state, near-infrared	Soft tissue procedures, endoscopic procedures	Neodymium-doped yttrium aluminum perovskite (**Nd:YAP**)	1340	FRP
Solid state, mid-infrared	Soft tissue procedures, hard tissue procedures	Erbium, chromium-doped yttrium scandium gallium garnet (**Er,Cr:YSGG**)	2780	FRP
Solid state, mid-infrared	Soft tissue procedures, hard tissue procedures	Erbium-doped yttrium aluminum garnet (**Er:YAG**)	2940	FRP
Gas, far infrared	Soft tissue procedures, hard tissue procedures	Carbon dioxide (CO_2) laser, with an active medium isotopic gas	9300	FRP
Gas, far-infrared	Soft tissue procedures	Carbon dioxide (CO_2) laser with an active medium of a mixture of gases	10,600	CW, GP, FRP

CW continuous wave, *GP* acquired or gated pulse, *FRP* free running pulse

5.6.3 Erbium Laser

The family of erbium lasers has two distinct wavelengths, Er, Cr: YSGG lasers and Er: YAG lasers. Erbium wavelengths have a secondary affinity for hydroxyapatite crystals and the most powerful absorption of water in any dental laser wavelength. It is the laser of selection for treatment of dental hard tissues, and can be used for soft tissue ablation because the dental soft tissue comprises a large percentage of water.

5.6.4   Diode Laser

The diode laser is a solid-state semiconductor containing various combinations of aluminum, gallium, arsenide, and occasionally indium producing different laser wavelengths, varying from approximately 445 to 1064 nm. These wavelengths are absorbed principally by tissue pigment melanin and hemoglobin, and inadequately absorbed by hydroxyapatite and water.

Dental lasers have a number of its applications in dentistry as given in Table 5.3. Considering that the light emitted serves both the goals of removing or shaping tissue, a number of functions can be performed.

5.7   Soft Tissue Application

5.7.1   Photobiomodulation

It is also known as "soft laser therapy" and is based on the concept that low level of doses of specific coherent wavelengths can turn on or turn off certain cellular components or functions. At low laser doses (2 J/cm^2), laser utilization stimulates proliferation, while at large doses (16 J/cm^2) it is suppressive [43, 44]. This technique induces analgesic, anti-inflammatory, and biomodulation effects at molecular level

Table 5.3 Uses of lasers in dentistry

Specialty	Uses
Oral surgery	Major or minor surgical procedures such as flap surgeries, frenectomies, removal of hyperplastic tissues, operculectomy, excisional biopsy, root end resection, gingivectomy procedures, exposure of impacted teeth, and vestibuloplasty
	Treatment of abscess, aphthous ulcer, granuloma, epulis, irritation fibroma
	Hemangioma and curettage
Periodontics	Flap surgery, frenectomy, gingival contouring/gingivectomy, pocket treatment
Orthodontics	Post orthodontic removal of residual cement
	Exposure of impacted teeth
Endodontics	Bleaching
	Canal irrigation
	Root resection in endodontic surgeries
Prosthetic and restorative dentistry	Caries removal
	Curing of material
	Removal of fractured restorations
	Etching of the tooth
	Sulcus deepening
	Crown contouring and lengthening
	Smile design
Pediatric dentistry	Removal of caries in deciduous teeth
	Pulpotomy and pulpectomy procedures

improving tissue healing processes and less postoperative discomfort for patients, without any negative effects [10, 45]. This technique is most useful in medically compromised patients where wound closure and tissue healing is of prime importance.

LLLT (low level laser) results in vasodilation of the cells, which causes increase in local blood flow, relaxation of smooth muscles, thus bringing in oxygen and further migration of immune cells to the targeted tissue. This in turn results in rapid maturation and regeneration [9, 46]. Accurate effects of PBM on the healing of lesions of recurrent aphthous stomatitis in humans have been recorded. Research has shown that LPL encourages healing and dentinogenesis following pulpotomy. This makes it useful in the healing of mucositis and oropharyngeal ulceration in patients enduring radiotherapy for head or neck cancer [47, 48].

Photostimulation of aphthous ulcers and recurrent herpetic lesions, with low power laser energy (He-Ne), can provide pain relief and accelerate the healing process. In recurrent herpes simplex labialis lesions, lesions get arrested before painful vesicles form, thus expediting the overall healing time, and minimizing the frequency of recurrence (Figs. 5.7 and 5.8) [49–51].

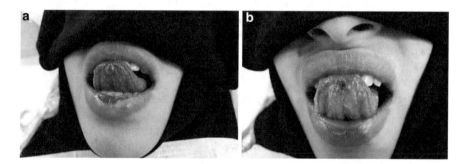

Fig. 5.7 Tongue mucosal using diode laser (980 nm). (**a**) Before laser treatment. (**b**) After laser treatment

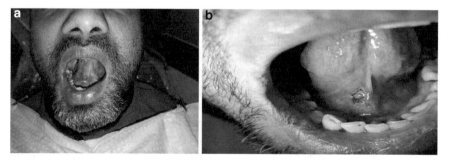

Fig. 5.8 Lingual papilloma using diode laser (980 nm). (**a**) Before laser treatment. (**b**) After laser treatment

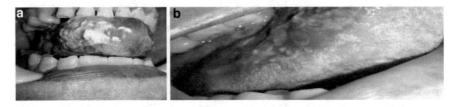

Fig. 5.9 Laser-assisted surgery for removing tongue leukoplakia using diode laser (980 nm). (**a**) Before laser treatment. (**b**) After laser treatment

Low-level laser energy is beneficial for photochemical activation of oxygen, releasing dyes, creating membrane and DNA damage to the microorganisms [52]. Photoactivated dye technique can be engaged with a system utilizing low power laser (100 mill watts) in visible red (semiconductor diode lasers) and toluidine blue dye. Studies have shown photoactivated disinfection (PAD) to be effective in killing bacteria: gram-positive bacteria including methicillin-resistant *Staphylococcus aureus*, gram-negative bacteria, fungi, viruses in complicated biofilms like subgingival plaque (Fig. 5.9) [53, 54].

The clinical applications of PAD involve disinfection of root canals, periodontal pockets, deep carious lesions, and sites of peri-implantitis. Tolonium chloride is practiced in high concentrations for screening patients, for malignancies of the oral mucosa and oropharynx [55, 56].

5.7.2 Photodynamic Therapy for Malignancies

Clinical investigations have published positive effects for the photodynamic therapy (PDT) of carcinoma in situ and squamous cell carcinoma, with the oral cavity, with acknowledgement rates approximating up to 90% [8, 57].

5.7.3 Soft Tissue Surgery

Soft tissue excisions can easily be performed using lasers. The targeted lesion is grasped with forceps or a similar instrument, with the laser beam directed towards the healthy tissue peripheral to the lesion. Care is needed not to tear any structures but rather allow the laser energy to do the work [58, 59]. Fig. 5.10 depicts an erbium laser removal of an irritation fibroma.

Low average power laser is used in *endodontic therapy procedures* such as post pulpotomy (with the laser beam applied directly to the remaining pulp and on the mucosa toward the root canal pulp); post pulpectomy (with the irradiation of the apical region); and periapical surgery (irradiating the mucosa of the area corresponding to the apical lesion and the sutures) [60, 61].

A fiber-supported laser delivery system with appropriate diameter tips (such as erbium lasers) and capable of delivering laser energy laterally is used for intracanal

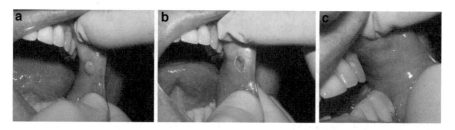

Fig. 5.10 (**a**) An irritation fibroma on the left mucosa, preoperative view. (**b**) An erbium laser was used to remove the fibroma, immediate postoperative view. There is minimal thermal tissue damage and good hemostasis. (**c**) One week postoperative view of surgical site with good healing

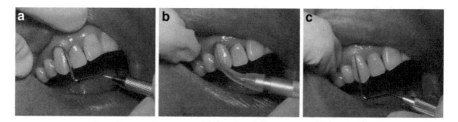

Fig. 5.11 (**a**) A single periodontal pocket with inflammatory tissue. (**b**) After the removal of biofilm, the diode laser is used to remove the diseased epithelial lining, reduce the bacterial population, and provide hemostasis. (**c**) Six month postoperative view shows periodontal health with no tissue recession

application [62]. However, the currently available laser energy output cannot shape the sides of canals. The ability to significantly reduce the bacterial contamination of the root canal system by disinfection, via the bactericidal effect of thermal interaction, is an advantage of the laser, and further development will enhance the use of lasers in endodontic therapy [63].

In *Periodontics,* depending on absorption characteristics, different lasers can be used in procedures such as gingivectomy, gingivoplasty, scaling and root planning, and removal of sulcular epithelium. While comparing lasers with conventional periodontal surgical procedures, reduction in plaque index, bleeding index, pocket depth, and better reattachment was observed [64, 65]. The devices used should be of thin fiber so that it can be easy on the soft tissue lining of the pocket. The energy used would be less than one-half that employed for surgical excision.

Figure 5.11 demonstrates a diode laser used adjunctively for treatment of gingivitis. Figure 5.12 shows a diode laser adjunctively treating peri-implant mucositis.

Another use of the laser in periodontics is for soft tissue management for impressions of indirect restorations. Fig. 5.13 depicts the use of a diode laser for tissue retraction and hemostasis prior to impression taking for two ceramic anterior crowns.

All dental wavelengths, including diode and Er,Cr:YSGG, can be used in removal of hyperplastic gingival tissues, due to its characteristic of less postoperative pain and absence of scarring etc., as opposed to conventional methods [66, 67].

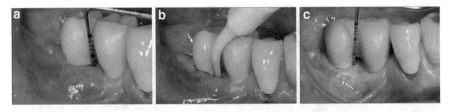

Fig. 5.12 (a) View of peri-implant mucositis on the lower right second molar implant fixture. (b) Prior to diode laser use, biofilm and other accretions removed from the implant with hand instruments. View shows diode laser is use to remove the diseased soft tissue, offer bacterial reduction, and provide hemostasis. (c) Four month postoperative probing demonstrates healthy tissue and implant stability

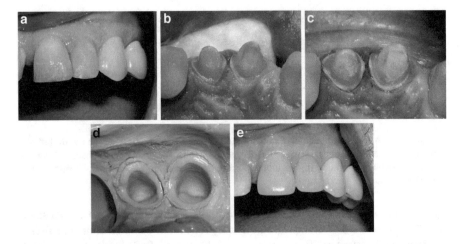

Fig. 5.13 (a) Maxillary left central and lateral incisors that will receive full porcelain crown restorations. (b) Completed preparations before any gingival tissue manipulation. (c) Diode laser used for tissue retraction and hemostasis, immediate postoperative view. Note completely dry field. No conventional retraction cord was used. (d) Immediately after laser use, an impression was taken. There is no debris and excellent detail. (e) Restorations placed 2 weeks later. The tissue height and tone responded well to the laser tissue retraction

Figure 5.14 shows preoperative gingival enlargement and immediate postoperative tissue removal using diode laser.

Gingivectomy with Er:YAG, Er,Cr:YSGG laser is advised for immunocompromised patients and in the removal of plaque/calculus from root surface with sufficient water cooling [68, 69]. A diode laser can also be used, although hyperplastic tissue can be very challenging to remove with the diode. However, normal tissue can be excised with good results. Fig. 5.15 shows the uncovering of a fully integrated implant fixture, and Fig. 5.16 shows soft tissue gingivectomy for an aesthetic procedure.

Crown lengthening procedures can also be done using a laser. Diode lasers and Nd:YAG have proven useful in removing soft tissue effectively without damage to

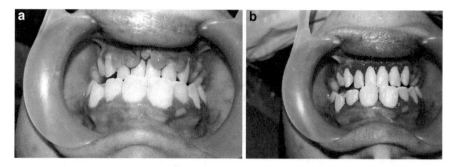

Fig. 5.14 Gingival enlargement using diode laser (980 nm). (**a**) Before laser treatment. (**b**) After laser treatment

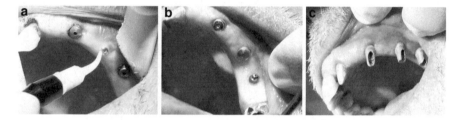

Fig. 5.15 (**a**) Uncovering of implant fixture using a diode laser. (**b**) Two week postoperative view of the tissue around the implant fixtures. The healing cap from the most distal fixture has been removed, showing the excellent tissue tone. (**c**) One week later, the final abutment copings are placed. Note the excellent soft tissue tone and contour

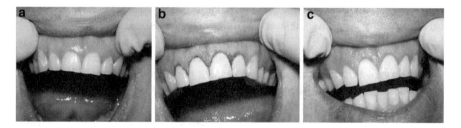

Fig. 5.16 (**a**) Preoperative view of excessive gingival tissue with shortened clinical crown display. (**b**) Biologic width was measured to ensure that adequate tissue was available for excision. A diode laser performed gingivectomy and gingivoplasty. The desired contours are easily placed with the laser and hemostasis is excellent. Immediate postoperative view. (**c**) Good tissue tone and contour are shown with an acceptable aesthetic result. Six month postoperative view

the surrounding tissues, while erbium lasers can be used to expose root structure [70]. The tissue removal should be done in such a way that biological width is always maintained. Water cooling should be used when working with erbium lasers on hard tissues [71]. Figure 5.17 shows osseous crown lengthening performed with an erbium laser.

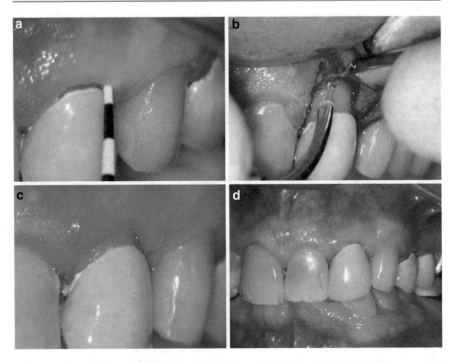

Fig. 5.17 (**a**) A new crown is necessary on an endodontically treated maxillary left central incisor because of a fracture of half of the remaining tooth structure. Periodontal probing shows inadequate biologic width for the proposed new subgingival margin placement. (**b**) After the tooth structure was built up, an open flap procedure and an erbium laser was used to remove labial bone and establish a new osseous contour. (**c**) The periodontal tissue has healed and adequate tooth structure is now available for a restoration. Six weeks postoperative. Note good soft tissue tone and contour. (**d**) Eight weeks postoperatively, the new crown has just been cemented

In *orthodontics*, an unerupted or partly erupted tooth can be revealed for bonding via conservative tissue removal, for reasonable positioning of a bracket or button. Using lasers for such treatment offers the advantages of no bleeding, less painful, and immediate fixing of the accessory [72, 73].

Insular areas of transient tissue hypertrophy can simply be removed with the diode laser. The diode laser is very beneficial for a number of isolated treatments, such as removing tissue that has disproportionate mini-screws, springs, and tools, as well as for compensating a tissue punch if required, when placing mini-screws in the unattached gingiva [74, 75]. Figure 5.18 shows this procedure using diode laser (980 nm).

5.7.4 Frenectomies

A laser-assisted frenectomy is a simple procedure that is best proposed after the diastema is closed as much as probable. Ankyloglossia can lead to problems with deglutition, speech, malocclusion, and periodontal problems. Frenectomies achieved

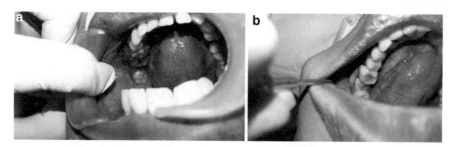

Fig. 5.18 Elimination of hyperplastic tissue using diode laser (980 nm). (**a**) Pretreatment. (**b**) After laser application

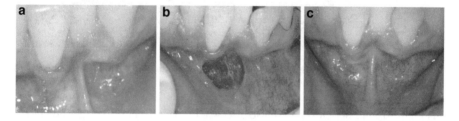

Fig. 5.19 (**a**) Mandibular anterior frenum impinging on attached gingiva, preoperative view. (**b**) Nd:YAG laser used to revise the frenal attachment, immediate postoperative view. Note good hemostasis and minimal thermal damage. (**c**) Two week postoperative view of surgical site with good healing

with laser favor excision of the frena painlessly, less bleeding, sutures, or surgical packing with no requirement for special postoperative care [76, 77]. Figures 5.19 and 5.20 demonstrate laser frenectomy procedures.

Lasers are also used for soft tissue retraction and its removal in restorative and implant dentistry. But the absorption characteristics of different lasers, and depth of penetration, play significant roles in treatment planning [78].

Prescription medications such as phenytoin and cyclosporine can cause fibrous gingival overgrowth, the removal of which can be accomplished by using the shorter wavelength lasers. This has minimal effects on enamel and cementum [79]. Conversely, removal of the gingival tissue to uncover an implant is best accomplished with the longer wavelength devices, such as erbium and carbon dioxide lasers, since their energy is absorbed on or near the surface. This prevents or minimizes heat buildup and transfer to the metallic implant fixture [72, 80].

5.8 Hard Tissue Applications

Argon laser (488 nm) provides high-intensity visible blue light, which is capable to initiate photopolymerization of light-cured dental materials such as composite resins resulting in a deeper cure and improved physical properties of the restorative

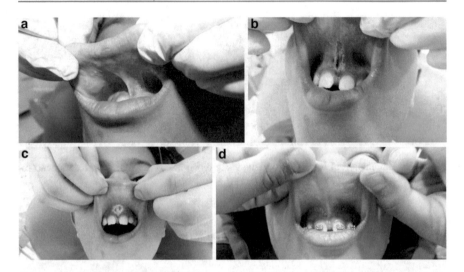

Fig. 5.20 Labial frenectomy using diode laser. (**a**) Before treatment. (**b**) After laser treatment. (**c**) After 5 days from laser treatment. (**d**) After 30 days

material. Argon laser emission is also effective to reconstruct the surface chemistry of both enamel and root surface dentine, which decreases the probability of recurrent caries [81].

Tooth discoloration is the change in color of teeth as compared with adjacent teeth. Bleaching of discolored teeth has become common and has decreased the need for more invasive treatment approaches [82]. Bleaching process, which involves the use of energy sources to increase the rate of release of bleaching radicals, can be accelerated by various laser wavelengths. Different lasers produce different wavelengths, hence not all lasers are suitable for bleaching as wavelengths absorbed, scattered, or transmitted through tooth structure can damage enamel, dentin and pulp [83, 84]. The bleaching impression relies on the specific absorption of a narrow spectral range of green light between 510 and 554 nm within the chelate compounds. Diode wavelengths (940 nm), for example, can also be used for bleaching with a different chemical catalyst [85]. The catalyst interacts with the light, whether visible or invisible to the human eye. $KTiOPO_4$, KTP, argon, and diode lasers can accomplish a positive outcome in office bleaching [86, 87].

5.9 Laser Fluorescence

Enamel demineralization with white spot forming on the buccal surfaces of the teeth is a comparatively common side influence from orthodontic treatment with fixed appliances. Studies have shown that such tiny areas of superficial enamel demineralization may remineralize.

5.10   Cavity Preparation, Caries, and Restorative Removal

Numerous studies describe the use of Er:YAG lasers, since 1988, for removing caries in the enamel and dentine by ablation, tooth preparation for a restoration, and removal of defective composite filling material (cement, composite resins, and glass ionomers). Figures 5.21 and 5.22 demonstrate an erbium laser for restorative dentistry.

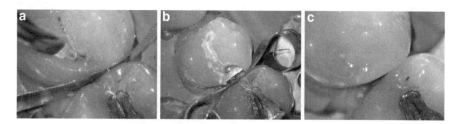

Fig. 5.21 (**a**) An erbium laser with a glass tip beginning to remove a carious lesion. (**b**) The completed preparation with the enamel surface etched. (**c**) The finished restoration in place

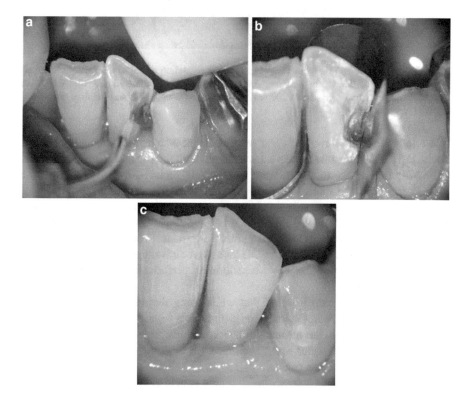

Fig. 5.22 (**a**) The erbium laser is aimed at the carious lesion. (**b**) The carious material is removed and the preparation completed. (**c**) The tooth is restored

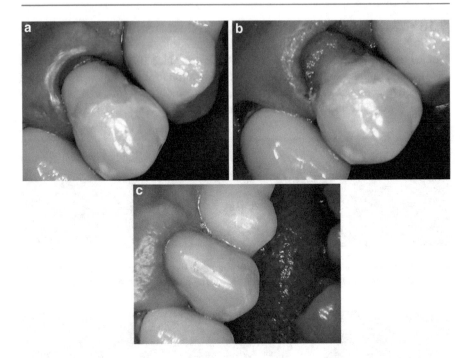

Fig. 5.23 (a) A preoperative view of a carious lesion extending apical to the existing inflamed marginal gingiva. (b) Shows the final preparation as well as the recontoured gingival tissue, both accomplished with the superpulsed 9300 nm carbon dioxide laser. (c) Depicts the final restoration and gingival contour

Carious tooth structure has higher water content than healthy enamel or dentin, so the laser would be able to interact selectively with the caries. On the other hand, if fluoride ions in the tooth structure have widely replaced hydroxyl groups, the laser energy must be increased to be effective [88]. The ablation mechanism of erbium lasers enhances the adhesion between the restorative material and the cavity. It also causes obliteration of the dentinal tubules [89]. However, removal of enamel and dentin by means of laser leads to thermal side effects. In contrast to this Er:YAG, superpulsed CO_2 laser and Er,Cr:YSGG lasers have advantage of reducing thermal effects [90, 91]. Figure 5.23 shows a restoration performed with the superpulsed CO_2 laser.

Clinicians should keep in mind that while using this type of laser for caries removal, cooling with water is indicated with no loss in laser intensity. Laser treatment is contact-free and has advantages over rotary instruments such as direct cooling of the area with water spray; absence of drilling sound, pressure, pain, temperature, and anesthesia can be omitted.

Laser etching has been assessed as an option to acid etching of enamel and dentine. Enamel and dentine surfaces etched with lasers expose micro-irregularities and no smear layer. CO_2, Nd:YAG, Er:YAG and the equivalent Er,Cr:YSGG laser are both an alternative for enamel conditioning and have proven to be more effective than phosphoric acid [92]. For etching with lasers, the surface is covered with accelerator and irradiated until the accelerator evaporates fully. Fracture of enamel is a common incident after ceramic brackets are detached from the tooth surface. This can be avoided by thermal detaching of brackets using CO_2 and YAG lasers [93, 94].

5.11 Treatment of Dentinal Hypersensitivity

Dentinal hypersensitivity is one of the numerous prevalent illnesses in clinical dental practices. Identification of the desensitizing influences of Er:YAG lasers with those of a traditional desensitizing system on cervically endangered hypersensitive dentine demonstrated a positive outcome than with other agents [95, 96].

5.12 Research

Lasers have been used for diagnostic and other research purposes as shown in Table 5.4.

5.13 3D Laser Scanner for E-Model Preparation

A laser scanner can be employed as a soft tissue scanner and is a priceless tool for its efficiency of treatment and formulation of 3D images of oral dental structures. There is no necessity of cast preparation as e-models are provided from scanned impressions. Images have been performed to establish databases for normative populations and cross-sectional growth changes and furthermore to estimate the clinical consequences in surgical and nonsurgical operations in the head and neck areas [97, 98].

Table 5.4 Laser applications used as research tools in dentistry

Laser type	Wavelength	Clinical application/research
Argon	488 and 515 nm	Detection of caries (laser fluorescence)
		Confocal microscopic imaging of soft and hard tissues
		Flow cytometric analysis of cells and cell sorting
Helium neon	633 nm	Scanning of phosphor plate radiographs
		Scanning of conventional radiographs for tele-radiology
		Profiling of tooth surfaces and dental restorations
Diode	633 nm	Laser Doppler flowmetry (LDF) to assess pulpal blood flow
	655 nm	Detection of caries (laser fluorescence)
	670 nm	Profiling of tooth surfaces and dental restorations
		Detection of subgingival calculus (laser fluorescence)
CO_2	10,600 nm	Detection of fissure caries by optical changes
Nd:YAG	1064 nm	Spectroscopic analysis of tooth structure
		Imaging of internal tooth structure
Er:YAG	2940 nm	Breakdown spectroscopic analysis of tooth structure

5.14   Benefits and Drawbacks of Dental Lasers

One of the main benefits of using dental lasers is its ability to accurately and precisely interact with target tissues. Lasers allows the clinician to achieve good hemostasis and reduce the need for sutures at the surgical site, during soft tissue procedures. There are less chances of metastasis associated with laser systems use and they also increase the chances of initial healing and rapid regeneration.

The hard tissue laser devices can selectively remove diseased tooth structure because a carious lesion has much higher water content than healthy tissue. In addition, use of lasers can minimize the need for anesthesia, while postoperative edema and scarring are markedly reduced. Osseous tissue removal and contouring proceed easily with the erbium family of instruments. Some of the other significant benefits to laser use are sterilization of the treatment site, relief of pain and anxiety for the patient, and laser exposure to enamel causes a reduction in caries activity.

There are some disadvantages to the current dental laser instruments. They are relatively high in cost and there is a need for additional training or qualified personnel. Although there are some laser tips that have side-firing capabilities, most of the laser energy is delivered in a circular spot at the end of the tip or handpiece. Because majorities of dental instruments are both side- and end-cutting, a modification of clinical technique will be required. Accessibility to the surgical area can sometimes pose a problem with the current available delivery system, and the clinician must prevent overheating the tissue. One additional drawback of the all tissue lasers is the inability to remove metallic restorations. Also, no single wavelength will optimally treat all dental disease.

5.15   Laser Safety

According to *The American National Standards Institute (ANSI),* lasers used in dentistry for bacterial decontamination or ablation techniques are considered to be class 4 lasers. This requires adequate control measures, laser safety officer (LSO), engineering controls, and training. The LSO is an individual who has been trained in laser safety, and does not necessarily have to be a clinician. That person provides all the necessary information, inspects, and maintains the laser and its accessories, and insures that all procedures for safety are carried out. All laser devices come with instructions on the safe use of the machine provided by the manufacturer. Clinicians using the laser devices should be aware of the fundamentals of laser physics.

Class 4 lasers are considered high-powered and can pose a hazard to the eye or skin from direct beam exposure. Protective eyewear for the patient and the entire surgical team along with proper clothing must be worn when the laser is under operation. The surgical environment should have a warning sign and limited access. High volume suction and normal infection control protocol must be followed. Use of screen and curtains should be promoted. The laser itself must be in good working order so that the manufactured safeguards prevent accidental laser exposure. Foot pedal control switch with protective hood prevents accidental depression by surgical staff.

The laser plume, also known as laser-generated air contaminates (LGAC,) is a visible or invisible biologic hazard of gas fumes created when the target tissue is ablated or vaporized. Proper management of laser plume is imperative as the laser plume has the ability to carry viruses, bacteria and other organisms that can be hazardous to the laser operator and assisting personnel. Use of laser filtration masks prevents airborne contamination.

Other important safety considerations include potential fire hazards and management of the laser plume. The fiber-optic tips should be steam sterilized. Combustible materials, such as alcohol, should never come in contact with the working beam of the laser and should be kept as far away as possible. Nitrous Oxide/Oxygen can be used in conjunction with a laser procedure as long as the scavenging system is operating properly.

5.16 Conclusion

Lasers technology for hard and soft tissue surgery application is at an extraordinary state of discrimination, having had individual decades of development, up to the modern time, and additional improvements can transpire. The field of laser-based photochemical reactions carries surpassing guarantee for supplementary applications, especially for targeting specific cells, pathogens, and molecules.

A moreover area of future germination is anticipated to be a unification of diagnostic and therapeutic laser techniques. Regarding the future, it is presumed that specific laser technologies will grow indispensable ingredients of contemporary dental patients beyond the next decade.

References

1. Parker S. Surgical lasers and hard dental tissue. Br Dent J. 2007;202:445–54.
2. Strauss RA, Fallon SD. Lasers in contemporary oral and maxillofacial surgery. Dent Clin N Am. 2004;48:861–88.
3. de Freitas LF, Hamblin MR. Proposed mechanisms of Photobiomodulation or low-level light therapy. IEEE J Sel Top Quantum Electron. 2016;22:348–64.
4. Bennaim M, Porato M, Jarleton A, Hamon M, Carroll JD, Gommeren K, Balligand M. Preliminary evaluation of the effects of photobiomodulation therapy and physical rehabilitation on early postoperative recovery of dogs undergoing hemilaminectomy for treatment of thoracolumbar intervertebral disk disease. Am J Vet Res. 2017;78:195–206.
5. Jassim Mohammed Al Timimi Z, Saleem Ismail Alhabeel M. Laser dental treatment techniques. In: Prev. Detect. Manag. Oral Cancer. IntechOpen 2019; 1–16.
6. Zahara AT. Clinical evaluation of scalpel Er: YAG Laser 2940nm and conventional surgery incisions wound after Oral soft tissue biopsy. Bangladesh Med Res Counc Bull. 2018; 43:149.
7. Houssein HAA, Jaafar MSS, Ali Z, Timimi ZA, Mustafa FHH. Study of Hematocrit in relation with age and gender using low power helium—neon laser irradiation. In: Ting H-N, editor. 5th Kuala Lumpur Int. Conf. Biomed . Eng. 2011. Berlin, Heidelberg: IFMBE Proc. Springer; 2011. p. 463–6.
8. Al Timimi Z, Jaafar M, Zubir Mat Jafri M. Photodynamic therapy and green laser blood therapy. Glob J Med Res. 2011;11:22–8.

9. Houssein HAA, Jaafar MS, Ali Z, Timimi ZA, Mustafa FH. Study of Hematocrit in relation with age and gender using low power helium—neon laser irradiation. In: Osman NAA, Abas WABW, Wahab AKA, Ting HN, editors. 5th Kuala Lumpur Int. Conf. Biomed. Eng ; 2011. p. 463–6.

10. Al-Timimi Z, Mustafa F. Recognizing the effectiveness of the diode laser 850nm on stimulate the proliferation and viability of mice mesenchymal stem cells derived from bone marrow and adipose tissue. Iraqi J Vet Sci. 2019;32:285–90.

11. Zahra A-T. Biological effects of yellow laser-induced of cell survival: structural DNA damage comparison is undergoing ultraviolet radiation photocoagulation. Int J Eng Res Gen Sci. 2014;2:544–8.

12. Eells JT, Wong-Riley MTT, VerHoeve J, Henry M, Buchman EV, Kane MP, Gould LJ, Das R, Jett M, Hodgson BD. Mitochondrial signal transduction in accelerated wound and retinal healing by near-infrared light therapy. Mitochondrion. 2004;4:559–67.

13. Chiari S. Photobiomodulation and lasers. Front Oral Biol 2015; 118–123.

14. Tang E, Arany P. Photobiomodulation and implants: implications for dentistry. J Periodontal Implant Sci. 2013; https://doi.org/10.5051/jpis.2013.43.6.262.

15. Myers TD, Sulewski JG. Evaluating dental lasers: what the clinician should know. Dent Clin N Am. 2004;48:1127–44.

16. Özcan A, Sevimay M. Laser in dentistry: review. Turkiye Klin J Dent Sci. 2016;22:122–9.

17. Najeeb S, Khurshid Z, Zafar MS, Ajlal S. Applications of light amplification by stimulated emission of radiation (lasers) for restorative dentistry. Med Princ Pract. 2016;25:201–11.

18. Zahra A-T. A comparative study of determination the spectral characteristics of serum total protein among laser system and spectrophotometric: advantage and limitation of suggested methods. Curr Anal Chem. 2019;15:583–90.

19. Aït-Ameur K, Passilly N, de Saint DR, Fromager M, Amara E-H, Boudjemai S, Doumaz D. Laser beam shaping. In: AIP Conf. Proc. AIP, pp 59–67; 2008.

20. Sargent M, Scully MO, Lamb WE. Laser physics. Laser Phys. 2018; https://doi.org/10.1201/9780429493515.

21. Coluzzi DJ, Convissar RA. Laser fundamentals. In: Princ. Pract. Laser Dent. Elsevier 2011; 12–26.

22. Svelto O. Principles of lasers. Princ Lasers. 2010; https://doi.org/10.1007/978-1-4419-1302-9.

23. Brückner F, Lepski D. Laser Cladding. In: Springer Ser. Mater. Sci. 2017;263–306.

24. Eichler HJ, Eichler J, Lux O. Optical Resonators. In: Springer Ser. Opt. Sci. 2018;231–244.

25. Dutta Majumdar J, Manna I. Laser processing of materials. Sadhana. 2003;28:495–562.

26. Sciamanna M, Shore KA. Physics and applications of laser diode chaos. Nat Photonics. 2015;9:151–62.

27. Nazemisalman B, Farsadeghi M, Sokhansanj M. Types of lasers and their applications in pediatric dentistry. J Lasers Med Sci. 2015;6:96–101.

28. Stopp S, Deppe H, Lueth T. A new concept for navigated laser surgery. Lasers Med Sci. 2008;23:261–6.

29. George R, Walsh LJ. Performance assessment of novel side firing flexible optical fibers for dental applications. Lasers Surg Med. 2009;41:214–21.

30. George R, Walsh LJ. Performance assessment of novel side firing safe tips for endodontic applications. J Biomed Opt. 2011;16:048004.

31. Verma S, Chaudhari P, Maheshwari S, Singh R. Laser in dentistry: an innovative tool in modern dental practice. Natl J Maxillofac Surg. 2012;3:124.

32. Kim C, Jeon MJ, Jung JH, Yang JD, Park H, Kang HW, Lee H. Fabrication of novel bundled fiber and performance assessment for clinical applications. Lasers Surg Med. 2014;46:718–25.

33. Vertucci FJ. Root canal morphology and its relationship to endodontic procedures. Endod Top. 2005;10:3–29.

34. Coluzzi DJ. Fundamentals of dental lasers: science and instruments. Dent Clin N Am. 2004;48:751–70.

35. Azevedo Rodrigues LK, Nobre dos Santos M, Pereira D, Videira Assaf A, Pardi V. Carbon dioxide laser in dental caries prevention. J Dent. 2004;32:531–40.

36. Coluzzi F, Ruggeri M. Clinical and economic evaluation of tapentadol extended release and oxycodone/naloxone extended release in comparison with controlled release oxycodone in musculoskeletal pain. Curr Med Res Opin. 2014;30:1139–51.
37. Chung SH, Mazur E. Surgical applications of femtosecond lasers. J Biophotonics. 2009; https://doi.org/10.1002/jbio.200910053.
38. Romanos GE, Gupta B, Yunker M, Romanos EB, Malmstrom H. Lasers use in dental implantology. Implant Dent. 2013; https://doi.org/10.1097/ID.0b013e3182885fcc.
39. Martens LC. Laser physics and a review of laser applications in dentistry for children. Eur Arch Paediatr Dent. 2011;12:61–7.
40. Carroll JD, Milward MR, Cooper PR, Hadis M, Palin WM. Developments in low level light therapy (LLLT) for dentistry. Dent Mater. 2014; https://doi.org/10.1016/j.dental.2014.02.006.
41. Smiley CJ, Tracy SL, Abt E, et al. Systematic review and meta-analysis on the nonsurgical treatment of chronic periodontitis by means of scaling and root planning with or without adjuncts. J Am Dent Assoc. 2015;146:508–24.e5
42. Plotino G, Cortese T, Grande NM, Leonardi DP, Di Giorgio G, Testarelli L, Gambarini G. New technologies to improve root canal disinfection. Braz Dent J. 2016; https://doi.org/10.1590/0103-6440201600726.
43. Kuffler DP. Photobiomodulation in promoting wound healing: a review. Regen Med. 2016;11:107–22.
44. Houssein HAA, Jaafar MS, Ali Z, Timimi ZA, Mustafa FH. Study of hematocrit in relation with age and gender using low power Helium—Neon laser irradiation. In: IFMBE Proc. 2011;463–466.
45. Diam WA, Zahra A-T (2019) Characterization and fabrication of Nd:YVO4 disc laser system. In: AIP Conf. Proc. p 020009.
46. Zahra JMA. Impact of laser (Nd: YVO4 Crystals, 532nm) radiation on white blood cells. Iraqi Laser Scientists Journal. 2019;1(3):1–6.
47. Maria OM, Eliopoulos N, Muanza T. Radiation-induced Oral mucositis. Front Oncol. 2017; https://doi.org/10.3389/fonc.2017.00089.
48. Rodríguez-Caballero A, Torres-Lagares D, Robles-García M, Pachón-Ibáñez J, González-Padilla D, Gutiérrez-Pérez JL. Cancer treatment-induced oral mucositis: a critical review. Int J Oral Maxillofac Surg. 2012;41:225–38.
49. Messadi DV, Younai F. Aphthous ulcers. Dermatol Ther. 2010;23:281–90.
50. Cui RZ, Bruce AJ, Rogers RS. Recurrent aphthous stomatitis. Clin Dermatol. 2016;34:475–81.
51. Najeeb S, Khurshid Z, Zohaib S, Najeeb B, Bin QS, Zafar MS. Management of recurrent aphthous ulcers using low-level lasers: a systematic review. Medicina (B Aires). 2016;52:263–8.
52. Rola P, Doroszko A, Derkacz A. The use of low-level energy laser radiation in basic and clinical research. Adv Clin Exp Med. 2014;23:835–42.
53. Pelaez M, Nolan NT, Pillai SC, et al. A review on the visible light active titanium dioxide photocatalysts for environmental applications. Appl Catal B Environ. 2012;125:331–49.
54. Labat-gest V, Tomasi S. Photothrombotic ischemia: a minimally invasive and reproducible photochemical cortical lesion model for mouse stroke studies. J Vis Exp. 2013; https://doi.org/10.3791/50370.
55. Jamil TS, Ghaly MY, Fathy NA, Abd el-halim TA, Österlund L. Enhancement of TiO2 behavior on photocatalytic oxidation of MO dye using TiO2/AC under visible irradiation and sunlight radiation. Sep Purif Technol. 2012;98:270–9.
56. Bartl MH, Boettcher SW, Frindell KL, Stucky GD. 3-D molecular assembly of function in Titania-based composite material systems. Acc Chem Res. 2005;38:263–71.
57. Eber AE, Perper M, Verne SH, Magno R, IAO ALO, ALHarbi M, Nouri K. Photodynamic therapy. In: Lasers dermatology med. Cham: Springer International Publishing; 2018. p. 261–73.
58. Pretell-Mazzini J, Barton MD, Conway SA, Temple HT. Unplanned excision of soft-tissue sarcomas. J Bone Joint Surg-Am. 2015;97:597–603.
59. Thacker MM, Potter BK, Pitcher JD, Temple HT. Soft tissue sarcomas of the foot and ankle: impact of unplanned excision, limb salvage, and multimodality therapy. Foot Ankle Int. 2008; https://doi.org/10.3113/FAI.2008.0690.

60. Del Fabbro M, Corbella S, Sequeira-Byron P, Tsesis I, Rosen E, Lolato A, Taschieri S. Endodontic procedures for retreatment of periapical lesions. Cochrane Database Syst Rev. 2016; https://doi.org/10.1002/14651858.CD005511.pub3.
61. De Paula EC, Gouw-Soares S. The use of lasers for endodontic applications in dentistry. Med Laser Appl. 2001; https://doi.org/10.1078/1615-1615-00027.
62. Asnaashari M, Safavi N. Disinfection of contaminated canals by different laser wavelengths, while performing root canal therapy. J Lasers Med Sci. 2013; https://doi.org/10.22037/2010. v4i1.3869.
63. Quinto J, Amaral MM, Francci CE, Ana PA, Moritz A, Zezell DM. Evaluation of intra root canal Er,Cr:YSGG laser irradiation on prosthetic post adherence. J Prosthodont. 2019; https://doi.org/10.1111/jopr.12609.
64. Okamoto CB, Bussadori SK, Prates RA, da Mota ACC, Tempestini Horliana ACR, Fernandes KPS, Motta LJ. Photodynamic therapy for endodontic treatment of primary teeth: a randomized controlled clinical trial. Photodiagn Photodyn Ther. 2020; https://doi.org/10.1016/j.pdpdt.2020.101732.
65. Chen M. The development of laser surgery and medicine in China. 2004 Shanghai Int Conf Laser Med Surg. 2005. doi:https://doi.org/10.1117/12.639086.
66. Jhingan P, Sandhu M, Jindal G, Goel D, Sachdev V. An in-vitro evaluation of the effect of 980 nm diode laser irradiation on intra-canal dentin surface and dentinal tubule openings after biomechanical preparation: scanning electron microscopic study. Indian J Dent. 2015; https://doi.org/10.4103/0975-962x.155889.
67. Janani M, Jafari F, Samiei M, Lotfipour F, Nakhlband A, Ghasemi N, Salari T. Evaluation of antibacterial efficacy of photodynamic therapy vs. 2.5% NaOCl against E. faecalis-infected root canals using real-time PCR technique. J Clin Exp Dent. 2017; https://doi.org/10.4317/jced.53526.
68. Asnaashari M, Ghorbanzadeh S, Azari-Marhabi S, Mojahedi SM. Laser assisted treatment of extra oral cutaneous sinus tract of endodontic origin: a case report. J Lasers Med Sci. 2017; https://doi.org/10.15171/jlms.2017.s13.
69. Wang HM, Zhou MQ, Hong J. Histological evaluations on periapical tissues after irradiation by erbium-doped yttrium aluminum garnet laser in Labradors dogs. Shanghai Kou Qiang Yi Xue. 2016;25:657.
70. Marzadori M, Stefanini M, Sangiorgi M, Mounssif I, Monaco C, Zucchelli G. Crown lengthening and restorative procedures in the esthetic zone. Periodontol 2000. 2018; https://doi.org/10.1111/prd.12208.
71. Chen C-K, Wu Y-T, Chang N-J, Lan W-H, Ke J-H, Fu E, Yuh D-Y. Er:YAG Laser for surgical crown lengthening: a 6-month clinical study. Int J Periodontics Restorative Dent. 2017; https://doi.org/10.11607/prd.2551.
72. Kang Y, Rabie AB, Wong RW. A review of laser applications in orthodontics. International journal of orthodontics (Milwaukee, Wis.). 2014;25(1): 47–56.
73. Fornaini C, Merigo E, Vescovi P, Lagori G, Rocca JP. Use of laser in orthodontics: applications and perspectives. Laser Ther. 2013; https://doi.org/10.5978/islsm.13-OR-10.
74. Üşümez S, Orhan M, Üşümez A. Laser etching of enamel for direct bonding with an Er, Cr:YSGG hydrokinetic laser system. Am J Orthod Dentofac Orthop. 2002; https://doi.org/10.1067/mod.2002.127294.
75. Giannelli M, Formigli L, Bani D. Comparative evaluation of Photoablative efficacy of erbium: yttrium-aluminium-garnet and diode laser for the treatment of gingival hyperpigmentation. A Randomized Split-Mouth Clinical Trial. J Periodontol. 2014; https://doi.org/10.1902/jop.2013.130219.
76. Kafas P, Stavrianos C, Jerjes W, Upile T, Vourvachis M, Theodoridis M, Stavrianou I. Upper-lip laser frenectomy without infiltrated anaesthesia in a paediatric patient: a case report. Cases J. 2009; https://doi.org/10.1186/1757-1626-2-7138.
77. Pié-Sánchez J, España-Tost AJ, Arnabat-Domínguez J, Gay-Escoda C. Comparative study of upper lip frenectomy with the CO 2 laser versus the Er, Cr: YSGG laser. Med Oral Patol Oral Cir Bucal. 2012; https://doi.org/10.4317/medoral.17373.

78. Gontijo I, Navarro RS, Haypek P, Ciamponi AL, Haddad AE. The applications of diode and Er:YAG lasers in labial frenectomy in infant patients. J Dent Child. 2005;72:10.
79. Azma E, Safavi N. Diode laser application in soft tissue oral surgery. J Lasers Med Sci. 2013;4:206–11.
80. Fiorotti RC, Bertolini MM, Nicola JH, Nicola EMD. Early lingual frenectomy assisted by CO2 laser helps prevention and treatment of functional alterations caused by ankyloglossia. Int J Orofacial Myology. 2004;30:64.
81. Koh RU, Oh T-J, Rudek I, Neiva GF, Misch CE, Rothman ED, Wang H-L. Hard and soft tissue changes after Crestal and Subcrestal immediate implant placement. J Periodontol. 2011; https://doi.org/10.1902/jop.2011.100541.
82. Ivanenko M, Werner M, Afilal S, Klasing M, Hering P. Ablation of hard bone tissue with pulsed CO2 lasers. Med Laser Appl. 2005; https://doi.org/10.1016/j.mla.2005.02.007.
83. Buchalla W, Attin T. External bleaching therapy with activation by heat, light or laser—a systematic review. Dent Mater. 2007; https://doi.org/10.1016/j.dental.2006.03.018.
84. Dostalova T, Jelinkova H, Housova D, Sulc J, Nemec M, Miyagi M, Brugnera Junior A, Zanin F. Diode laser-activated bleaching. Braz. Dent. J. 2004;15:SI3.
85. Fekrazad R, Alimazandarani S, Kalhori KAM, Assadian H, Mirmohammadi SM. Comparison of laser and power bleaching techniques in tooth color change. J Clin Exp Dent. 2017; https://doi.org/10.4317/jced.53435.
86. De Moor RJG, Verheyen J, Diachuk A, Verheyen P, Meire MA, De Coster PJ, Keulemans F, De Bruyne M, Walsh LJ. Insight in the chemistry of laser-activated dental bleaching. Sci World J. 2015; https://doi.org/10.1155/2015/650492.
87. Kalies S, Kuetemeyer K, Heisterkamp A. Mechanisms of high-order photobleaching and its relationship to intracellular ablation. Biomed Opt Express. 2011; https://doi.org/10.1364/boe.2.000805.
88. Yang J, Dutra V. Utility of radiology, laser fluorescence, and transillumination. Dent Clin N Am. 2005; https://doi.org/10.1016/j.cden.2005.05.010.
89. Thareja RK, Sharma AK, Shukla S. Spectroscopic investigations of carious tooth decay. Med Eng Phys. 2008; https://doi.org/10.1016/j.medengphy.2008.02.005.
90. Al-Batayneh OB, Seow WK, Walsh LJ (2014) Assessment of Er:YAG laser for cavity preparation in primary and permanent teeth: a scanning electron microscopy and thermographic study. Pediatr Dent 36 90.
91. Ciaramicoli MT, Carvalho RCR, Eduardo CP. Treatment of cervical dentin hypersensitivity using neodymium: Yttrium-Aluminum-Garnet laser. Clin Eval Lasers Surg Med. 2003; https://doi.org/10.1002/lsm.10232.
92. Eguro T, Maeda T, Tanabe M, Otsuki M, Tanaka H. Adhesion of composite resins to enamel irradiated by the Er:YAG laser: application of the ultrasonic scaler on irradiated surface. Lasers Surg Med. 2001; https://doi.org/10.1002/lsm.1063.
93. Strobl K, Bahns TL, Wiliham L, Bishara SE, Stwalley WC. Laser-aided debonding of orthodontic ceramic brackets. Am J Orthod Dentofac Orthop. 1992; https://doi.org/10.1016/0889-5406(92)70007-W.
94. Tocchio RM, Williams PT, Mayer FJ, Standing KG. Laser debonding of ceramic orthodontic brackets. Am J Orthod Dentofac Orthop. 1993; https://doi.org/10.1016/S0889-5406(05)81765-2.
95. Sgolastra F, Petrucci A, Gatto R, Monaco A. Effectiveness of laser in dentinal hypersensitivity treatment: a systematic review. J Endod. 2011; https://doi.org/10.1016/j.joen.2010.11.034.
96. Kara C, Orbak R. Comparative evaluation of Nd:YAG laser and fluoride varnish for the treatment of dentinal hypersensitivity. J Endod. 2009; https://doi.org/10.1016/j.joen.2009.04.004.
97. Persson A, Andersson M, Oden A, Sandborgh-Englund G. A three-dimensional evaluation of a laser scanner and a touch-probe scanner. J Prosthet Dent. 2006; https://doi.org/10.1016/j.prosdent.2006.01.003.
98. Kovacs L, Zimmermann A, Brockmann G, Baurecht H, Schwenzer-Zimmerer K, Papadopulos NA, Papadopoulos MA, Sader R, Biemer E, Zeilhofer HF. Accuracy and precision of the three-dimensional assessment of the facial surface using a 3-D laser scanner. IEEE Trans Med Imaging. 2006; https://doi.org/10.1109/TMI.2006.873624.

Digital Impressions

6

Nadia Khalifa

6.1   Introduction

Due to the advancement of digital technology, conventional dental impressions are rapidly being replaced by digital impressions using intraoral scanners (IOS) and may be totally replaced within the next decade. Intraoral scanners (IOS) are devices for capturing direct optical impressions in dentistry. They project a light source onto the dental arches, and prepared tooth surfaces with the images being captured by imaging sensors.

Many dental laboratories scan casts or impressions and design their restorations digitally using computers, ensuring an efficient and cost-effective workflow.

There are many questions to consider when choosing an IOS:

- What is the cost of purchase? (ranges between $20,000 and $40,000).
- Is the scanner small, light, and easy to use? Would it be comfortable for the patients?
- Does it require powder, display images in color, perform chairside milling, or continue the same workflow to computer-aided design/computer-aided manufacturing (CAD/CAM) lab(s)?
- Are there costs involved for image export and storage, upgrades?
- Are there licensing/usage fees (can reach up to $3500/year)?
- Is the scanner compatible with the practice management software, is it portable, is touch screen, and can it be plugged into USB and laptop?

This chapter attempts to address all these concerns. In addition, the benefits of digital impressions along with its limitations are also discussed.

N. Khalifa (✉)
Department of Preventive and Restorative Dentistry, College of Dental Medicine,
Sharjah, UAE
e-mail: n.khalifa@sharjah.ac.ae

© Springer Nature Switzerland AG 2021
P. Jain, M. Gupta (eds.), *Digitization in Dentistry*,
https://doi.org/10.1007/978-3-030-65169-5_6

Table 6.1 Differences between digital impressions and CAD CAM systems

Digital impressions	CAD-CAM (Chairside)
A scanner wand is used intraorally to record a digital image of the preparation	Chairside CAD/CAM systems include both a scanner and a mill for fabricating a restoration. With these systems, clinicians can scan, design, and mill a full-contour restoration in-office
These can be reviewed instantly, and changes made. Practitioner can even re-scan the image if needed	This system offers methods and tools to modify the restoration, such as adjusting contacts, height, color, and occlusion
The data file is electronically transmitted to the dental laboratory or the manufacturing company (open or closed system) along with a prescription	As opposed to electronically sending the data to the laboratory, *computer-aided design (CAD)* can be done and completed chairside. The file is sent to an in-office milling machine, for *computer-aided manufacturing (CAM)* for the final prosthesis. The finished restoration can be cemented during the same appointment
Significantly lower cost than CAD CAM system	Higher economics than a scanner alone, and require training for the entire staff
Any type of restoration can be created using a digital impression, from all ceramic crowns to gold inlays	Final prosthesis is milled from a ceramic or composite block

6.2 History

Digital technology was introduced to dentistry by Dr. Duret in the 1970s. In 1987, Dr. Mormann introduced the concept of computer-aided design/computer-aided manufacturing (CAD/CAM) technology. Currently, two types of digital systems are available: CAD/CAM systems and three-dimensional (3D) digital impression systems (Table 6.1).

Digital impression systems can be further be divided into either direct digitalization (intraoral scanners) or indirect digitalization (extraoral scanners) depending on the requirement. Intraoral scanners were introduced as stand-alone devices that capture a digital impression and send the file to a dental laboratory for prosthesis fabrication. They were originally a part of CAD/CAM systems which produce a digital impression of prepared teeth.

When using extraoral scanners, there is no need for any change to the clinical workflow for taking conventional impressions. Either the impression itself is scanned, the impression is poured with stone and scanned, or a model is printed and scanned, to create a digital 3D file.

6.3 Comparison between Conventional and Digital Impressions

A meta-analysis and systematic review found most of the studies included in their study to be in vitro studies that gained better marginal and internal fit of fixed restorations with digital rather than conventional impression techniques [1]. They also concluded that restorations produced from digital dies had smaller marginal and internal discrepancy compared to stereolithography apparatus (SLA) polyurethane dies.

Recently, less deviation for short span restorations were observed using current IOS compared to conventional impressions, but this does not apply for long span restorations where conventional impression techniques still provide the lowest deviation [2, 3] Consequently, a recent systematic review investigating accuracy of digital impressions in fixed prosthodontics concluded that conventional impressions performed using high-precision impression materials showed greater accuracy than digital impressions [4].

6.4   Technology of Digital Impression Systems

Intraoral scanning systems use different imaging technologies (either a laser or a video) to capture their 3D images. Some systems such as CEREC base its imaging on *triangulation*, a technique in which a light source is reflected off an object. Light triangulation limits accuracy when scanning curved surfaces especially those that do not reflect light evenly, such as teeth with amalgam restorations. Therefore, some systems require the use of titanium dioxide powder as a contrast medium to correct the problem of light triangulation, whereas others do not.

Current systems use different light source technologies, including laser, structured (striped) light, or LED illumination.

Digital impression data transfer systems using IOS can be classified in different ways. If the IOS allows the digital impression to be sent directly via export of source files such as STL (Standard Tessellation Language or "send-to-lab"), PLY (Polygon File Format), and OBJ (Object File Format) to different laboratory units giving the desired flexibility [5], it is known as an **open system**, and if not, it is a **closed system**.

Open systems allow practitioners to work with different laboratories and maximize the potential of their investment with options. The STL file format is simple and small, thus making its processing faster, but without representation of color or texture. On the other hand, OBJ and PLY formats can store properties such as color and texture and benefit from improved 3D printers.

In a closed system, the digital impressions are sent to the manufacturing company, at a fee. The advantage is that since the configuration, collection, and manipulation of the data is by the same manufacturer, it provides security and a single place for delivery. Some scanners allow only acquisition of data, which is then sent to the laboratory for further processing and manufacturing. On the other hand, there are scanners that besides acquisition are able to mill or print same day, thereby allowing the patient to have a dental restoration in a single sitting.

Data collection methods, transfer of images, strategies for tracking, and size of scanner head may vary between different types of scanners, but each procedure produces a digital model of the patient's dentition.

6.5 Advantages of Digital Impressions

Advantages of digital impressions include eliminating the need of materials for making impressions, leading to better patient comfort [6, 7], with little or no gagging. This avoids the pouring of casts, and adjustments are easier due to the positive image of tooth preparation being visible on the computer screen. Similarly, it does not require temporization or retraction-cord packing, the rubber dam can be used with digital impressions, does not need to be disinfected except for the tip, is easier to store, and most importantly, the dental restoration can be delivered on the same day of digital scanning using CAD/ CAM technology.

It also allows for better communication with patients as well as dental technicians. Scanners can capture the prepared teeth, the neighboring teeth, and at times, the whole arch. Opposing arch scans and simulation movements in a virtual articulator are also possible [8].

6.6 Disadvantages of Digital Impressions

As with every novel technology, there is a learning curve, and nonexperts might require additional time to take the digital images. Other disadvantages include the inability to detect subgingivally prepared margins of teeth and the high initial investment cost of IOS.

6.7 Clinical Indications and Contraindications of Digital Impressions and IOS

In *Prosthodontics*, digital impressions can be used to design and mill single tooth crowns, endodontic crowns, resin onlays and inlays, veneers, fixed partial dentures, removable partial denture frameworks, implant bridges post and cores, temporary restorations, and digital smile design. Contraindications include long span fixed partial dentures, long span implant supported fixed partial dentures, and complete removable dentures.

In *Orthodontics*, they can be used for diagnosis and treatment planning, to fabricate orthodontic aligners, custom-made devices and retainers. They can also be used for guided implant surgery.

General contraindications include inability of the patient to sit still and restricted access to area as in case of the head of the intraoral scanner being too large or if there are interferences by the tongue or an orthodontic appliance [9]. It is important to control bleeding prior to scanning to obtain an acceptable image.

6.8 Accuracy of Intraoral Scanners

A variety of IOSs are used by dentists these days (Figs. 6.1 and 6.2), and with it researchers started reviewing the literature on the use of these devices [10]. The important question to ask is if the accuracy of digital dental models generated

Fig. 6.1 Intraoral scanning in process (*Courtesy* Dr. Tariq Saadi)

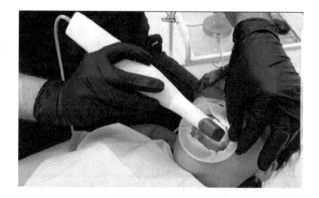

Fig. 6.2 Viewing of scanned image (*Courtesy* of Dr. Tariq Saadi)

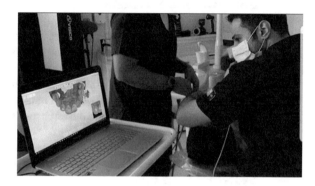

Table 6.2 Ideal characteristics of an intraoral scanner

Feature	Requirement
Trueness	High
Precision	High
Resolution	High
Need for powder	Not needed
Scanning speed	Fast
Tip of the scanner	Small
Colored images	Yes
System	Open

from an IOS is equivalent to that of dental plaster models [11]. Accuracy of the device encompasses "trueness (closeness of agreement between the experimental dataset and the real object) and precision (closeness of agreement among different scans performed by the same scanner)" [12] (Table 6.2). An important limitation of studies investigating the accuracy of scans is their conduction in vitro, because it has been observed that intraoral conditions can influence their accuracy [9].

A systematic review [13] investigating the mean accuracy of digital technologies including intraoral tissues observed that scanning of a dentate arch by laboratory and IOS ranged between 17 and 378 μm. For prepared teeth, the minimal accuracy was 23 μm, but when the complete arch was scanned it was 60 μm. Scanning of single tooth preparations showed an accuracy between 20 and 40 μm, and that of digital implant scanning had an accuracy of 19–112 μm. Accuracy for partially and completely edentulous arches ranged between 30–220 μm while for completely edentulous arches alone the range was between 44 and 591 μm. Authors of the review concluded that current digital technologies are accurate for specific applications but the scanning of edentulous arches still represents a challenge [13]. Other researchers similarly commented this to be due to the mobility of the tissues and a lack of reference landmarks in edentulous arches [14]. Overall, there are variable outcomes among the different IOS systems [15].

6.9   Comparison of Accuracy between Intraoral Scanners and Extraoral Scanners

When comparing accuracy of IOS with extraoral scanners (EOS), there have been many conflicting reports [9, 16–18]. It has been suggested that intraoral conditions such as saliva and limited spacing can contribute to the inaccuracy of a scan. It is noteworthy to mention that EOS, due to the many steps required to manufacture a restoration, can also have error introduced in the stages of impression taking, gypsum or SLA polyurethane model-making, in addition to the error resulting from digitization [19].

6.10   Common Commercially Available Intraoral Scanning Systems (Table 6.3)

The following intraoral scanners are not ranked in any specific order.

6.10.1 CEREC

In 1983, Prof. Mörmann pioneered the concept of in-office CAD/CAM by introducing the CEREC 1 unit (Sirona Dental Systems GmbH, Bensheim, Germany) [20]. Software capability improved from 2D to 3D imaging in early 2000 with *CEREC 3 Redcam,* which used infrared light to scan objects and needed an even layer of opaque powder to capture a 3D image of the preparation, the antagonist, as well as functional registration.

Bluecam became available in 2009, using blue light with shorter wavelength and needing only a thin layer of powder. Its newer mode recorded images automatically, while the camera was held in front of the tooth, leading to much faster image acquisition. *Bluecam* combined several single images to create a 3D model.

Omnicam, which was introduced in 2012, was the first CAD system from Sirona that did not require powder, and unlike *Bluecam*, it used for continuous image capturing to generate a 3D model allowing for colored full-arch and half-arch scans.

Primescan is the most recent of the CEREC IOS. Its many advantages are that it can scan up to a depth of 20 mm, has a touchscreen, is powder-free, is able to scan

Table 6.3 Comparison of different types of IOS

Scanner	Technology	System	Contrast medium required (powder)	User interface	Weight (approx.) Wand tip (approx.)
CEREC Bluecam	Visible blue light	Closed	Yes	Simple and intuitive, compact tool bars, menus, use of mouse	280 g 22 mm × 17 mm
CEREC Omnicam	Continuous 3D color capture	Closed	No	Simple and intuitive, compact tool bars, menus, use of mouse	15 mm × 15 mm
CEREC Primescan	Blue laser	Open	No	Touch-enabled and intuitive user interface	10 mm × 11 mm
3 M true definition	Video scanning	Open	Yes (light)	Touch screen tablet	200 g 14.4 mm × 16.2 mm
3Shape Trios	Confocal microscopy	Open	No	Touch screen	1 kg
Align iTero element	Parallel confocal laser scanning	Open	No	Interactive	470 g 50 mm × 68 mm
Planmeca PlanScan	Blue laser projected pattern triangulation	PlanScan and other open systems	No	Cable interface, icons, mouse	544 g 48 mm × 53 mm
Emerald TM	Blue laser projected pattern triangulation	Open	No	Cable interface	235 g 41 mm × 45 mm
Carestream	LED of amber, blue, and green with active triangulation	Carestream solutions and other open systems	No	Cable interface	316 g 13 mm × 13 mm
Medit i500	Continuous video capture	Open	No	Cable interface	276 g 18 mm × 152 mm
Dental wings Virtuo vivo	Multiscan imaging	Open	No	Touch screen Integrated voice and gesture control	213 g

reflective surfaces, can scan color photo-realistically, gives shade detection, prevents fogging, is very fast (performs a full arch scan of upper and lower jaw, bite registration, model calculation in approximately 50–180 s), is disinfectable with wipes and is autoclavable, can undergo dry heat sterilization, and has single-use sleeves and mirror sleeves. Primescan software also has design functions. Figure 6.3 shows the comparisons between the different CEREC systems available.

Fig. 6.3 Different CEREC
systems (Courtesy
"Dentsply Sirona")

CAMERA	SYSTEM	CART
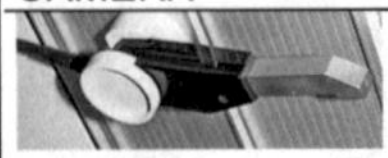	CEREC 1	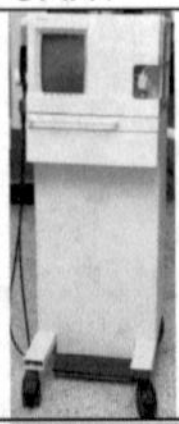
	CEREC 2	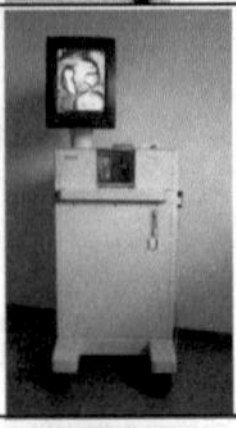
	CEREC 3 *Redcam*	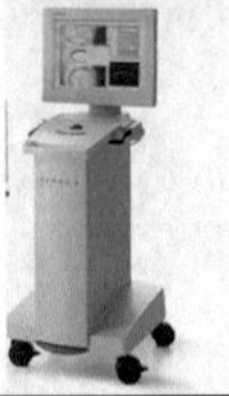
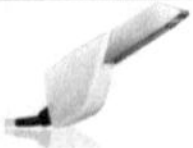	CEREC *Bluecam*	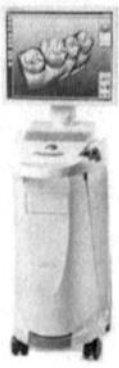
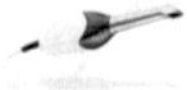	CEREC *Omnicam*	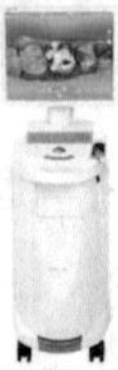
	CEREC *Primescan*	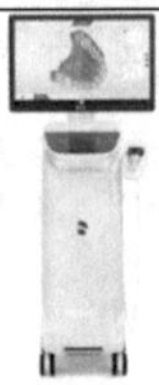

6.10.2 Midmark Mobile True Definition Scanner

Midmark acquired the 3 M™ True Definition Scanner in 2019 and renamed it the *Midmark Mobile True Definition Scanner,* which is a mobile intraoral scanner operating on a tablet (Fig. 6.4).

It uses video scanning technology instead of laser, but it still requires a light coating of scanning spray to capture the image. It is an open system producing STL files and does not require field calibrations. Two full arch scans or four quadrant scans can be done before requiring a recharge. The entire console weighs 2.75 kg and weight of wand with cable is 253 g. The length and width of wand are 254 and 16.2 mm, respectively.

Acquisition Method Trinocular is stereo-proprietary 3D in motion reconstruction, with a capture rate of 20 image triplets per second. Its average processing and upload time for the following are: (a) Quadrant: 2-min acquisition (upper/lower/buccal bite) ~30 min (presuming 10 Mbps measured upload performance from office Wi-Fi), (b) Full arch: 6-min acquisition (upper/lower/3 bite scans) ~90 min (presuming 10 Mbps measured upload performance from office Wi-Fi).

The *Midmark Mobile True Definition Scanner* can be used to create crowns, bridges, inlays, onlays, veneers, partials, clear aligners, mouth guards, and orthodontic appliances and models.

6.10.3 Trios®4 Scanner

This IOS (3shape, Copenhagen, Denmark) produces colored images and does not require powder, has a touch screen, and has an open format as it produces DCM and

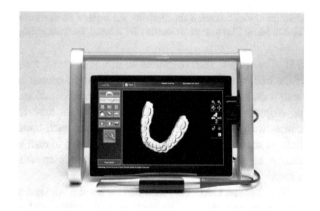

Fig. 6.4 Midmark MobileTrue Definition Scanner (Courtesy "Midmark")

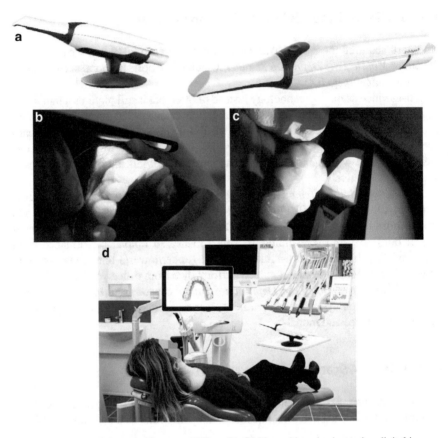

Fig. 6.5 (a) Trios 4 scanner *(Courtesy "3Shape")*. (b) Normal imaging/capturing digital impression. (c) Caries detection functionality via built-in fluorescence technology. (d) Full arch scan, TRIOS Move Plus scanner *(Courtesy Dr. Ahmad, Institute of Digital Dentistry, NZ)*

STL files (Fig. 6.5). It measures 42 mm × 274 mm, weighs 345 g if wired and 375 g if the battery is included. It has an LED light source and has caries diagnostic aid with a dedicated tip for detection of interproximal caries using infrared scans in development, and has smart tips with instant heat technology. *Trios®4 wireless* comes with three rechargeable batteries and each battery provides 45 min of continuous scanning. It takes approximately 2–4 h to charge fully depending on battery charge level, and its wireless range extends to within 5 m. *Trios®4* requires subscription charges.

The 3Shape CAD software can be used to design several kinds of restorations and frameworks such as crowns, bridges, inlays, onlays, veneers, implants, three-unit implant bridges, and posts and cores.

Trios Move+, which is the newest version of an ergonomic cart by 3Shape, now comes with an even larger 15.6-inch full HD touch screen, a 36% larger working

Fig. 6.6 Trios Move + *(Courtesy "3Shape")*

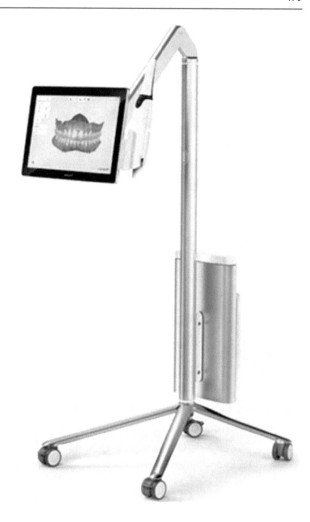

area than the previous models and a USB 2.0 port at the back of the screen for the import and export of scans (Fig. 6.6).

6.10.4 iTero Element 5D

It comes as a wheeled stand or laptop configuration (Figs. 6.7 and 6.8). The wand emits red laser light (680 nm Class 1), as well as white or 850 nm LED emissions. The length, width, and depth of the wand are 346, 50, and 68 mm, respectively, and its weight is 470 g (without cable). It simultaneously records 3D, intraoral color, and near-infrared imaging and enables comparison over time using *iTero* time-lapse technology.

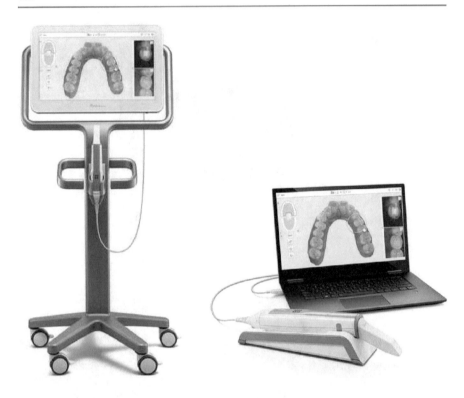

Fig. 6.7 iTero Element 5D *(Adapted from iTero.com)*

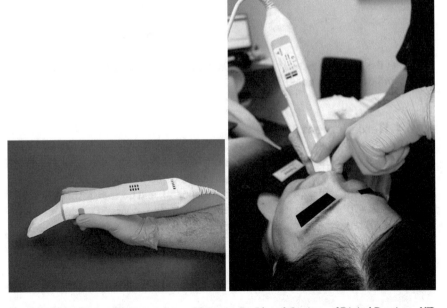

Fig. 6.8 iTero element 5D scanner in use *(Courtesy Dr. Ahmad, Institute of Digital Dentistry, NZ)*

It has an interactive interface, and as an open system, *iTero* is compatible with software that accepts STL images. Its use requires subscription charges. It is useful in restorative work involving crowns, FPDs, veneers, implants, aligners, and retainers.

6.10.5 Planmeca PlanScan®

Planscan can be integrated into a *Planmeca* dental unit or connected to a PC. The scans of the lower and upper arches in occlusion can be exported as open STL and PLY files, and there are scanning options of color and grayscale. There are four scanning tips available, namely, grayscale standard, landscape, portrait, and color. These are autoclavable, have antifogging technology, and a cable interface firewire 800 or thunderbolt (via adapter). Its light source is blue laser, and scanning technology is through projected pattern triangulation. Its dimensions (scanner with tip) are $48 \times 53 \times 276$ mm, with a weight of (scanner with tip) 544 g. The scanner is shown in Fig. 6.9.

6.10.6 Emerald™

This IOS is similar to the above scanners in that it can be integrated into a *Planmeca* dental unit or connected to a PC (Fig. 6.10). The scans of lower and upper arches in occlusion are exported as open STL and PLY files. It scans in true color and has two autoclavable scanning tip options: standard and slimline. The autoclavable "cariosity tip" is for caries detection, has **antifogging technology**, uses red, green, and blue lasers as light source and uses projected pattern triangulation as the scanning

Fig. 6.9 PlanScan®
Scanner *(Courtesy Planmeca)*

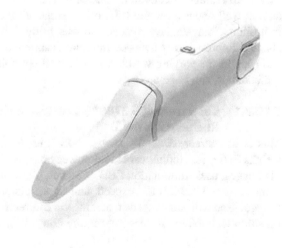

Fig. 6.10 Emerald™
Scanner *(Courtesy
Planmeca)*

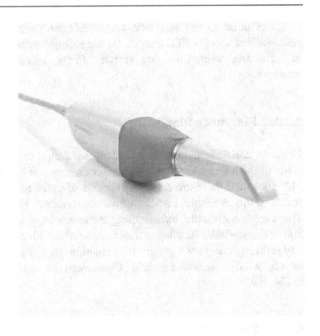

technology. Its dimensions (scanner with tip) are 41 × 45 × 249 mm and weighs (scanner with tip) 235 g. The cable interface is USB A type connection on the laptop and USB C type connection on the scanner. All cables are designed to transmit data via USB 3.0.

Indications: Inlays/onlays, veneers, crowns, bridges, full arches, scan bodies, models, and impressions.

6.10.7 Emerald™ S

This is an enhanced version of *Emerald*™, and a practiced user can scan an entire arch in well under a minute (Fig. 6.11). It has all the features of the *Emerald*™. Indications: inlays/onlays, veneers, crowns, bridges, full arches, scan bodies, models, and impressions. *Planmeca* intraoral scanners have built-in design functions and support the varying workflows of several specialties, such as prosthodontics, orthodontics, and implantology.

6.10.7.1 Carestream CS 3700® (Carestream Health, Rochester, NY, US)

This is Carestream Dental's newest IOS (Fig. 6.12) after Carestream 3500. It weighs 316 g (excluding cable and power box), is able to capture full color HD 3D images, uses illumination LED of amber, blue, and green colors. Its computer connection is USB 2.0 high speed, and its acquisition method is through active triangulation with smart shade matching via Bidirectional Reflectance Distribution Function technology. It does not require contrast medium, scans in true color in

Fig. 6.11 Emerald™ S Scanner *(Courtesy Planmeca)*

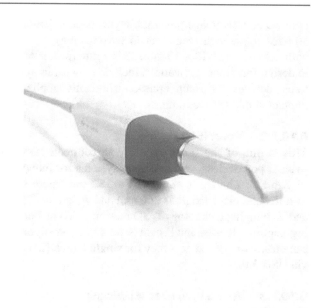

Fig. 6.12 (**a**) Carestream CS 3700® automatically detects the enamel color of the scan area to help identify the correct position for restorative outcomes *(Adapted from Carestream Dental LLC)*. (**b**) Intraoral imaging of Carestream CS 3700®

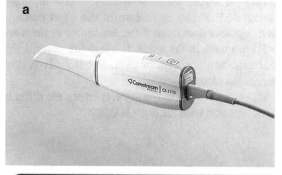

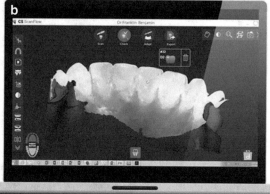

both 2D and 3D image plus multilayer shade information, and has scan speed of 30 s for single arch scans (per in vitro testing), and 10 frames per second (fps) with fields of view 13 × 13 mm, 13 × 7 mm (posterior tip). The scanner has built-in design functions. Indications include crowns, inlays, onlays, bridges, and dentures, devices for sleep apnea, orthodontic appliances, surgical guides, and implant-supported restorations.

6.10.7.2 Medit i500

This is one of the more recently introduced IOS. They are competitively priced, powderless, and are open systems for integrated CAD/CAM workflow (Fig. 6.13). **The tip is small (18 × 152 mm)** *with* **single button control.** The overall hand piece length is 266 mm and weight is 276 g. It has a high resolution, and its imaging technology is 3D motion video technology with fill color streaming capture. It uses intelligent scan-detecting algorithm with two high-speed cameras, with a good accuracy for single crown [21] and data can be transmitted via USB 3.0.

6.10.7.3 Virtuo Vivo (Dental Wings)

These IOS are ergonomically designed with pen grip hold and have removable sleeves that are autoclavable (Fig. 6.14). The wand is light and weighs only 213 g. It uses motion control technology such as gesture and voice controls, allowing for touch-free manipulation of screen. It also has a touchscreen. It has an integrated air mouse feature in the hand piece. It uses multiscan imaging, which captures data from different angles at the same time. It has the power of two 3D scanners in the wand, has real life color, a light on wand, and an audible signal give confirmation of data. It has built-in design functions and requires subscription charges.

Table 6.3 gives the comparison between the different IOS, and Fig. 6.15 shows images captured with different IOS.

Fig. 6.13 Medit i500 scanner *(Courtesy Dr. Ahmad, Institute of Digital Dentistry, NZ)*

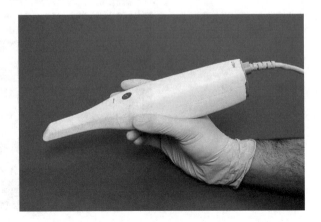

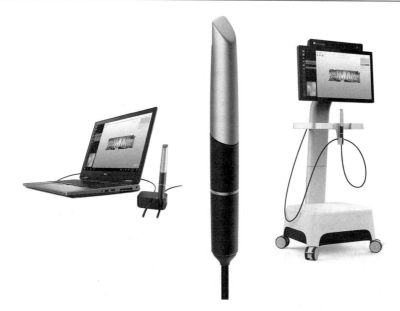

Fig. 6.14 Virtuo vivo scanner *(Reproduced with permission from Dental wings)*

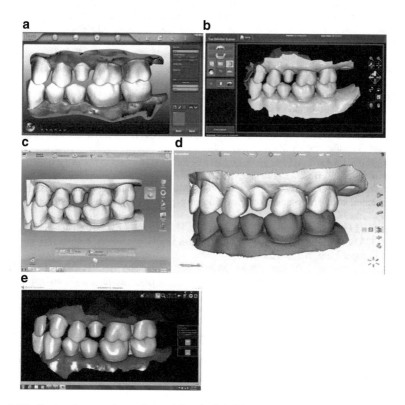

Fig. 6.15 Captured screenshots of a partial arch digital impression done with the iTero (**a**), the 3 M True Definition Scanner (**b**), the CEREC AC with Bluecam (**c**), the PlanScan (**d**), and the CareStream CS 3500 (**e**). *(Reproduced with permission from John Wiley and Sons)*

6.11   Conclusion

Systems are constantly improving and moving from single images to live video streaming. More IOS systems are constantly being introduced into the market (Vatech-Ezscan, GC Aadva IOS etc.), and might rival other IOS in the future. With the rapid advancement of digital technology in dental clinics, procedures that previously needed a highly skilled workforce are being replaced by an easier, faster, and more predictable digital workflows.

References

1. Chochlidakis KM, Papaspyridakos P, Geminiani A, Chen CJ, Feng IJ, Ercoli C. Digital versus conventional impressions for fixed prosthodontics: a systematic review and meta-analysis. J Prosthet Dent. 2016; https://doi.org/10.1016/j.prosdent.2015.12.017.
2. Schmidt A, Klussmann L, Wöstmann B, Schlenz MA. Accuracy of digital and conventional full-arch impressions in patients : an update; 2020 doi:https://doi.org/10.3390/jcm9030688.
3. Atieh MA, Ritter AV, Ko CC, Duqum I. Accuracy evaluation of intraoral optical impressions: a clinical study using a reference appliance. J Prosthet Dent. 2017;118:400–5.
4. Giachetti L, Sarti C, Cinelli F, Russo D. Accuracy of digital impressions in fixed prosthodontics: a systematic review of clinical studies. Int J Prosthodont. 2020;33:192–201.
5. Van Noort R. The future of dental devices is digital. Dent Mater. 2012;28:3–12.
6. Mangano A, Beretta M, Luongo G, Mangano C, Mangano F. Conventional vs digital impressions: acceptability, treatment comfort and stress among young orthodontic patients. Open Dent J. 2018; https://doi.org/10.2174/1874210601812010118.
7. Burhardt L, Livas C, Kerdijk W, van der Meer WJ, Ren Y. Treatment comfort, time perception, and preference for conventional and digital impression techniques: a comparative study in young patients. Am J Orthod Dentofac Orthop. 2016;150:261–7.
8. Porter JL, Carrico CK, Lindauer SJ, Tüfekçi E. Comparison of intraoral and extraoral scanners on the accuracy of digital model articulation. J Orthod. 2018;45(4):275–82.
9. Flügge TV, Schlager S, Nelson K, Nahles S, Metzger MC. Precision of intraoral digital dental impressions with iTero and extraoral digitization with the iTero and a model scanner. Am J Orthod Dentofac Orthop. 2013;144:471–8.
10. Mangano F, Gandolfi A, Luongo G, Logozzo S. Intraoral scanners in dentistry: a review of the current literature. BMC Oral Health. 2017;17:149.
11. Aragón MLC, Pontes LF, Bichara LM, Flores-Mir C, Normando D. Validity and reliability of intraoral scanners compared to conventional gypsum models measurements: a systematic review. Eur J Orthod. 2016;38:429–34.
12. Tapie L, Lebon N, Mawussi B, Fron-Chabouis H, Duret F, Attal J-P. Understanding dental CAD/CAM for restorations – the digital workflow from a mechanical engineering viewpoint. Int J Comput Dent. 2015;18:21–44.
13. Bohner L, Gamba DD, Hanisch M, Marcio BS, Tortamano Neto P, Laganá DC, Sesma N. Accuracy of digital technologies for the scanning of facial, skeletal, and intraoral tissues: a systematic review. J Prosthet Dent. 2019; https://doi.org/10.1016/j.prosdent.2018.01.015.
14. Patzelt SBM, Vonau S, Stampf S, Att W. Assessing the feasibility and accuracy of digitizing edentulous jaws. J Am Dent Assoc. 2013;144:914–20.
15. Aswani K, Wankhade S, Khalikar A, Deogade S. Accuracy of an intraoral digital impression: a review. J Indian Prosthodont Soc. 2020;20:27–37.
16. Sason G, Mistry G, Tabassum R, Shetty O. A comparative evaluation of intraoral and extraoral digital impressions: an in vivo study. J Indian Prosthodont Soc. 2018;18:108–16.

17. Bohner LOL, De Luca Canto G, Marció BS, Laganá DC, Sesma N, Tortamano Neto P. Computer-aided analysis of digital dental impressions obtained from intraoral and extraoral scanners. J Prosthet Dent 2017; doi:https://doi.org/10.1016/j.prosdent.2016.11.018.
18. Flügge T, Att W, Metzger M, Nelson K. Precision of dental implant digitization using intraoral scanners. Int J Prosthodont. 2016; https://doi.org/10.11607/ijp.4417.
19. Moldan M, Wöstmann B, Rudolph H. Accuracy of intraoral and extraoral digital data acquisition for dental restorations. doi:https://doi.org/10.1590/1678-775720150266.
20. Mörmann WH (2006) The evolution of the CEREC system. doi:https://doi.org/10.14219/jada.archive.2006.0398.
21. Hack GD, Patzelt SBM. Evaluation of the accuracy of six intraoral scanning. Am Dent Assoc. 2015;10:1–5.

Digital Orthodontics

7

Lana Dalbah

7.1 Digital Imaging

7.1.1 History

For years, 2D imaging modalities like panoramic, cephalometric radiography, and dental photography have been used routinely by orthodontists to do basic orthodontic diagnosis, treatment planning, and monitoring of case progress. Certain cases, though, would require 3D investigation, like impacted canines and TMJ pathology, and the only option for 3D imaging and analysis in the past was medical-grade Computed Tomography (CT), but the radiation dose associated with it was so high to justify its use by orthodontists, especially because of the age of the orthodontic patient population [1]. Details about the imaging technologies is given in Chap. 3. CBCT and its use in orthodontics will be touched upon briefly in this section.

7.2 Cone Beam Computed Tomography (CBCT)

The advancement in technology and the invention of Cone Beam Computed Tomography (CBCT) provided a great alternative to CT. Some of the key advantages of CBCT over CT are that CBCT has a relatively lower radiation dose and cost, a significantly smaller footprint, and the acquisition and reconstruction time is lesser. All this made CBCT gradually replace 2D imaging, particularly in cases with impacted teeth (Fig. 7.1) [2], eruption problems, root proximities, root resorption, TMJ issues, complex orthognathic surgery cases, and to locate and diagnose maxillofacial pathologic structures [3].

L. Dalbah (✉)
European University College, Dubai, UAE

© Springer Nature Switzerland AG 2021
P. Jain, M. Gupta (eds.), *Digitization in Dentistry*,
https://doi.org/10.1007/978-3-030-65169-5_7

Fig. 7.1 CBCT
demonstrating the location
of the impacted canine [2]

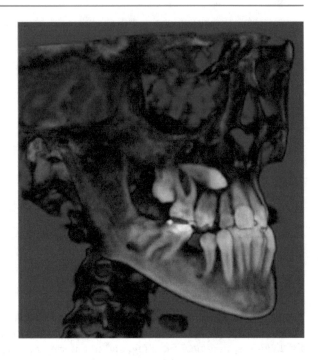

7.2.1   Additional Benefits of CBCT in the Orthodontic Practice

Apart from the additional advantages of CBCT for accurate diagnosis and treatment
planning, CBCT data can be used to [1]:

1. Design 3D guides for miniscrews placement which will help orthodontists avoid
   any damage to anatomical structures and reduce patient discomfort (Fig. 7.2) [4].
2. Analyze and monitor airway volume (Fig. 7.3) [2].
3. Monitor and study very accurately the skeletal and dental effects of rapid maxillary expansion or any treatment modality that expands the teeth transversely.

7.3   3D Facial Photography

Facial scanners provide a 3D topography of a patient's facial surface anatomy,
which when combined with digital study model and CBCT image will give a complete 3D virtual representation of the patient [3, 5].

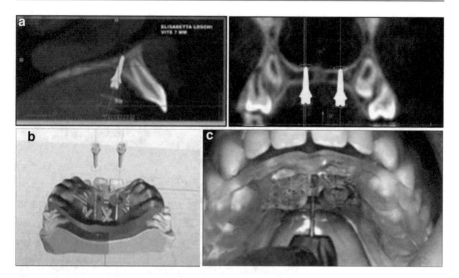

Fig. 7.2 (**a**) CBCT scan of tooth 21 superimposed on digital model of upper arch to identify ideal palatal insertion sites for two miniscrews (Reproduced with permission from [4]). (**b**). Three-dimensional surgical guide design. (**c**) Cylindrical guide removed with dental bur after miniscrew insertion. (Reproduced with Permission from Maino BG, Paoletto E, Lombardo L, Siciliani G. A Three-Dimensional Digital Insertion Guide for Palatal Miniscrew Placement. J Clin Orthod. 2016;50(1):12–22)

Fig. 7.3 3D image of the airway obtained from CBCT data [2]

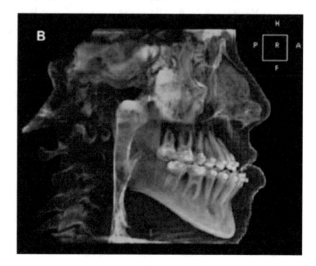

Fig. 7.4 Vectra M3
Imaging system (Adopted
from http://www.
canfieldsci.com/)

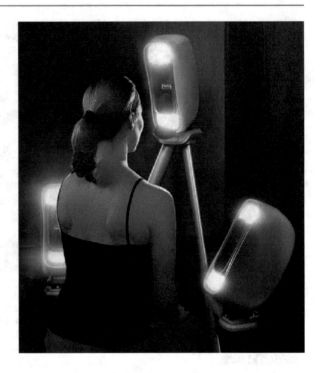

Facial scan can be generated within seconds either with a facial scanning machine like the Vectra M3 (Fig. 7.4), Artec Eva, and Arc Bellus 3D (Fig. 7.5), or can be created from the same CBCT scan like Planmeca ProFace, or simply using a smart phone app like Bellus 3D face app.

Clinicians and dental labs can use the 3D face as an integral part of diagnostic, surgical, and restorative smile design planning to accelerate high-value case acceptance and clinician approval. It is also a highly effective tool for preoperative planning and postoperative comparisons and superimpositions [6].

7.4   4D Facial Photography

There are certain limitations to 2D which are well documented. Using videos, evaluation of the motion of facial muscles mainly during talking and smiling was undertaken with some benefits but the main drawback is again 2D capture.

For this purpose, the motion capture stereophotogrammetry has recently been introduced to overcome the errors obtained from 2D and 3D still photography. 4D imaging allows clinicians to gain information and treatment plan based on a patient's facial animations and expressions rather than the static views. 3dMD-face™ dynamic system (3dMD, Atlanta, GA) and 4D capture system (DI3D™, Dimensional Imaging, Glasgow) are examples of commercially available 4D imaging systems [6].

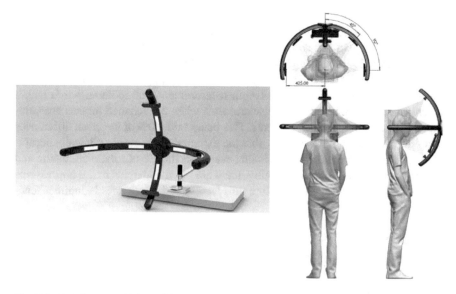

Fig. 7.5   Facial scanner (Adopted from https://www.bellus3d.com/arc)

7.5   Digital Model Acquisition

A digital model of a patient's teeth and oral structures can be acquired using three different methods:

1. Extraoral scanners.
2. Intraoral scanners.
3. Cone Beam Computer Tomography.

7.5.1   Extraoral Scanners

7.5.1.1 History

The primary purpose of digital model was to allow for easier storage of patient's study models. In the 1990s, Ortho CAD™ introduced digital model fabrication into dentistry. Ortho CAD™ was primarily a scanning center where stone models or PVS impressions were sent and processed into digital file that was downloaded to an orthodontist's office network. This has significantly reduced the need for large physical storage areas. By 2014, digital models were commonly used for diagnostic purposes in 21–55% of the US orthodontic practices [7].

Extraoral (EO) scanners offer an indirect method of obtaining a 3D digital model. Components of an extraoral scanner include: (a) a chamber with a platform, (b) a laser light source, and (c) a digital camera. Laser or white light technology is used to scan the impression or plaster model. The scanner is usually used in a laboratory setting where the impression or model, and bite registration is placed inside the chamber on the platform and rotates 360° allowing different angles to be recorded by a specialized sensor that gathers reflected surface data points from the object.

In terms of precision and accuracy, some studies [8, 9] showed significant differences in mesiodistal widths, arch length measurement, and tooth size-arch length discrepancy (TSALD) analysis measurements when 3D scanned models are compared to plaster model measurements. This being said, 90% of the mean differences were less than 0.20 mm, verifying that the extraoral scanners are clinically acceptable. One reason for inaccuracies is that even with the use of rotational feature and multiple angle views during scanning, there are often undercuts in the impressions or models that are difficult to capture thus leading to inaccuracies in indirect scanning techniques.

How to Choose an Appropriate EO Scanner

The different models differ mainly in resolutions and speeds. Accuracy of scans range from 15–200 microns, and speed for plaster model and impression scan range from 1 min 30 s to 7 min. Each scanner comes with a software that provides different features like digital storage of patient records, 3D cast analysis, and treatment planning features, such as tooth size measurements, landmark identification, arch length analysis, tooth segmentation, and evaluation of occlusion and occlusal contacts. Some software like Ortho analyzer feature sculpt and rebase applications with collision control, tooth movement simulation, superimposition of study models with photographs or DICOM data from CBCT images, and digital manufacture of appliances and restorations.

7.6   Intraoral Scanner

The intraoral scanner is an electronic device that emits a light source (which can be laser or structured) that captures the anatomical structures of the teeth and surrounding gum and creates a digital document of it in the form of 3D images (Fig. 7.6) [10]. This topic is covered in detail in Chap. 6.

7.6.1   Scanners in Orthodontics Today

7.6.1.1 Precision and Accuracy

Modern scanners' precision is equal to or even better than alginate impressions converted to stone casts. One reason can be the elimination of error during impression taking and handling and the other reason is the elimination of error that can occur during pouring and manipulation in the lab. The less steps we have, the less error we get [6, 11].

Fig. 7.6 Scan of the
occlusion (3Shape)
(Reproduced with
permission from John
Wiley and Sons) [10]

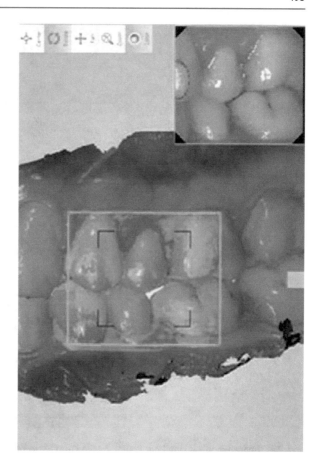

7.6.1.2 Advantages

Digitally scanned occlusal records have several advantages over traditional study casts, in that they are [3, 6, 12]:

- Accurate and simple to produce.
- Easy to detect and correct defects immediately which reduces the time lost in retake due to impression inaccuracies and distortion.
- Cause minimal patient discomfort, mainly in patients with gag reflex or kids who are apprehensive towards impressions or their taste.
- Eliminate the need to maintain the materials required for conventional impressions.
- Minimize disinfection and cross-contamination issues.
- Avoid the storage problems of plaster casts, the possibility of breakage or misplacement.

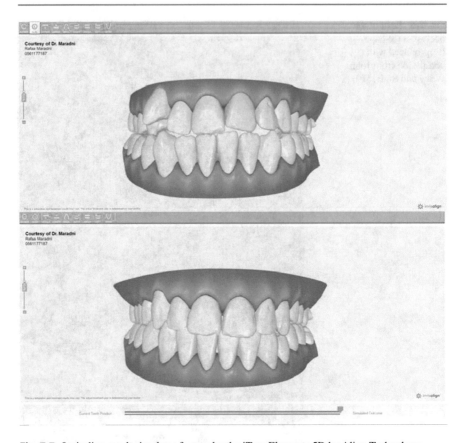

Fig. 7.7 Invisalign result simulator feature by the iTero Elements 5D by Align Technology

- Easily shared worldwide without the need for packing and shipping, which will save on time and shipping cost.
- Immediately available chairside for analysis and viewing.
- Faster to start treatment planning and model analysis like arch length, arch width, and tooth size Bolton analysis in speedy and more accurate method.
- Can be used in various orthodontic software to perform virtual treatment plans within minutes as opposed to diagnostic wax up. One example is the iTero Element 5D by Align Technology that provides Invisalign result simulator feature in which within 1 min after a full scan of the mouth is performed, the patient can see an example of a possible result after orthodontic treatment (Fig. 7.7).
- Facilitates better communication with other professionals mainly in multidisciplinary cases that needs restorative planning.
- Perfect marketing tool as it facilitates virtual treatment objective (VTO) communication with patient, visualization of treatment outcome, and help the patient better understand the treatment process.

With an intraoral scanner, orthodontists report improved diagnosis and treatment planning abilities, increased case acceptance, faster records submission to insurance companies, fewer retakes, reduced chair time, reduced storage requirements, quicker lab turnaround times, improved appliance accuracy and fit, lower inventory expenses, and reduced treatment times [13].

7.6.1.3 Disadvantages
• High initial and maintenance cost.
• Taking the bite registration can be an issue with certain types of malocclusion like posterior cross bite or open bite.

7.7 CBCT

The image of the dentition from CBCT can be used in certain cases, like (orthognathic surgery, dental impaction, and craniofacial syndromic cases) that require CBCT for diagnosis and treatment planning, or if the clinic adapted a protocol of replacing the 2D imaging (panoramic/cephalometric) by CBCT.

If one does acquire a CBCT scanned image, the CBCT images can be merged with the STL files from digital intraoral scans to create a 3D image of the dentition as well as the corresponding bone and root. This will allow the clinician to monitor the roots movement during treatment by retaking IO scans and superimposing them on the initial scan to monitor root movement [14]. The merged CBCT and STL files can also facilitate the creation of surgical guides, placement of temporary anchorage devices (TADs), and exposure of impacted teeth.

7.8 3D Printing

3D printing or additive manufacturing is a process of making three-dimensional solid objects from a digital file. It is the opposite of subtractive manufacturing, in which a block of material is carved away to form the object (as with milling units such as the chairside economical restoration of aesthetic ceramics, or CEREC).

7.8.1 History

In 1984, Chuck Hull developed 3D printing, also known as additive manufacturing, when he was using ultraviolet light to cure tabletop coatings. He established the 3D Systems Company in 1986 and created the first machine for rapid prototyping, which he called stereolithography (SLA) [15].

7.8.2 3D Printing Technologies

The most common technologies used for 3D printing today are stereolithography (SLA) and digital light processing (DLP) [16]. Some of the materials that are used in 3D printers are plastic, cobalt, nickel, steel, aluminum, and titanium. The print medium is either in liquid form or unwound from a spool.

7.9   Digitization and Direct Appliance Manufacture

Over the course of the past decade, the dental industry has been revolutionized by computer-aided design/computer-aided manufacturing (CAD/CAM) and 3D printing technology. Used in conjunction with intraoral scanning, 3D printing offers more efficiency in orthodontic practices and laboratories through fabrication of study models, aligners, acrylic and metal appliances, and indirect bonding trays. All this brought a new level of speed and ease to old procedures [13, 16].

The digitization process requires the dentition and soft tissues to be accurately captured by an intraoral scan or produced with a lab scanner from the impression tray/gypsum cast directly, allowing the acquired 3D data to be used to design and manufacture any type of appliance. The output from IO/EO scanners is usually saved in stereo lithographic (STL) format. Most software systems allow access to these files, enabling import and manipulation of the 3D data to design the appliance as desired.

7.10   Study Models

A rapidly advancing digital technology in orthodontics is 3D modelling and printing, prompting a transition from a more traditional clinical workflow toward an almost exclusively digital format. Digital models of the patient dentition and oral structures can be created either indirectly from a patient's models or impressions using an extraoral scanner, or directly from the patient's oral cavity using an intraoral scanner.

Most clinicians are satisfied with manipulating and analyzing digital models and will not request a printed 3D model for case study except in complex cases or in a teaching environment where it can be challenging to manipulate the digital models to discuss and explain treatment plans to students or patients [17] (Fig. 7.8).

7.11   Aligners

Clear aligner therapy (Fig. 7.9) with Invisalign introduced by Align Technology in the late 1990s led the way in using a virtual model, creating a virtual treatment plan (Fig. 7.10), and manufacturing appliances from digital models. Nowadays, many companies, like clear correct, 3 M™ Clarity™ Aligners, Eon aligners, and many

Fig. 7.8   3D printed
study model

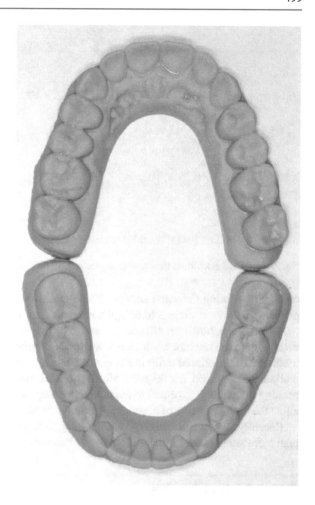

Fig. 7.9   Clear aligner

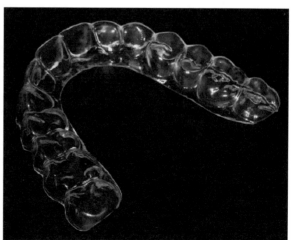

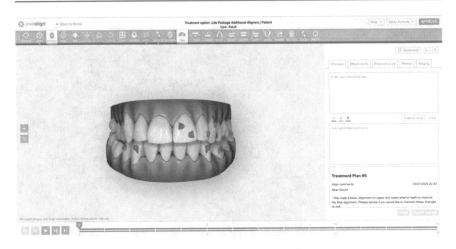

Fig. 7.10 ClinCheck virtual treatment plan platform by Invisalign

others are offering the same service. The digital workflow of CAD/CAM and 3D printer will allow clinicians to design and create their own in-house aligners [3].

At this stage, however, aligners are still molded on individual printed models of every step in the sequence, which is a waste of 3D printed material, as thousands of tooth arches are printed daily in many orthodontic clinics and laboratories, without a stipulated regimen for disposal afterwards. Advancement in biocompatible 3D printing materials is expected to overcome this step in the very near future as it will allow the direct printing of aligners without the need for printed models.

Recently, digital smile design is being integrated with virtual aligners' treatment plan software in order to plan the treatment based on the best smile for the patient.

7.12 Custom Brackets

7.12.1 Lingual Brackets

Customization of brackets started with lingual appliances over 15 years ago when Dr. Wiechmann created a fully customized lingual appliance Incognito (3 M Unitek, Monrovia, CA) (Fig. 7.11).

A virtual setup is created to achieve the treatment outcome, then fully customized brackets are digitally designed to fit the lingual surface of the teeth, then they are 3D printed in wax, and then cast in gold. The wires are then robotically bent to fit the individual arch form and to achieve the desired treatment outcome. The result is a fully customized lingual appliance with a low profile that closely mimics the lingual tooth surfaces, with a high degree of precision, and reduced tongue discomfort [18].

The orthodontist has the option to either do direct bonding of the brackets, due to the extended customized base, which permits clear-cut positioning on the tooth, or

Fig. 7.11 Lingual
orthodontic treatment

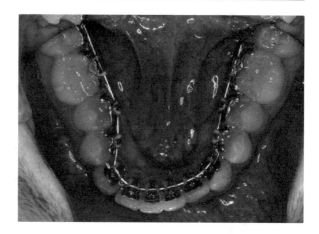

Fig. 7.12 Two-phase
silicone bonding tray with
pre-coated lingual
brackets. (Reproduced with
permission from Am J
Orthod Dentofac Orthop,
American Association of
Orthodontists) [18]

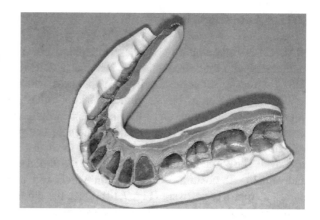

to do indirect bonding with the two-phase silicon bonding trays (Fig. 7.12) [18], which is the more time-saving option and will reduce the possibility of saliva contamination. This technology has overcome the many disadvantages that orthodontists faced with lingual braces like the substantially higher bracket loss compared to labial cases, the complexity and imprecision of indirect rebonding technique, the time-consuming finishing process, and the overall less quality compared to labial cases [19].

When accuracy in tooth positioning with a fully customized lingual orthodontic appliance, Incognito (3 M Unitek, Monrovia, CA), was studied it showed accuracy in achieving the goals planned at the initial setup, except for the full amount of planned expansion and the inclination at the second molars [20, 21]. Several other fully customizable lingual appliances have since been developed around the world and in popular use among orthodontists today, such as SureSmile (Orametrix, Inc., Richardson, TX), STb (Scuzzo-Takemoto bracket; Ormco, Orange, CA), in-Ovation L (Dentsply Sirona GAC, York, PA), and even self-ligating systems such as Harmony (American Orthodontics Corporation, Sheboygan, WI) and Alias (Ormco).

Fig. 7.13 INBRACE
looped round archwires
(Adopted from https://
inbrace.com)

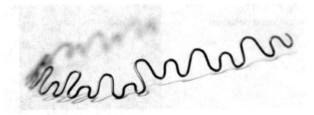

The newest fully customized lingual appliance today, INBRACE (Swift Health Systems, Inc., Irvine, CA), is a unique and innovative lingual orthodontic solution consisting of looped round arch wires (Fig. 7.13). The loops at the interproximal extend gingivally, allowing patients to floss freely and maintain a healthy periodontal condition.

7.12.2 Labial Brackets

CAD/CAM orthodontic appliances technology has also been utilized for labial appliances with the introduction of Insignia by ORMCO (Ormco, Glendora, CA, USA) as a system of customized labial appliances, which are then indirectly bonded.

The process begins by the clinician taking either a polyvinyl siloxane (PVS) impression or intraoral scan of the patient's dentition, which is sent to Ormco® for creation of digital models of the dental arches. The technicians then complete a virtual setup for ideal occlusion and arch form that is sent to the clinician for approval. The clinician can then manipulate the digital setup to achieve the intended individual tooth position, occlusion, smile arch, and arch form utilizing Ormco®'s Insignia Approver software (Fig. 7.14). Once the clinician approves the treatment virtual setup, then they select their preferred bracket system [22, 23].

The Insignia system is then reverse engineered, to achieve the final result, in one of several ways depending on the clinician's choice of bracket. If metal twin brackets are selected, then they are individualized by precision-cutting the slots in the milled-in faces, while metal self-ligating brackets are customized by varying the thickness and angulations of the bracket base. The selection of ceramic twin or self-ligating brackets limits the amount of customization that can be achieved; however, this can be overcome by matching the prescriptions of stock brackets as closely as possible to the Insignia virtual prescriptions and compensating for any differences with adjustments to the positioning jigs and custom-formed arch wires [22].

The final step of the Insignia system is milling bracket transfer jigs to fit the occlusal surfaces of the teeth, allowing for simple and reliable placement of the appliances and to ensure maximum effectiveness of the appliance (Fig. 7.15) [22]. The jigs allow for three-quarters of the bracket pad edges to be exposed during bonding so that the majority of excess composite can be removed prior to polymerization, which minimizes composite flash cleanup time after the jigs are removed.

The system allows first-order compensation bends to be made in all types of metal wires, including copper nickel titanium, nickel titanium, stainless steel, and

Fig. 7.14 Insignia
pre- and posttreatment
virtual setups

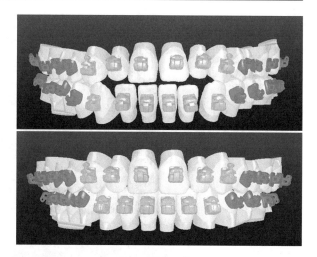

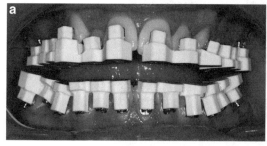
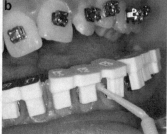

Fig. 7.15 (**a**). Insignia bonding jigs placed on groups of teeth. (**b**) Micro-brush used to remove excess composite before light curing. (Reproduced with permission from JCO. Gracco A, Tracey S. The insignia system of customized orthodontics. J Clin Orthod. 2011;45(8):442–51) [22]

titanium molybdenum (Fig. 7.16) [22]. The Insignia system True Roots offers superimposition of the patient's intraoral scan data and Dicom data from CBCT imaging, thereby enabling the doctor to see the root positions more clearly, which can be very valuable for treatment planning [24] (Fig. 7.17).

Ormco's Insignia system effectiveness and efficiency compared to the traditional twin appliances was investigated. In one study [25], the Insignia cases showed significantly lower ABO scores, a reduced number of arch wire appointments, and shorter overall treatment times. Whereas, in another study [26] CAD/CAM orthodontic appliances produce similar treatment outcomes compared with direct and indirect bonded appliances, CAD/CAM group had minimal shorter treatment times.

A recent randomized controlled trial (RCT) [27] evaluated the efficiency of the Insignia appliance and found no difference in the treatment time and final Peer Assessment Rating (PAR) score between the Insignia group and the control group. They concluded that "treatment duration and quality were affected by the orthodontist and the severity of malocclusion at the start of treatment rather than by the orthodontic system used".

Fig. 7.16 Customized arch wires with first-order compensation bends in upper and lower arches. (Reproduced with permission from JCO. Gracco A, Tracey S. The insignia system of customized orthodontics. J Clin Orthod. 2011;45(8): 442–51) [22]

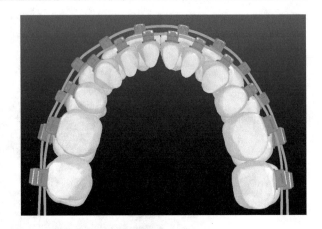

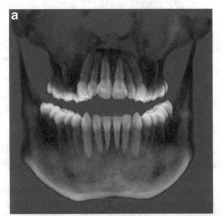

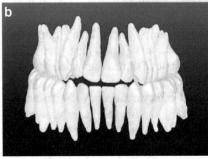
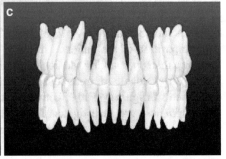

Fig. 7.17 (**a**) CBCT rendering. (**b**) Insignia system with Tru Roots (**c**). Setup with Tru Roots. (Reproduced with permission from Elsevier Publishing) [24]

7.13   Custom Wires

Although most orthodontists nowadays utilize a form of straight wire appliance, wire bending is still required sometimes during finishing and detailing stages of treatment. Many of the newer orthodontists, who have been trained exclusively on straight wire appliance, feel they lack the skills for accurate wire bending.

SureSmile system (Orametrix, Richardson TX) offers a unique approach to CAD/CAM orthodontics by providing robotically bent arch wires (Fig. 7.18) [3], which can be ordered at any time during the treatment to help finish the case to the desired outcome. Also, the fact that it can be ordered in any arch wire dimension makes it compatible with any conventional bracket system [28].

The process starts with an intraoral scan or CBCT of the dentition. The clinician has the option to either order the wires during treatment to help finish the case, or to order it before the bonding appointment, in which case a customized indirect bonding tray (Elemetrix IDB) can be ordered.

The data from the intraoral scan is used to construct a digital model of the patient's dentition. The teeth can then be moved to their desired final position. Once the clinician approves the digital dental setup, the software calculates the arch wire

Fig. 7.18 SureSmile System (Orametrix, Richardson TX) wire-bending robot (Reproduced with permission from Elsevier Publishing) [3]

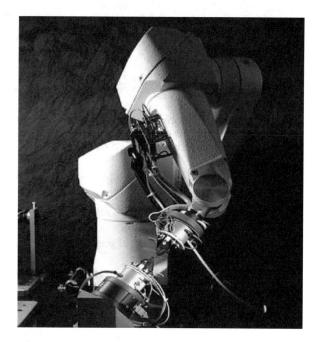

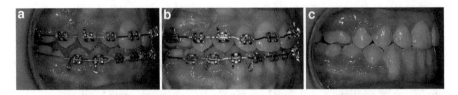

Fig. 7.19 Customized wires can be used to refine and detail a case (**a–c**). (Reproduced with permission from Elsevier Publishing) [23]

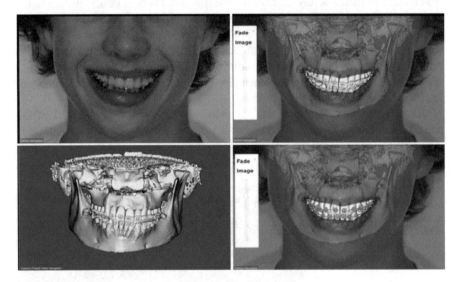

Fig. 7.20 Merging of the facial smile photos, intraoral scan, and CBCT data to create a model that can simulate treatment outcomes and mechanics. SureSmile System (Orametrix, Richardson TX). (Reproduced with permission from Elsevier Publishing) [3]

bends needed to create the final dental setup using the precise location of the bracket slot on each individual tooth [23] (Fig. 7.19).

Another advantage of the system is that CBCT data can be merged to give accurate root positioning and to enable working within the bony envelope of the individual patient. The incorporation of the facial photographs allows the smile design to be done in 3D [3] (Fig. 7.20).

Clinical effectiveness of SureSmile was studies by many researchers. One study found that SureSmile reduced treatment time by 7 months with better ABO score for alignment and rotations. However, the second order root angulation was worse when compared to conventional treatment [29]. Another study showed that mesiodistal and vertical tooth positions were found to be the most accurate movements with the SureSmile system, while crown torque, tip, and rotation movements were less predictable [30].

7.14   Indirect Bonding

Indirect bonding has been advocated for many years as a way to improve speed and outcome of orthodontic treatment; however, the technique is still only used by a minority of orthodontists. The reasons for this are sensitive clinical and laboratory techniques, additional step that takes time, cost, excessive cleaning of adhesive is needed, and the one heard most frequently is "fear of increased bracket failures." The latest advances in digital technology, such as intraoral scanning, 3D printing, and bracket placement software, made indirect bonding much easier and predictable procedure that is worthwhile for clinicians to explore.

The initial step after scanning and segmentation of teeth is to place the brackets on the virtual model (Fig. 7.21). The various software packages usually carry a multitude of bracket libraries that the clinician can choose from and allows different bracket

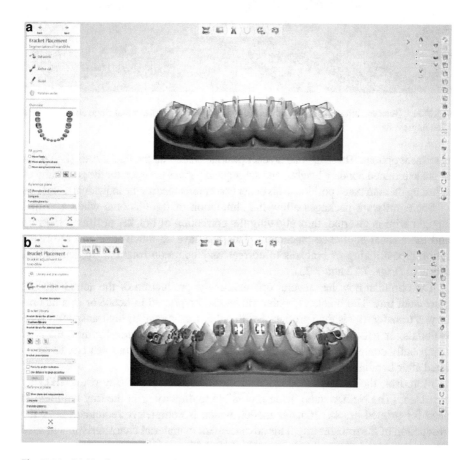

Fig. 7.21 (**a**) Teeth segments and FA points located by OrthoAnalyzer software. (**b**) Brackets placed on virtual models using FA points as guide

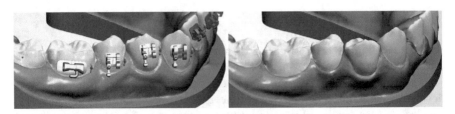

Fig. 7.22 Initial bracket using calculated FA points on the left. On the right estimated outcome with 0.019 × 0.025 wire in place showing incorrect marginal ridge relationships between second bicuspid and first bicuspid and molar

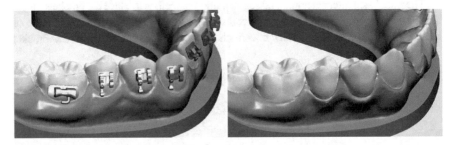

Fig. 7.23 Outcome after manual correction of bracket placement. Marginal ridge adaptation has been improved

placement options. These include bracket positions based on the Facial Axis (FA) point or predetermined bonding heights, and subsequently gives the operator the possibility of adjusting the automated position to his or her exact preference for the individual teeth [24].

Some software packages allow the simulation of the outcome when a virtual straight wire is inserted, thus allowing the correction of bracket positioning errors and more ideal appliance placement. This can save so much time and effort for future repositioning of brackets to correct very common rotation, tip, and height mistakes (Figs. 7.22 and 7.23).

The clinician now has several options for the production of the actual bracket placement tray. The bracket transfer model can be printed in-house or in a laboratory. A transfer tray is then produced with either transparent or nontransparent PVS materials, or with a commercially available pressure or vacuum-forming material that usually comprises an inner soft layer with an outer hard tray that can be separated after bonding to facilitate tray removal [31] (Fig. 7.24).

Moreover, the recent introduction of the indirect bonding tray resin (IBT) by NextDent (The Netherlands) made it possible to directly print the tray without the need for printed bracket transfer model, which is completely redundant after the production of the transfer tray. This advancement in material characteristic will save time and material cost and reduce waste (Fig. 7.25).

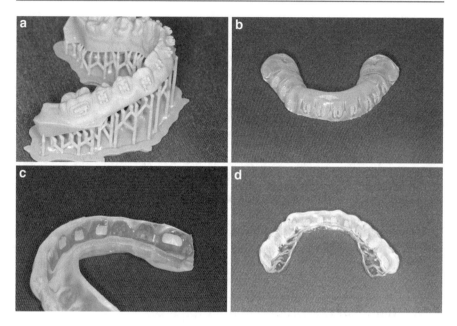

Fig. 7.24 (a) Bracket-positioning model, (b) Pressure-formed bracket-transfer tray fabricated in soft mouth guard material, (c) Metal brackets in transfer tray, (d) Two-tray method (Reproduced with permission from JCO. Christensen LR. Digital workflows in orthodontics. J Clin Orthod. 2018;52(1):34–44) [31]

Fig. 7.25 Internal view of the virtual indirect bonding tray with gingival open architecture for easy transfer tray removal

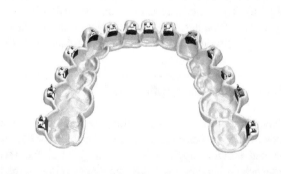

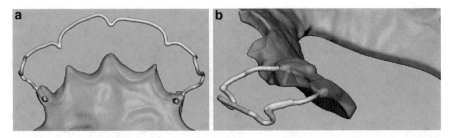

Fig. 7.26 The incorporation of metal components in removable appliances (**a**) Clay of the fitting surface of the base plate is shown in green. The tips of the fitted labial bow are inserted in the tubes. (**b**) The tags of the Adams clasp are fitted in the base plate (green). (Reproduced with permission from Am J Orthod Dentofac Orthop, American Association of Orthodontists) [11]

In summary, indirect bonding with this digital method is simple, predictable, and thought to increase bracket positioning accuracy and thus reduce overall treatment times.

7.15 Removable and Functional Appliances

The introduction of biocompatible resins as 3D printing material made it possible to directly print and manufacture removable appliances without the need for plaster casts. Appliances that are usually made from acrylic can either be milled from polymethyl methacrylate (PMMA) or printed in biocompatible resin on a dedicated 3D printer. Appliances can be supplemented with ball hooks or other retentive clasps if necessary [11, 31] (Fig. 7.26) [11]. Functional appliances can also be manufactured digitally. The dental arches in normal occlusion is captured by IO scanner, followed by a scan of the desired postured position of the mandible. Those two registrations enable the production of a functional appliance [31] (Fig. 7.27).

7.16 Metallic Appliances

Recently introduced laser melting technology [32] made the direct printing of metallic appliances by either cobalt chromium or titanium a reality. Commonly used banded metallic appliances such as Quad Helix, Hyrax expander, lingual arch, transpalatal bar, and the Herbst appliance required the placement of separators followed by bands fitting and analogue impression. This process can be more efficient with digital technology.

The process starts by the STL file of the dentition being imported from IO/EO scanner to a software where it is possible to manipulate three-dimensional files. In this virtual space, the orthodontic appliance can be designed as desired. Molar bands can have the same shape as a classic molar band, just not passing through the contact points to the neighboring tooth (Fig. 7.28), or like a C-clasp shape from partial prosthodontics (Fig. 7.29) [32]. In order to join metal pieces of an appliance, laser welding is preferable to soldering because the precise placement of the energy spot and low

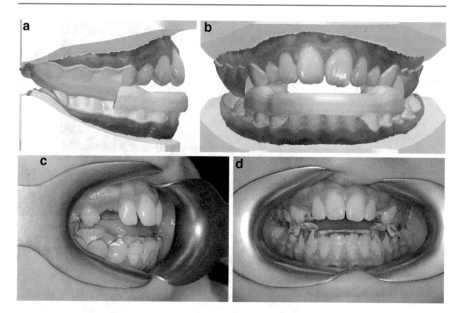

Fig. 7.27 (**a**) Side view appliance design. (**b**) Frontal view appliance design. (**c**) Side view 3D printed appliance. (**d**) Frontal view 3D printed appliance. Twin block style appliance designed using Appliance Designer (Reproduced with permission from JCO. Christensen LR. Digital workflows in orthodontics. J Clin Orthod. 2018;52(1):34–44) [31]

Fig. 7.28 Design of a banded tongue crib

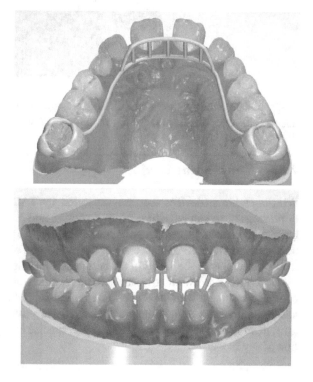

Fig. 7.29 Lingual arch with open molar-band design for improved cleaning. (Reproduced with Permission from Elsevier Publishing) [32]

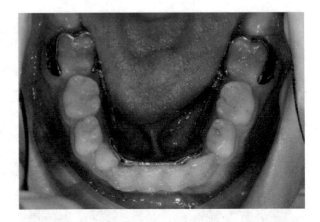

Fig. 7.30 Laser welding done directly on printed model (Reproduced with permission from JCO) (Groth C, Kravitz ND, Shirck JM. Incorporating three-dimensional printing in orthodontics. J Clin Orthod. 2018;52(1): 28–33) [33]

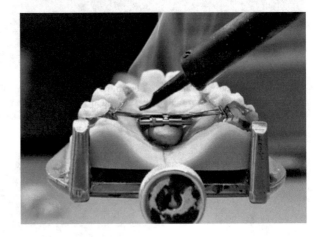

heat application reduce the chance of model distortion, so that the printed model does not need to be replicated in gypsum [32, 33] (Fig. 7.30 [33] & Fig. 7.31 [32]).

7.17 Bone-Borne Devices

With bone-borne devices that are supported by TADs, an intraoral scan/digital printer workflow can be used not only to design and produce the palatal appliance, but also to create a placement guide that simplifies the procedure. Also, combining intraoral scans and CBCT data enables the production of implant insertion guides to insure placement of the TADs in the best possible locations [31] (Fig. 7.32).

There are a number of advantages to this digital workflow; it eliminates the discomfort associated with separation and impression taking and reduces chair time and the number of appointments. Moreover, the virtual appliance design allows great flexibility in appliance design with very precise fitting and without the production of any models.

Fig. 7.31 Hyrax close-up after laser melting and sintering (Reproduced with Permission from Elsevier Publishing) [32]

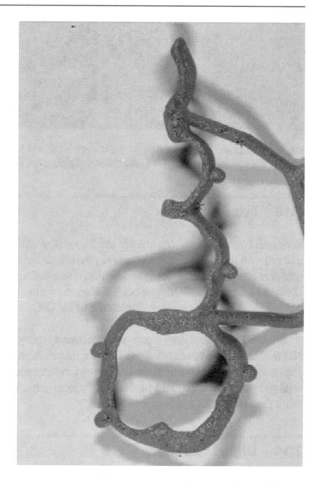

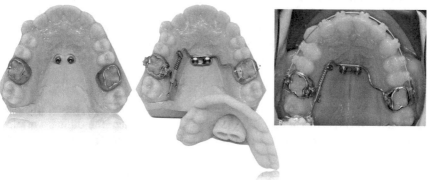

Fig. 7.32 Three-dimensionally designed and manufactured hybrid molar distalization appliance and drill guide for placement of two supporting Benefit temporary anchorage devices. (Reproduced with permission from JCO. Christensen LR. Digital work flows in orthodontics. J Clin Orthod. 2018;52(1):34–44) [31]

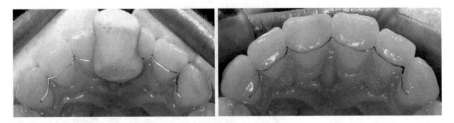

Fig. 7.33 Indirect bonding jig with MEMOTAIN CAD/CAM retainer before and after cementation showing optimal fit (Adopted from https://ca-digit.com/en/products/memotain/)

7.18 Fixed Retainers

Permanent retainers are commonly used by many clinicians to stabilize treatment outcomes in the anterior teeth. It is now possible to design and fabricate CAD/CAM retainers based on a scan from the dentition either before or after braces are removed. If the scan is taken with lingual braces, then the software has the feature of removal of the braces virtually and the fabrication of CAD/CAM retainer to be ready on the day of the debond [34].

MEMOTAIN® retainers are manufactured using the shape-memory alloy NITINOL and as a result are much thinner, more adapted to the tooth surface, allow physiologic tooth movement, and are more comfortable in contrast to conventional retainers. Once it is brought to shape, this innovative material cannot be bent any more [35] (Fig. 7.33).

7.19 Digital Workflow

There are numerous advantages to converting to a fully digital workflow. Elimination of traditional impressions and dental-cast production stages enhance practice efficiency, patient comfort, avoidance of impression redundancy and the need for band fitting, elimination of shipping expenses, delays, and model breakage; shorter laboratory turnaround time; improved office cleanliness; and better communication with the laboratory technician [17].

Patient digital impressions are stored in a more convenient way and can be easily transferred to any lab or an in-office milling machine for a simpler, faster, and more predictable appliance fabrication (Fig. 7.34). Simply stated, the digital workflow promotes both patient comfort and practice efficiency. Moreover, it meets the demand of multiple-doctor practices and multiple practice locations.

On the other hand, a limitation of digital dentistry is the high cost, not only in devices, but also in software subscription, updates, and trainings for the medical staff who work with them.

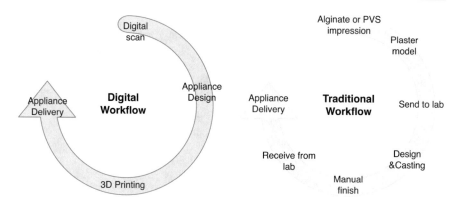

Fig. 7.34 Traditional versus digital workflow in the orthodontic office

7.20 Apps

As of the latest review in 2019, a total of 354 orthodontic apps exist across both the iOS and Android platforms. These apps could be classified as patient education apps, patient management apps, diagnostic apps, and updating apps [36]. These apps can either be paid or free (Table 7.1).

The currently available orthodontic apps are useful for clinicians as well as patients and are as varied as practice management, peer-reviewed journals, diagnostic apps, orthodontic education, patient reminder apps, progress trackers, model analysis apps, public awareness information, fun with braces, and many others [37–41].

7.21 Tele-Orthodontics and Remote Monitoring

Tele-orthodontics is a broad term that encompasses the use of information technology and telecommunications to provide remote orthodontic consultation, care, advice, or treatment virtually rather than direct personal contact. This could be especially important in areas with limited access to orthodontic care. Similarly, those who travel frequently or have busy schedules can benefit tremendously from remote monitoring. In this way, patients are not required to attend the office physically until an adjustment is necessary, which for the busy patient and family can make treatment less taxing on their time and transportation costs, and for the orthodontic office it can free up significant chair time commonly used for progress checks [42].

Other advantages of remote monitoring include earlier diagnoses, reduction of overall treatment time via early interception of problems such as non-tracking aligners, debonded brackets or broken appliances, allowing for such problems to be

Table 7.1 Orthodontic A

Category	Apps	Description
Patient education	BraceMate	Allows the patient to choose the color of their braces
	Teeth braces photo editor, Braces photo booth	Photo editor app to choose braces
	Braces help	Educates the patient to care for their braces
	Invisible braces scan	Patients can check whether they are suitable for invisible braces
	Orthoconnex	Allows patients to obtain consultations from orthodontists
Patient management	My orthodontist	Appointment app
	Skin n' smiles, milestone orthodontics	
	Smile-tastic!	Elastic change reminder app
	Remindalign	Aligner change reminder app
	Bracesetters orthodontics	Appointment, aligner change and orthodontic emergency app
	Brace off!	Progress tracking app
	Brace reminder	Appliance activation reminder app
	Smart smile	Aligner wear reminder app
Diagnostic apps	Ortho ruler, smart tooth	Tooth ratio calculating app
	CephNinja	Cephalometric analysis app
	One Ceph	
	MBT chart helper	Bracket positioning app
	Easy IOTN	App to calculate the index of orthodontic
	iModel Analysis 2	Model analysis app

addressed promptly. The dark side of tele-monitoring can be the loss of rapport between the patient and doctor, which might lead to loss of trust, and the legal issues of risking patient confidentiality due to communication of patient records over the Internet.

An important "application" (app) that facilitates this technology is Dental Monitoring (DM) (Dental Monitoring SAS Paris, France). It allows practitioners to remotely monitor patients' treatment progress. It consists of three integrated platforms: a mobile app for the patient, a patented movement tracking algorithm, and a web-based Doctor Dashboard where updates of the patients' progress are received [42, 43] (Fig. 7.35 [42]).

DM™ provides four tiers of monitoring, varying in their uses and monthly costs.

1. Pretreatment monitoring: aids in monitoring tooth eruption or Phase 1 cases.
2. Treatment monitoring: aids in monitoring all types of treatment including conventional, customized vestibular or lingual appliances and aligners [3] (Fig. 7.36).
3. Posttreatment monitoring: Allows for 2 years to monitor posttreatment stability.
4. DM GoLive™: DM GoLiveTM is a patented algorithm supervised by the DM™ clinical team that detects nontracking aligners.

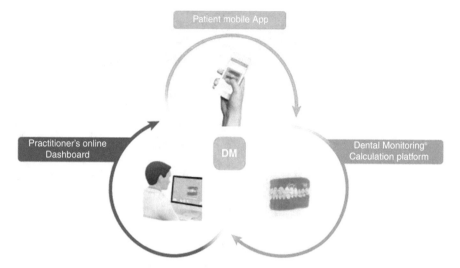

Fig. 7.35 Dental Monitoring consists of three integrated platforms: a mobile application for the patient, a patented movement tracking algorithm, and a web-based Doctor Dashboard. (Reproduced with Permission from Elsevier Publishing) [42]

Fig. 7.36 Dental Monitoring software analyzing tooth movement using artificial intelligence (Reproduced with Permission from Elsevier Publishing) [3]

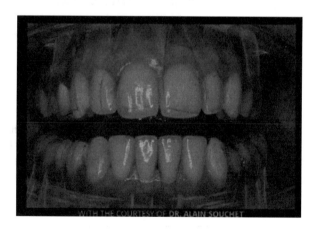

SuperPowerMe is another very innovative approach for monitoring facemask wear in children. It is composed of 3D-printed facemask, which makes the device customizable and comfortable to the child's face. It also incorporates sensors into the appliance that not only allows clinician to measure compliance but also to link up with a smart device application that turns to a computer game. By wearing the facemask, the child becomes a superhero who gains power by fighting against monsters and characters displayed on a smartphone application. This not only encourages compliance but makes wearing the facemask more fun and entertaining [44] (Fig. 7.37).

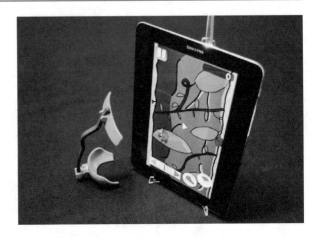

Fig. 7.37 SuperPowerMe facemask and game (Adopted from http://scfablab.unisi.it/?portfolio =superpowerme)

It is expected that the use of tele-orthodontics and tele-monitoring will increase during and after Covid-19 lockdown that affected most countries of the world and made it impossible for the clinician to meet face to face with their patient.

7.22 Do Yourself (DIY) Orthodontics

Digital technology is not without its dangers and negatives. The increased availability of 3D printers and digital tools made it easy for patients to attempt DIY orthodontics. There have been several new reports of patients attempting their own orthodontic treatment with homemade appliances.

Additionally, several companies are converting "patients" into "consumers" and establishing "direct-to-consumer" approach. These companies offer clear aligner treatment at a much cheaper rate than orthodontists and market directly to the "consumer". For example, in the UK, Your Smile Direct offers services that involve impression making at home with a DIY kit that arrives on request. This is followed by direct delivery of aligners without the patient needing to be properly assessed and diagnosed by orthodontists. This obviously involves high risk to the patient at multilevel [45].

7.23 Look into the Future

With the rapid increase in simplicity, availability, and reduction of cost of rapid prototyping and 3D printers, it is likely that future orthodontic offices will have desktop printers, and most appliances will be manufactured in-house with little need to pre-manufacture components. In-house robotic wire bending will also be common with wire bending robots becoming available commercially.

It is expected that every clinic will design and print their own aligners, mainly with the creation of direct printed shape memory plastics that will make the manufacturing more efficient and effective.

Smartphones are going to be able to perform accurate intraoral scans, maybe with an additional wireless small-size handle that fits intraorally, and it is likely that patients will be able to obtain scan of their mouths using their own handheld devices. This will facilitate simpler cases to be treated by either DIY orthodontic providers or automated services with mail order appliances and will make it possible to have retainers replaced remotely.

In the very near future, it can be expected that orthodontic specialists will only be required to be involved clinically in the management of complicated malocclusions, and that more work will be done in front of computers, tablets, and mobile phones than in the clinic.

7.24   Conclusion

Orthodontics is rapidly embracing new materials and advanced technologies, making the fully equipped 3D orthodontic office a reality. The incorporation of intraoral scanners and 3D printers enables an orthodontic office to transition to a completely digital laboratory workflow—a system that is not only more comfortable for the patient, but also more efficient for the practice. Furthermore, the software integration of digital models, 3D facial scans, and CBCT facilitate treatment simulations and establish a meaningful communication with patients.

The primary disadvantages of going digital is the significant investment, not only in devices, but also in software subscription, updates, and trainings for the medical staff who works with them. Nevertheless, new companies, scanner and printer models are emerging daily which result in significant decline of systems cost, and it is expected that 3D printers will become a standard piece of dental equipment in the near future.

References

1. Tadinada A, Schneider S, Yadav S. Role of cone beam computed tomography in contemporary orthodontics. Semin Orthod. [Internet. 2018;24(4):407–15. https://doi.org/10.1053/j.sodo.2018.10.005.
2. Ghoneima A, Allam E, Kula K, Windsor L. Three-dimensional imaging and software advances in orthodontics. In: Orthod Basic Asp Clin Considerations. 2012.
3. Tarraf NE, Ali DM. Present and the future of digital orthodontics☆. Semin Orthod. [Internet. 2018;24(4):376–85. https://doi.org/10.1053/j.sodo.2018.10.002.
4. Maino BG, Paoletto E, Lombardo L, Siciliani GA. Three-dimensional digital insertion guide for palatal Miniscrew placement. J Clin Orthod. 2016;50(1):12–22.
5. Almulla S, Premjani P, Vaid NR, Fadia DF, Ferguson DJ. Evaluating the accuracy of facial models obtained from volume wrapping: 2D images on CBCT versus 3D on CBCT. Semin Orthod. 2018;24(4):443–50. [Internet]. https://doi.org/10.1053/j.sodo.2018.10.008.
6. Starkey NE. The three-dimensional era of orthodontics: The past, present, and future of digital technology.
7. Starkey NE. The three-dimensional era of orthodontics: the past, present, and future of digital technology. University of Southern California Digital Library (USC.DL) 2017.

8. Cabral Correia GD, Lima Habib FA, Vogel CJ. Tooth-size discrepancy: a comparison between manual and digital methods. Dental Press J Orthod. 2014;19(4):107–13.
9. Kim J, Heo G, Lagravère MO. Accuracy of laser-scanned models compared to plaster models and cone-beam computed tomography. Angle Orthod. 2014;84(3):443–50.
10. Emilia Taneva, Budi Kusnoto and Carla A. Evans (September 3rd 2015). 3D Scanning, Imaging, and Printing in Orthodontics, Issues in Contemporary Orthodontics, Farid Bourzgui, IntechOpen. https://doi.org/10.5772/60010.
11. Al Mortadi N, Jones Q, Eggbeer D, Lewis J, Williams RJ. Fabrication of a resin appliance with alloy components using digital technology without an analog impression. Am J Orthod Dentofac Orthop. [Internet. 2015;148(5):862–7. https://doi.org/10.1016/j.ajodo.2015.06.014.
12. Baker SR. The cutting edge. Arch Otolaryngol Neck Surg. 1988;114(6):621.
13. Kravitz ND, Groth C, Jones PE, Graham JW, Redmond WR. Intraoral digital scanners. J Clin Orthod. 2014;48(6):337–47.
14. Lee RJ, Pham J, Choy M, Weissheimer A, Dougherty HL, Sameshima GT, et al. Monitoring of typodont root movement via crown superimposition of single cone-beam computed tomography and consecutive intraoral scans. Am J Orthod Dentofac Orthop. [Internet. 2014;145(3):399–409. https://doi.org/10.1016/j.ajodo.2013.12.011.
15. Hull CW. Arcadia, Calif. Apparatus for production of three-dimensional ob- jects by stereolithography, U.S. Patent No. 4,575,330, March 11, 1986. 1984.
16. Christian G, Kravitz ND, Jones PE, Graham JW, Redmond WR. OVERVIEW three-dimensional printing technology—JCO online. J Clin Orthod. 2014;XLVIII(8):475–85. https://www-jco-online-com.proxy.library.vcu.edu/archive/2014/08/475/
17. Evans C, Taneva E, Kusnoto B. 3D Scanning, Imaging, and Printing in Orthodontics. In 2015.
18. Wiechmann D, Rummel V, Thalheim A, Simon JS, Wiechmann L. Customized brackets and archwires for lingual orthodontic treatment. Am J Orthod Dentofac Orthop. 2003;124(5):593–9.
19. Rummel V, Wiechmann D, Sachdeva RC. Precision finishing in lingual orthodontics. J Clin Orthod. 1999;33(2):101–13.
20. Grauer D, Proffit WR. Accuracy in tooth positioning with a fully customized lingual orthodontic appliance. Am J Orthod Dentofac Orthop. 2011;140(3):433–43.
21. Awad MG, Ellouze S, Ashley S, Vaid N, Makki L, Ferguson DJ. Accuracy of digital predictions with CAD/CAM labial and lingual appliances: a retrospective cohort study. Semin Orthod. [Internet. 2018;24(4):393–406. https://doi.org/10.1053/j.sodo.2018.10.004.
22. Gracco A, Tracey S. The insignia system of customized orthodontics. J Clin Orthod. 2011;45(8):442–51.
23. Nguyen T, Jackson T. 3D technologies for precision in orthodontics. Semin Orthod. [Internet. 2018;24(4):386–92. https://doi.org/10.1053/j.sodo.2018.10.003.
24. Christensen LR, Cope JB. Digital technology for indirect bonding. Semin Orthod. [Internet. 2018;24(4):451–60. https://doi.org/10.1053/j.sodo.2018.10.009.
25. Weber DJ, Koroluk LD, Phillips C, Nguyen T, Proffit WR. Clinical effectiveness and efficiency of customized vs conventional preadjusted bracket systems. J Clin Orthod. 2013;47(4):261–6.
26. Brown MW, Koroluk L, Ko CC, Zhang K, Chen M, Nguyen T. Effectiveness and efficiency of a CAD/CAM orthodontic bracket system. Am J Orthod Dentofac Orthop. 2015;148(6):1067–74.
27. Penning EW, Peerlings RHJ, Govers JDM, Rischen RJ, Zinad K, Bronkhorst EM, et al. Orthodontics with customized versus noncustomized appliances: a randomized controlled clinical trial. J Dent Res. 2017;96(13):1498–504.
28. Sachdeva RC. SureSmile technology in a patient--centered orthodontic practice. J Clin Orthod. 2001;35(4):245–53.
29. Alford TJ, Roberts WE, Hartsfield JK, Eckert GJ, Snyder RJ. Clinical outcomes for patients finished with the SureSmile™ method compared with conventional fixed orthodontic therapy. Angle Orthod. 2011;81(3):383–8.
30. Larson BE, Vaubel CJ, Grünheid T. Effectiveness of computer-assisted orthodontic treatment technology to achieve predicted outcomes. Angle Orthod. 2013;83(4):557–62.
31. Christensen LR. Digital workflows in orthodontics. J Clin Orthod. 2018;52(1):34–44.

32. Graf S. Clinical guidelines for direct printed metal orthodontic appliances. Semin Orthod. [Internet. 2018;24(4):461–9. https://doi.org/10.1053/j.sodo.2018.10.010.
33. Groth C, Kravitz ND, Shirck JM. Incorporating three-dimensional printing in orthodontics. J Clin Orthod. 2018;52(1):28–33.
34. Wolf M, Schumacher P, Jäger F, Wego J, Fritz U, Korbmacher-Steiner H, et al. Novel lingual retainer created using CAD/CAM technology: evaluation of its positioning accuracy. J Orofac Orthop. 2015;76(2):164–74.
35. Breuning KH. Efficient tooth movement with new technologies for customized treatment. J Clin Orthod. 2011;45(5):257–62.
36. Phatak S, Daokar S. Orthodontic apps: a stairway to the future YR - 2019/4/1. Int J Orthod Rehabil.   (2 UL— http://www.orthodrehab.org/article.asp?issn=2349-5243;year=2019;vo lume=10;issue=2;spage=75;epage=81;aulast=Phatak;t=5):75 OP-81 VO – 10
37. Gupta G, Vaid NR. The world of orthodontic apps. APOS Trends Orthod. 2017;7:73–9.
38. Siddiqui NR, Hodges S, Sharif MO. Availability of orthodontic smartphone apps. J Orthod. 2019;46(3):235–41.
39. Singh P. Orthodontic apps for smartphones. J Orthod. 2013;40(3):249–55.
40. Pandey A, Mahajan S. Apps in orthodontics: a review. Int J Curr Adv Res. 2018;7
41. Sayar G, Kilinc DD. Manual tracing versus smartphone application (app) tracing: a comparative study. Acta Odontol Scand. [Internet. 2017;75(8):588–94. https://doi.org/10.108 0/00016357.2017.1364420.
42. Hansa I, Semaan SJ, Vaid NR, Ferguson DJ. Remote monitoring and "tele-orthodontics": concept, scope and applications. Semin Orthod. [Internet. 2018;24(4):470–81. https://doi. org/10.1053/j.sodo.2018.10.011.
43. John Wiley & Sons, Inc. Monitoring of tooth movement. Hoboken, NJ: John Wiley & Sons, Inc.; 2017. p. 55–63.
44. Fossati M, Marti P GCS. No title. 2018.; https://www.f6s.com/superpowerme.
45. Vaid NR. Commoditizing orthodontics: "being as good as your dumbest competitor?". APOS Trends Orthod. 2016;6:121–2.

Digital Occlusal Analysis and Force Finishing

8

Sushil Koirala

8.1   Introduction

Dentistry is one of the fastest-growing field in medical science due to the recent advancement in digital and materials science and technology. As dentistry progresses into the digital world, the successful integration of automation and new technology will continue to offer more competent, precise, and healthy treatment modalities for the patients. However, we need to understand clearly that any new science, technologies, and protocols in dentistry will only be successful if they are embraced and incorporated with a vision of achieving Quality of Life (QOL) through dentistry. In this regard, the contemporary dentistry demands well-considered concepts and treatment protocols that provide a simple, comprehensive, patients-centric, and minimally invasive methodology to achieve the long-term optimum results in terms of health, function, and aesthetics and high patient satisfaction at minimal biological cost. There are various practice philosophies in dentistry and, the author believes that the dentist has the full right to adopt the practice philosophy that he or she prefers. However, it is always advisable to apply oneself to understanding, analyzing, and comparing this philosophy with others.

Since early years of career, the author has been embracing the "Vedic Smile Dentistry," a holistic dental care and treatment approach, which is based on the Vedic philosophy of consciousness and natural harmony (Fig. 8.1), and the *Smile Design Wheel* (Fig. 8.2) protocol in daily practice. The Smile Design Wheel protocol [1] includes the components of psychology, health, function, and aesthetics (PHFA), which can guide clinicians to preserve tooth structure, prolong tooth

S. Koirala (✉)
Vedic Smile Pvt. Ltd, Kathmandu, Nepal

The Department of Vedic Smile Dentistry, National Dental Hospital Ltd, Kathmandu, Nepal

© Springer Nature Switzerland AG 2021
P. Jain, M. Gupta (eds.), *Digitization in Dentistry*,
https://doi.org/10.1007/978-3-030-65169-5_8

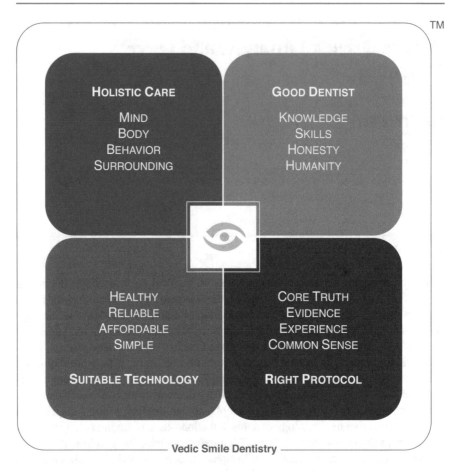

Fig. 8.1 Vedic Smile practice approach and its key components: holistic care, good dentist, right protocol, and suitable technology

longevity, reduce treatment cost, lessen the number of restoration replacement cycles in a lifetime, increase patient confidence and trust in the clinician, while enhancing the image of the profession during dental treatment. The wheel especially focuses on function as one of the critical factors for long-term clinical success, as it is directly related to the occlusion, which generates various forces and stresses that occur within the masticatory system of a patient.

This chapter focuses on the role of dental occlusion, occlusal forces, and occlusal forces diseases (OFD) that a dentist may encounter in daily clinical dentistry, and details how to integrate the Force Finishing concept and its protocol to diagnose, prevent, and manage the occlusal force disorders in clinical practice.

Fig. 8.2 Smile Design
Wheel protocol, suggesting
to consider psychology,
health, function, and
aesthetic components of
the patient during
diagnosis, treatment, and
follow-up visits

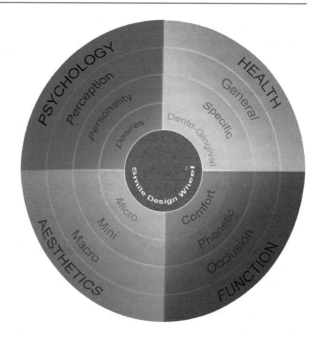

8.2   Dental Occlusion: The Foundation of Vedic Smile Dentistry (VSD) Approach

Dental occlusion has been, and is still to some extent, a controversial discipline, as there are numerous questions related to occlusion which have not yet been answered with scientific certainty [2]. There are many diverse and polarized opinions regarding this subject that are seldom based on current scientific evidences, such as the etiology of bruxism, the role of occlusion in Temporomandibular Disorders (TMD), orthodontic treatment, and its effects on TMD pain, and determining a correct mandibular position as a reference point for treatment [2]. When a dentist performs dental procedures like fillings, crowns, bridges, removable prosthesis, implant-supported restorations, full mouth reconstructions, orthodontics, occlusal therapy, tooth extraction, and so on, it may affect occlusion and bring some changes in occlusal force balance of the masticatory system of a patient.

The study of occlusion in dentistry has two components: the science and the art. Objective clinical issues like how teeth fit together, and how the forces or stresses generated within the masticatory system affect the teeth and supporting structures are addressed by the science component. However, the subjective response "feel" of the patient to their natural or therapeutic occlusion and its customized management by clinicians is more of an art than a science. Hence, the study of dental occlusion is always a mixture of science and art. With so many concepts and philosophies in clinical practice of occlusion, the question arises on *how to choose the best occlusal scheme for the patient?* Patients generally adapt to various occlusal schemes delivered by differing clinicians, which are based upon the clinician's knowledge, occlusal skill, and comfort rendering the occlusal treatment. Hence, in the clinical practice of occlusion in minimally invasive comprehensive dentistry, a clinician must follow the knowledge of scientific literature and research-based evidence, and use his or her clinical experiences and artistic skills to respect the patient's ability to physiologically adopt the new occlusal schemes.

Several reviews of the literature regarding the history of dental occlusion suggests that occlusion can be divided into three physiologic stages [3–6] and they are:

- Normal occlusion and commonly known as "physiologic" occlusion, which suggests that treatment is not required.
- Pathologic occlusion, also known as "non-physiologic," which suggests that treatment may be required.
- Therapeutic occlusion, often referred as to "treatment" or an "ideal" occlusion.

In clinical practice, there are three treatment categories routinely employed in occlusal treatment [2].

1. **Occlusal Maintenance**: This is the first category where the existing scheme of the occlusion is not changed, and only a limited number of restorations are introduced to a physiologically acceptable original occlusal scheme (Fig. 8.3).
2. **Occlusal Modification:** This is the second category where only minor or moderate changes or improvements are made to the original occlusal scheme but maintaining the original intercuspal position and vertical dimension of occlusion (VDO), that is either physiologically acceptable, or nonphysiologic and unacceptable (Fig. 8.4).
3. **Occlusal Reconstruction:** This is the third category where major occlusal scheme changes are made to improve a non-physiologic or unacceptable occlusion into physiologic occlusion by changing intercuspal position and/or establishment of new vertical dimension of occlusal (VDO) (Fig. 8.5).

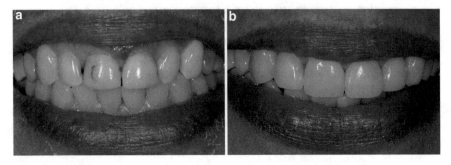

Fig. 8.3 (a–b) Example of occlusal maintenance category: anterior direct composite veneers with existing occlusion maintenance

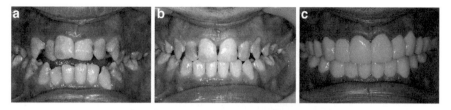

Fig. 8.4 (**a–c**) Example of occlusal modification but maintaining original vertical dimension of occlusion (VDO): orthodontics treatment followed by temporary restorations

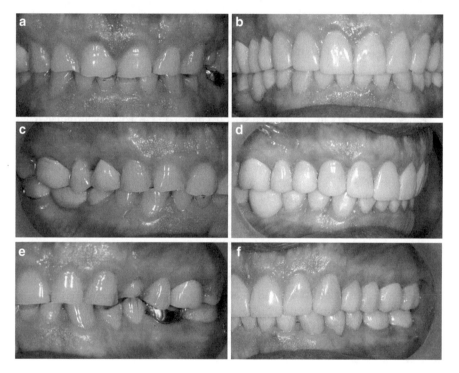

Fig. 8.5 (**a–f**) Example of occlusal reconstruction—non-prep restorations for dental occlusion reconstruction with VOD modification

Among three categories of occlusal treatment, the maintenance and modification types are considered easier to accomplish when compared to the reconstruction type, because the first two types are founded on preexisting intercuspal position (reference point) and the pretreatment vertical dimension of occlusion (VDO). However, when an occlusal treatment is required to convert pathologic occlusion into physiologic occlusion, then a new occlusal scheme needs to provide, requiring suitable changes on existing intercuspal position and/or vertical dimension.

At this stage, the original intercuspal position is no longer available for the clinician as the reference point. This is considered as a complex case in restorative dentistry and is one of the core clinical areas in the study of the art and science of

Table 8.1 Jaw position theories

Centric relation theory (Schuyler): The occlusion is determined by the manner in which the ligaments brace the components of the jaw joint, particularly the rearmost hinge axis [56]. There are various clinical techniques proposed to record centric relation (CR). The bimanual manipulation technique of Dawson [4], the Lucia jig, and the leaf-gauge technique, as reported by Long [149], are popular techniques for positioning the mandible in CR. Prior to this, chin-point guidance and swallowing techniques were used to locate and record CR
Neuromuscular theory (Jankelson): The occlusion is determined by gravity and based on the position in which the jaw muscles are most relaxed. Trans electric nerve stimulation (TENS) is employed to relax the muscles [150]
Intercuspal theory: The occlusion is determined by the habitual fit with the most tooth contact
Anterior protrusive position theory (Gelb 4/7 position): The occlusion is determined by the manner in which the muscles brace the components of the jaw joint. The Gelb 4/7 jaw position is found by using appliances to open the occlusion and reposition the mandible forwards and downwards of the true center of the glenoid fossa [150]

occlusion where many clinicians may become confused as to how to address different clinical situations with the best occlusal Scheme.

A new reference point needs to be selected based on the newly determined mandibular positions, which further adds to the confusion, based on the *Jaw Position Theories* (Table 8.1).

The newly selected mandibular position (position of mandibular condyle within the glenoid fossa of the temporal bone) directly affects the occlusion because the condyles and the teeth each occupy the opposite ends of the solid mandible. Every clinical case is different as it is related to a patient's status of health, their functional requirements, and their aesthetic needs and desires. Function is directly related to the forces that a patient generates within his/her stomatoganthic system.

There are four different theories that clinicians can view and think about occlusion. Each of these theories has its individual value, and treatments that are founded on each have been successful. These theories of occlusion differ in the consideration of where the jaw or temporomandibular joint should be positioned during the treatment. Despite their theoretical mandibular position differences, all of these theories have similar agreement on the following four concepts, which are related to occlusal contacts and occlusal forces [5, 7–9].

1. *How teeth should meet during mandibular closure*: All teeth should occlude simultaneously in mandibular closure movement.
2. *How the occlusal load should be distributed within the dental arch*: An equal percentage of occlusal forces should be shared between the right and left arch halves.
3. *How the occlusal load should be distributed on tooth*: An equal percentage of occlusal force should be distributed on each tooth's cross-arch counterpart tooth.
4. *Lateral excursive contacts*: Anterior teeth should immediately disclude the posterior teeth during excursive movements.

Based on the laterotrusive movements from centric occlusion, various concepts of functional occlusion were recognized and advocated as physiologic: balanced occlusion [10, 11] canine-protected occlusion [12–19], group function occlusion [20–24], mixed canine-protected and group function [25], flat plane (attrition) teeth occlusion [26, 27], biologic (multi-varied), physiologic occlusion [28]. However, no single type of functional occlusion has been found to predominate in nature, and there appears to be no scientific evidence to support one occlusal scheme over other [29]. It is, therefore, when selecting a suitable mandibular position for the treatment, the clinician must consider the possible clinical effects that the selected mandibular position will have on the final occlusion outcome, and the extent of the treatment required, and its biological cost to achieve the treatment goals. Hence, the Vedic Smile Dentistry (VSD) protocol advises to choose the most conservative occlusal treatment approach to lessen both the biological and financial cost of the treatment for the patient.

8.3   Occlusal Forces: Key to Occlusal Harmony

Dental occlusion should be observed as the relationship between teeth, masticatory muscles, and temporomandibular joints in a function and dysfunction that generates craniomandibular forces and stresses within the stomatoganthic system of a patient. If a clinician can appreciate the study of dental occlusion as an art and science of craniomandibular force balance, then it is much easy to apply practically in clinical dentistry to achieve optional oral health through occlusal harmony. The stomatoganthic system is a complex unit, consists of an interactive network of teeth, their occlusion and supporting mechanisms, the upper and lower jaws, the temporomandibular (jaw) joints, the muscles, the blood and nerve supplies, and the salivary glands, designed to carry out three major functions: mastication, swallowing, and speech. These functions are basic to life, but are also secondary functions that support in respiration, and the expression of human emotion. Utilizing coordinated muscle contraction, mandibular motion and craniomandibular forces are generated, which is then closely involved with the functioning of the dentition. The geometry of craniofacial skeleton with muscles attached, all are related to the tooth compressions that occur when the mandible is in motion, which generates occlusal forces between the mandible and the cranium.

8.4   Mastication and Occlusal Forces

Mastication is the act of chewing food [30] and is a complex function that utilizes not only the masticatory muscles, the teeth, and the periodontal supportive structures, but also the lips, cheeks, tongue, and the salivary glands. Mastication is made up of rhythmic, and well-controlled separations and closures of the maxillary and mandibular teeth. Studies have shown that during an act of mastication, tooth contact does occur, where few contacts occur when the food is initially introduced into the mouth, but then as the bolus is broken down, the frequency of tooth contacts increases [31, 32]. However, in the final stage of mastication just before swallowing,

Table 8.2 Function and tooth contact forces [34–37, 40]

Function	Occlusal force (kg)
Chewing	6.8–26.7
Swallowing	30.2
Maximum bite force	70–400
Parafunction	70–400

tooth contact occurs during every stroke but forces to the teeth are deemed minimal [33]. The amount of the force placed on the teeth during mastication varies greatly from individual to individual and multiple other factors, as shown in (Table 8.2) [34–39].

8.5 Swallowing and Occlusal Forces

The act of swallowing requires a series of coordinated muscular contractions that move a bolus of food from the oral cavity, through the esophagus, to the stomach and it consists of voluntary, involuntary, and reflex muscular activities. During swallowing, the teeth are brought up into their maximum intercuspal position (MIP), which well stabilizes the mandible by fixing its position against maxilla, so that contraction of the suprahyoid and infrahyoid muscles can control the hyoid bone during swallowing. There are two types of swallowing: somatic (adult) and visceral (infantile). In adult swallowing, the teeth are used to stabilize the mandible, but during infantile swallowing, the mandible is braced when the tongue is placed forward and between the dental arches or gum pads [40]. This type of swallowing remains with the child until the posterior teeth erupt. The occlusal forces produced during swallowing in asymptomatic adults are shown in (Table 8.2).

8.6 Speech and Occlusal Forces

Speech is the third major function of the stomatoganthic system. Controlled contraction and relaxation of the vocal cords and the bands of the larynx create sounds with the desired pitch. By varying the relationships of the lips and tongue to the palate and teeth, a human can produce a variety of sounds [41]. However, tooth contacts do not routinely occur during speech, such that no tooth contact force is generated during any act of speech.

8.7 Parafunctional and Occlusal Forces

As mentioned above mastication, swallowing, speaking, respiration, and expressing emotional expression are the vital functions of the stomatoganthic system. However, some activities are considered "nonfunctional" or parafunctional, and are popularly known as self-destructive oral habits. The following are the so-called parafunctional habits:

- Teeth clenching for long duration.
- Teeth grinding at night time as seen in bruxism.
- Sustained contractions of the muscles of mastication (without dental contact).
- Chewing of the lips, cheeks, or tongue.
- Tongue thrust.
- Nail chewing, cuticle chewing.
- Chewing foreign objects (e.g., pencil).
- Patient self-altering of their mandibular posture.

All these parafunctional habits produce some type of forces within the stomatoganthic system. However, their harmful effects depend upon the magnitude, direction, duration, and the frequency of the force applied to the system. Among these commonly observed oral parafunctional habits, bruxism and clenching are more important as they produce heavy occlusal forces within the stomatoganthic system, and these activities can occur subconsciously and the patients are often unaware about their active parafunction. In Vedic Smile Dentistry (VSD) protocol, the clinician must rule out and consider parafunctional activities such as bruxism and clenching during diagnosis, treatment planning, and execution. The occlusal forces comparison between functional and parafunctional activities (bruxism and clenching) is shown in Table 8.2.

8.8   Occlusal Force Harmony, Disharmony, and Disorders

When a person uses their stomatoganthic system for the above-mentioned activities and habits, masticatory forces generated are often disseminated through a series of complex physiological processes within the body. The physiological tolerance level (the resistive and adaptive capacities) of the patient plays a vital role in maintaining occlusal force harmony. If the ongoing disharmony of the occlusal forces exceed the physiologic tolerance limit of the patient, the system can breakdown, which usually begins with the "weakest link" like teeth, muscles, joints, or airway (TMJA complex) within the individual's stomatoganthic system, creating sign and symptoms of occlusal force disorder (Fig. 8.6). Hence, Occlusal Force Disorders (OFD) can be defined as "the disorders of teeth, muscles, temporomandibular joints, and airway (TMJA-Complex), resultant from excess occlusal force which is greater than the individual's adaptive capacity" [2]. There are four major occlusal force disharmony factors that directly or indirectly affect the force components of the masticatory system [2].
Morphological Factors:

- *Dental type:* Intercuspal position (ICP) contacts, the angle of tooth contacts, the type of tooth contacts presents in an excursive movement, the anterior-posterior contact location.
- *Condylar position:* The relation of mandibular condyles with the glenoid fossae.
- *Craniofacial type*: Dolichofacial, mesiofacial, or brachyfacial type affect the vertical dimension of occlusion (VDO) and directly affect the generation of occlusal force magnitude.

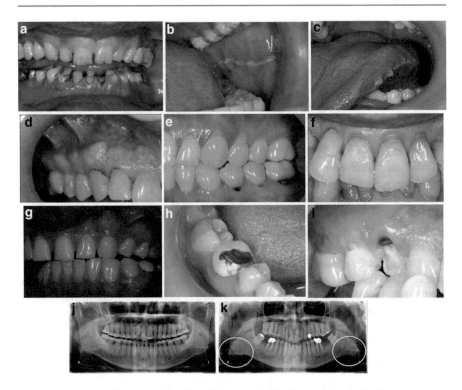

Fig. 8.6 (**a–j**) Some examples of Occlusal Force Disorders *(Image Courtesy Vedic Smile, Nepal)*.
(**a**) Severe attrition due to heavy bruxism. (**b**) Cheek marks (linea alba) resultant from heavy teeth
clenching. (**c**) Tongue indentation of a person with heavy clenching habit. (**d**) Exostoses formed
from heavy occlusal forces. (**e**) Cervical abfraction due to significant frictional forces on excursive
movement. (**f**) Cervical abfraction on anterior teeth due to deep bite and heavy forces. (**g**) Loss of
canine guidance and anterior teeth attrition. (**h**) Fracture of the ceramic layer of a PFM crown, due
to a concentrate of heavy occlusal force on the restoration. (**i**) Fracture tooth cusp due to high
excursive movement frictional forces. (**j**) Panoramic radiograph showing heavy bruxism. Note the
flat cusps and minimal enamel present on the posterior teeth. (**k**) Panoramic radiograph showing
prominent mandibular angles due to hyperactive masseter muscles

Pathophysiological Factors: Tooth decay and periodontal diseases affect occlusal
force balance due to the loss of tooth contact surface, periodontal supporting tissues,
and the tooth itself. Pathological conditions like upper airway obstruction may lead
to the various malocclusion, oral breathing, and sleep breathing disorders. Sleep
breathing disorders can promote parafunctional habits like teeth clenching and
grinding, which produce high occlusal force within the stomatoganthic system.

Parafunctional Habit and Psychosocial Factors: Parafunctional habits such as
bruxism and teeth clenching are thought to be closely related to various psychosocial factors like anxiety, depression, stress, emotional sensitivity, hyperactivity, and
personality type. These habits generate high occlusal forces within masticatory systems, leading to occlusal force disorders (OFD). However, in clinical dentistry, the
management of these parafunctional habits is the most neglected, thereby affecting
the long-term success of restorative dentistry.

Table 8.3   Clinical sign and symptoms of occlusal force disorders (OFD) [2]

	Teeth and periodontal complex
Type 1	**Teeth:** Excessive tooth wear (attrition), abfraction formation, tooth fracture, enamel cracking, tooth mobility, frequent restoration failure, implant prosthesis loosening, dentinal hypersensitivity, pulpitis, pulpal atrophy, pulpal dystrophic calcification, and tooth pain upon occluding **Periodontium:** Tooth hypermobility, gingival recession, thickening of the lamina dura, tooth migration **Alveolar bone:** Angular bone loss, the presence of tori and exostosis, and dehiscence
Type II	**Muscles complex** **Masticatory muscles:** Tender to palpation, masticatory muscle hypertrophy, muscle in coordination, muscle fatigue, muscle hyperactivity, pain, discomfort, and reduced range of mandibular motion, temporal headache, and earache **Lips, cheek, and tongue:** Cheek mark (linea alba), traumatic ulcers, tongue indentation
Type III	**Mandible and joint complex** **Mandible and TM joint**: Movement deviation, internal disk derangement, clicking sounds, structural deformation, maxilla-mandibular TM joint asymmetry, TM joint discomfort and pain, TM joint degenerative changes, and locking and dislocation
Type IV	**Airway complex** **Upper airway obstruction and breathing mode**: The main characteristics of a compromised airway complex (upper airway obstructions and breathing mode) are the presence of hypertrophied tonsils or adenoids, mouth breathing, anterior open occlusion, cross bite, excessive anterior facial height, incompetent lip posture, excessive appearance of maxillary anterior teeth, narrow external nares, and a V-shaped maxillary arch

In Vedic Smile Dentistry (VSD) practice, the early recognition, correct diagnosis, and suitable intervention of occlusal force diseases is given a high priority. Hence, a detailed clinical history, thorough clinical examination, and suitable diagnostic tests are recommended to recognize the "weakest link" (the teeth-periodontium, muscles, mandible and joints, and airway complex) within the patient's stomatognathic system to develop a suitable treatment plan for long-term health, function, and aesthetics at minimal biological cost. The sign and symptoms of OFD [2] are classified into four clinical categories as shown in Table 8.3 for better understanding. It should be noted that the sign and symptoms of the differing occlusal force disorder types are not mutually exclusive but are interrelated [2].

8.9   Dental Occlusion Analysis: The Digital Vs Nondigital Approach

A primary principle of comprehensive dentistry is that all of the components of the masticatory system (teeth, soft tissues, skeletal structures, occlusal force disharmony, muscles, and joints) are intimately related and dependent on one another for ideal function [42, 43], and address both function and esthetics [44–46]. The Vedic Smile Dentistry (VSD) practice follows the psychology, health, function, and aesthetics as orders of the treatment steps while approaching any clinical cases in dentistry. Therefore, some typical examples of dental disturbances linked to dental occlusion can be bruxism, attrition, erosion, abfraction, muscle pain dysfunction syndrome, and TMJ problems [47–55].

Occlusal concepts are developed together with advances in the dental technology enabling improved restorative options. Fully balanced occlusion is required for complete dentures and was initially used with fixed restorations for a short time. This was abandoned in favor of "mutual protection," "anterior guidance," and "anterior disclusion." However, current concepts create a paradigm shift from "mutual protection" with "anterior disclusion" to a "selective excursive guidance" with "selective disclusion" guided by "individual clinical determinates" [10, 22, 56–58, 59]. Decisions for patient-driven therapy will need to consider the best therapeutic options for the particular patient, their quality of life, comfort, age, and health, psychophysiological, and psychosocial conditions. Excessively rigid concepts need to be avoided and decisions tailored to patient-centered needs and expectations [60]. Comprehensive dental occlusion analysis has four key areas in clinical examination and documentation: teeth fit, muscles coordination, joints stability and airway pattern, also known as the TMJA components.

- *Airway Pattern:* The dysfunction of human airway and breathing pattern can cause malocclusion and skeletal deformation [61–66].
- *Joints Stability:* The morphology and relation of temporomandibular joints position with glenoid fosse guides the joints stability, its movements in coordination with muscles and neurons.
- *Muscles Coordination:* The masticatory muscles in coordination with the neural system controls the application of force or load (magnitude, duration, and direction) over the teeth and joints.
- *Teeth Stability:* The number of teeth, position, and their morphology guides the maximal intercuspal position (ICP) of teeth stability (occlusal stability).

Priority is given to examining the joint stability to recognize the level of occlusal instability. The information on existing joints and occlusal stability quality is very important in establishing a correct diagnosis and suitable treatment plan. Hence, during dental occlusal analysis, it is necessary to find out the patient's true occlusion relation (CR) with joints, as occlusal contacts on a small number of teeth create discomfort, causing the patient to subconsciously shift the jaw to a habitual bite (Centric Occlusion) position where the upper and lower teeth are in maximum intercuspation. This subconscious mechanism is called the "Neuromuscular Avoidance Pattern" [67]. This mechanism prevents clinicians from seeing CO-CR discrepancies in the mouth at the time of the initial examination [68–71] and makes the clinician to believe that it is the patient's true occlusion relationship.

Various scientific studies have already proven that occlusal instability (malfunction) causes deflective temporomandibular joints (TMJ) positioning [71], which can lead to the development of tissue damage, such as the loosening of the ligamentous apparatus [72], inflammation of the capsular components, displacement of the condyle and articular cartilage [73], or in the worst case, resorption of the bony structures of the TMJs [74]. These kinds of tissue injuries can lead to symptoms such as muscle hyperactivity, neck pain, headaches, and other neurological symptoms such as muscle or joint pain and/or decreased range of motion of the mandibular movements in a very high percentage of cases [75–84]. Hence, dental occlusion seems to be a "fine-tuning" neurologic feedback system that guides mandibular movements against maxillary dentition [85–88]. At the same time, occlusal contacts (occlusal stability) seem to be responsible for maintaining the condylar position within a physiological range [89–92]. The extent of the dental occlusion examination will vary from patient to patient.

In Vedic Smile Dentistry (VSD) approach, a comprehensive occlusal examination (TMJA Complex Analysis) is advisable when a patient present with complex problems requires a planning of major restorative works with the change in the existing occlusal scheme and vertical dimension of occlusion. The comprehensive occlusal examination process begins with careful history taking and meticulous clinical examination. All sign and symptoms of OFD should be recorded, and any necessary investigations such as articulated study casts, vitality test, dental radiograph, and imaging (CBCT, MRI) and sleep analysis test may be prescribed for additional information. The patient's existing occlusal indicators should be documented as well as this assists in case monitoring and follow-up.

The chapter has introduced the concept of occlusion and its importance in diagnosis till now. The next segment of the chapter deals with performing occlusal analysis using digital and nondigital approach.

8.10   The Nondigital Approach in Occlusion Analysis

1. In nondigital approach, the status of existing static and dynamic dental occlusion is examined via different static dental materials such as articulating paper strips, shimstock foils, elastomeric impression materials; occlusal wax sheets are placed between opposing teeth to imprint, or mark with color, the occlusal contacts. These nondigital occlusal indicators are often combined with the patient's verbal feedback based on proprioception occlusal "feel," to guide a clinician in detecting heavy occlusal contact points. It is interesting to note that articulating paper mark size is widely used and accepted as an indicator of forceful tooth contact. This has been advocated in textbooks on occlusion [53, 93–96] as the paper mark area being representative of the occlusal load. The darker paper marks ("bull's-eye") indicate heavy load or excessive forces, and smaller lighter marks indicate lesser loads [53, 93, 94]. Additionally, the presence of many similar-sized paper marks spread around the contacting arches are indicative of equal occlusal contact intensity, and evenness, and simultaneity [96, 97].

However, recent studies have shown that markings seen on the teeth do not quantify occlusal forces or time sequence of the occlusal contact order, and that the ink substrate left on the teeth is not an accurate indicator with which to judge a tooth contact's relative force levels [52, 98–100]. To date, the literature offers no evidence to suggest that variable articulation paper mark shape and size can describe varying occlusal contact forces in any predictable way [52, 98–102]. Articulators may be the most useful tools for the production of dental restorations, but they cannot simulate the neuromuscular mechanism [103].

In summary, occlusal indicators such as articulating paper strips, shimstock foils, elastomeric impression materials, occlusal wax sheets marks specifically only indicate occlusal contact location and contact size, not occlusal force levels and contact timing durations [52, 98]. In addition, although, they print of the end of the occlusion, they cannot provide significant information such as which tooth is the first one in occlusion, which one is second, or which one is the last, and the force differences between these contact points. Hence, in contemporary clinical practice, reliability on only on a manual approach to occlusion analysis is questionable.

8.11   The Digital Approach to Occlusion Analysis

Digital occlusal analysis systems are the fastest and safest way to analyze the dental occlusion. If not intervened, all occlusal contacts can be controlled in detail and tied in sequentially together with relative force information. Analysis of the occlusion can be performed under maximum physiological conditions. Each intervention will be perceived by the neuromuscular mechanism, and the movement will not be a physiological function.

Digital occlusal analysis systems give the clinician control of extreme physiologic occlusion [104–109]. Digital Occlusion, started with the use of first T-Scan I system in 1984 (T-Scan 200, Tekscan, Inc., Boston, MA, USA). The earliest publication about T-Scan I system appeared in the dental literature in 1987 [110]. The development of this technology has required many iterations over the past decades beginning with T-Scan I, T-Scan II for Windows®, T-Scan III with turbo recording, to a simplified desktop version introduced in T-Scan 8, to the present-day version known as *T-Scan 10* (Fig. 8.7).

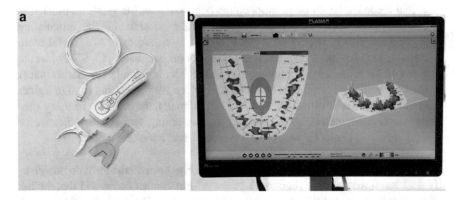

Fig. 8.7 (**a, b**) The T-Scan 10 recording hardware components include the Novus recording handle, two sizes of plastic molded sensor supports and two sizes of the High Definition (HD) Novus-specific sensors *(Photos Courtesy of Tekscan™, Inc.)*

Since mid-1985, numerous authors have studied the various T-Scan versions and have clinically validated the T-Scan sensor's occlusal force reproduction and its timing quantification in literatures [111–120], which inspired the manufacturer to improve the hardware components and the system's recording sensors, to be more accurate, repeatable, and precise. A reliable recording methodology and definitive treatment protocols have been developed and tested in research environments [2, 121–132]. With the popularity of digital occlusion concept in dental medicine, now there is a high demand for simple and cost-effective, yet predictable digital occlusion product in the global market. This led to the development of a new digital occlusion product in 2019, **OccluSense®** by Bausch GmbH & Co. KG (Fig. 8.8).

The new system developed by Bausch combines the traditional tooth marking and digital registration of the pressure distribution on occlusal surfaces together. The device is being used in combination with a 60 microns thin single-use pressure sensor color coated in red, which is applied exactly like a conventional occlusion test foil. The patient masticatory pressure distribution is recorded digitally in 256 pressure levels and later transmitted to the OccluSense application software for further evaluation. The recordings are being stored in the patient management system of the application software and can be reviewed or exported at any time. The company has marketed the device as electronic articulating paper.

However, the author prefers to categorize it as digital articulating paper as the device can provide tooth contact location with red ink mark on the tooth and with relative pressure. Furthermore, there is no need to use another set of conventional articulating paper to correlate the digital tooth contacts location. The author believes that, due to its ability to provide only two basic occlusion information, that is, tooth contact location and tooth contact relative pressure, it could be very useful for day-to-day simple to moderate cases of checking teeth contact location and their relative

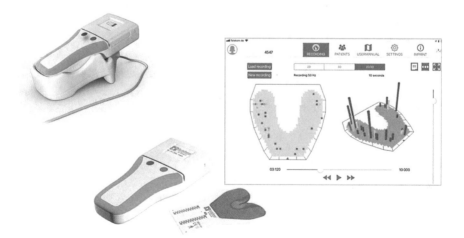

Fig. 8.8 The Occlusense recording handle and an unused recording sensor *(Image Courtesy by Bausch GmbH & Co. KG, Germany)*

pressure. OccluScense system is a relatively new invention with not much research or evidence base to its credit.

For complex occlusal treatment cases, a clinician may need to gather all fundamental occlusal information during diagnosis, treatment, and follow-up to maintain, modify, or reconstruct new occlusal scheme to enhance the occlusal harmony. T-Scan system is capable of providing the clinician all such occlusal information if required. With more than three-decades-long history, the T-Scan system's has progressed incredibly, with rigorous testing, criticisms, and improvements of its different versions [60, 113, 114, 133–142]. The current version that is available in the market, T-Scan 10, can record 256 levels of relative occlusal force presented in a multiple spectrum of colors, while simultaneously registering the time sequence of occlusal contacts in 0.003 s increments.

Practicing digital occlusion by using precise objective data to isolate problem occlusal contacts is very different from practicing subjective interpretation, which uses ink marking materials and subjectivity to isolate occlusal contacts. For ease to understand the clinical capabilities of both digital occlusal-related devices presently available in the market, and to select them as per clinical requirement in the practice, a simple comparison between conventional articulating paper, digital articulating paper (OccluSense), and digital occlusion scanner (T-Scan 10) is shown in Table. 8.4.

The next section discusses the Force Finishing concept using conventional articulating paper and digital occlusal scanner (T-Scan 10), because the OccluSense device available in the market at present is not designed to measure *maximum bite force, occlusion time and path, disclusion time and path, a center of occlusal forces distribution, and habitual multibite pattern,* like occlusal parameters that are required for Force Finishing of complex cases.

Table 8.4 Comparison between conventional articulating paper, digital articulating paper (**OccluSense),** and digital occlusion scanner (**T-Scan 10**)

Dental occlusal analysis parameters	Conventional articulating paper	Digital articulating paper (OccluSense)	Digital occlusion scanner (T-Scan 10)
Tooth contact location	Yes	Yes	Yes
Tooth contact size	Yes	Yes	Yes
Tooth contact relative forces (pressure)	No	Yes	Yes
Tooth contact sequences	No	Yes	Yes
Occlusal force distribution	No	Yes	Yes
Maximum bite force	No	No	Yes
Occlusal time and path	No	No	Yes
Disclusion time and path	No	No	Yes
Center of occlusal forces distribution	No	No	Yes
Habitual multibite pattern	No	No	Yes

8.12   Force Finishing Concept and Protocol

The concept of Force Finishing (FF) and its clinical protocol was introduced by the author in 2011 to simplify the clinical approach of obtaining occlusal harmony in dentistry. Force Finishing is defined as a clinical concept and technique employed to optimize the occlusal force components of the masticatory system, using objective measurements of dental occlusal forces and timing. The goal is to obtain harmonized occlusal force and timing parameters, so that long-term health, function, and craniofacial aesthetics are maintained [2]. Fig. 8.9 explains the occlusal force harmony cycle and role of Force Finishing in reestablishing occlusal force harmony within masticatory system.

Case finishing is one of the important clinical steps in dentistry. The overall aesthetics, functional forces, and oral health are the three fundamental components that need to be considered during case finishing. Clinicians spend significant clinical time and effort on the aesthetic results, because aesthetic components are visible to the naked eye to both the clinician and the patient, where the outcome can immediately be appreciated. However, the force components are invisible, and their negative effects are not easily appreciated clinically, until the effects become chronic. Reliability solely on articulating paper marks for occlusal forces is common practice. Therefore, the occlusal forces and their harmony are the most neglected components in clinical dentistry. It should be noted that when the force components are not addressed properly during the treatment, clinicians may encounter various signs and symptoms of occlusal force disorders (OFD). Force Finishing should not be confused with conventional occlusal equilibration [43] or unmeasured occlusal adjustment procedures [126].

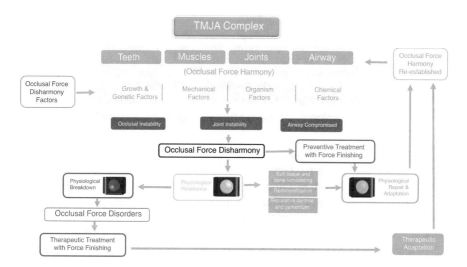

Fig. 8.9 Occlusal force harmony cycle: This schematic diagram shows the flow of occlusal force harmony and disharmony, occlusal force disorders, and the role of Force Finishing in re-establishing occlusal force harmony

Table 8.5 Force finishing clinical facts [5, 7–9, 15, 60, 137–148]

- Unilateral tooth contacts increase force in the opposite joint.
- Bilateral even tooth contacts during ICP give more stability to the teeth, muscles, and joints.
- When the number of occluding teeth increases, the total percentage of forces to each tooth decreases.
- The vertical forces created by tooth contacts are well accepted by the periodontal ligament, but horizontal forces cannot be effectively dissipated.
- Horizontal occlusal force should be directed through the long axis of the tooth (axial loading) as a goal of force finishing in the posterior teeth.
- Axial loading can be accomplished by cusp tip to flat surface contacts or by creating reciprocal incline contacts (also known as tripodization).
- The amount of the force that can be generated between teeth depends on the distance of the teeth from the temporomandibular joint, combined with applied muscular force vectors (fulcrum principle).
- The anterior teeth are not positioned well in the arches to accept heavy axial force. They are normally positioned at a labial angle to the direction of closure, so loading them axially is nearly impossible.
- The anterior teeth, unlike the posterior teeth, are in proper position to accept horizontal forces of eccentric mandibular movements.
- The anterior teeth should immediately disocclude the posterior teeth during excursive movements resulting in friction-free excursive movements that limit wear on teeth and activate low levels of excursive muscle function.
- The canines are best suited to accepting the horizontal forces that occur during eccentric movements.
- The canines have the longest and the largest roots and therefore the best crown/root ratio.
- The canines have surrounded by dense compact bone, which tolerates the forces better than the medullary bone found around the posterior teeth
- The canines are centered on sensory input and the resultant effect on the muscles of mastication. Apparently, fewer muscles are active when the canines contact during eccentric movements than when posterior teeth contact
- During force finishing of left or right laterotrusive excursive movements, canine guidance is the preferred excursive control in order to best dissipate any damaging horizontal forces
- When canine guidance cannot be achieved during case finishing, the most favorable alternative to canine guidance is group function
- The most desirable group function consisting of the canines, premolars, and sometimes the mesiobuccal cusp of the first molar
- Any laterotrusive contacts other than the mesial portion of the first molar are not desirable because of the increased amount of muscle force that can be created as the contact nears the fulcrum (temporomandibular joint)

The concept of Force Finishing is based upon normal human masticatory physiology and the occlusal force facts and the figures that were derived from various scientific studies as shown in Table 8.5. Force finishing plays a major role in establishing structural stability, by optimizing the occlusal force distribution during any dental treatment such as during a restorative case, or periodontal therapy, in prosthodontic reconstruction, after orthodontic tooth movement, or when using therapeutic oral appliances [2]. Among various occlusal components parameters, Force Finishing emphasizes on tooth contact location, tooth contact size, tooth contact relative forces, tooth contact sequences, maximum bite force, occlusal force distribution, occlusion time and path, disclusion time and path, center of occlusal forces distribution, and lastly the habitual bite pattern, as the key dental occlusion parameters, to be recorded and analyzed in establishing healthy, functional, and comfortable dental occlusion.

Based on the dental treatment categories (occlusal, maintenance, modification, and reconstruction) and the need of the patient, Force Finishing can be divided into two clinical types.

Preventive Force Finishing (PFF) (Table 8.6): It aims to protect and maintain a patient's physiologically accepted, original occlusal scheme, while preventing existing restorations and prosthesis, as well as any newly installed restorations, from failure by optimizing the occlusal force components of the stomatoganthic system.

Table 8.6   Preventive force finishing: Clinical protocol

Clinical steps	Dental occlusal parameter guiding tools	Dental contouring finishing and polishing tools
Step 1: During centric closure movement		
1. Bring all the teeth into occlusal contact by selective contouring (using additive or reductive methods)	Articulating paper	Force finishing kit (regular and smooth diamond points for reductive contouring)
2. Measure tooth-contact forces and timing sequences	Digital occlusion scanner (T-scan 10)	
3. Correlate the intraoral conventional articulating paper marks with the digital force and timing scan. Now by playing the recorded force movie frame-by-frame adjust early high-pressure points, one by one, based upon the digital force scan on occlusal contact timing sequence data		Direct composite resin for additive contouring
4. Equalize right and left arch-half force percentages		
5. Distribute nearly equal force percentage on each posterior tooth counterpart (i.e., left first molar region should nearly equal right first molar region force percentage), one by one		
6. Keep light tooth contacts (lower force percentage) in the anterior region, but there should be definitive anterior contact where possible		
7. Check the location of Center of Occlusal Forces (COF) distribution and bring it down the midline and to the center of the distribution of all contacting teeth		
8. Achieve simultaneous contacts of all teeth during mandibular closure and check occlusion time and path		
9. In case of implant restorations, selectively adjust the natural tooth contact timing and the implant-supported prosthesis from making contact until the teeth nearby to the implants, reach moderate occlusal contact force		
10. Check habitual bite pattern and changes you have made		

(continued)

Table 8.6 (continued)

Clinical steps	Dental occlusal parameter guiding tools	Dental contouring finishing and polishing tools
Step 2. During excursive and protrusive movements		
1. Check for opposing excursive frictional contacts using digital scan and record the right and left excursive movements, and the protrusive movements. Playback the recorded scan frame by frame and determine where prolonged excursive frictional contacts are present. Then use different colored conventional articulating paper to mark the located areas of opposing surface prolonged excursive contacts	Articulating paper Digital occlusion scanner (T-Scan 10)	Force finishing kit (regular and smooth diamond points for reductive contouring) Direct composite resin for additive contouring
2. Remove all prolonged frictional contacts on the restorations and/or teeth, so that the disclusion time is reduced and the excursive movement (disclusion path) becomes smooth and fast for the patient to accomplish		
3. Achieve canine-protected guidance whenever possible with minor selective coronoplasty, or by bonding composite resin to the lingual surface of the maxillary canines		
Step 3. Aesthetic finishing		
1. Aesthetic touch-up: Achieve natural surface details with necessary minor surface adjustments by placing texture, grooves, pits, and other special surface effects into the restorations.		– Force finishing kit (silicon finishing and polishing points)
2. Polishing sequence: *Pre-polishing:* Remove any remaining surface scratches that result from aesthetic touch-up process *Polishing:* Establish a blemish-free and smooth surface with no visible scratches present on the restoration. *Super Polishing:* Polish the restoration to an enamel-like luster		
Step 4. Finishing evaluation		
1. Evaluate the aesthetics, the health of the teeth, and the gingiva, and the overall patient comfort status	Dental loupe Digital photographic images Digital occlusion scanner (T-scan 10)	
2. Confirm the force finishing end results (tooth contact location, tooth contact size, tooth contact relative forces, tooth contact sequences, maximum bite force, occlusal force distribution, occlusion time and path, disclusion time and path, center of occlusal forces distribution, and habitual multibite pattern) by using digital force scan		
3. Document the final case finishing result with the digital force scan and digital photography.		

Table 8.7   Therapeutic Force Finishing: Clinical protocol

General clinical steps	Dental occlusal parameter guiding tools	Dental contouring, finishing and polishing tools
1. The occlusal load (force percentage) must be distributed as per the periodontal health, root and occlusal surface area available, and the available numbers of load-bearing teeth	Articulating paper Digital occlusion scanner (T-scan 10)	Force finishing kit (regular and smooth diamond points for reductive contouring) Direct composite resin for additive contouring
2. Reduce the occlusal load percentage on weak teeth that present with compromised periodontal bone support, are mobile, and/or present as painful or hypersensitive teeth, so as to support the natural healing process		
3. Remove excursive frictional forces on painful, mobile, and hypersensitive teeth		
4. In cases of masticatory muscle pain symptoms, reduce the disclusion time, and balance the occlusal forces by using minimally invasive tooth contouring methods (combining bonding and coronoplasty)		
5. If conservative methods are not possible to safely accomplish the needed occlusal changes, use a therapeutic oral appliance and reduce on its occlusal table the disclusion time, while also balancing the closure occlusal forces		
6. Lastly, finish and polish all the tooth or prosthetic surfaces, evaluate final case finishing result, and document the force finishing result with digital occlusal scanner and digital photography	Dental loupe Digital photographic images	Force finishing kit (silicon finishing and polishing points)

Therapeutic Force Finishing (TFF) (Table 8.7): It aims to customize the occlusal force components to treat or manage the specific occlusal force disorders. The concept of Force Finishing is based on do no harm dentistry approach and follows three core principles, while completing occlusal treatment to achieve harmonized occlusal forces for long-term clinical success:

- **Recognize** the "weakest link" in a patient's stomatoganthic system, based on existing occlusal force disorders (OFD) signs and symptoms.
- **Decide** to maintain, modify, or reconstruct the existing occlusion as per the patient's need and demand.
- **Optimize** the fundamental occlusal components (tooth contact location, tooth contact size, tooth contact relative forces, tooth contact sequences, maximum bite force, occlusal force distribution, occlusion time and path, disclusion time and path, center of occlusal forces distribution, and habitual

Table 8.8 Aesthetic finishing clinical Facts

1. A rough restoration surface allows dental plaque to adhere, which can promote secondary caries and periodontal diseases. As the free surface energy of uneven surfaces is lower than that of smooth surfaces, microorganisms can easily adhere and colonize. As a result, susceptibility to soft-tissue infection and caries can increase [151–154]
2. The rough surface of the final restoration promotes marginal restoration discoloration, which can decrease the aesthetic quality of the restorations [155–159]
3. Surface gloss plays an important role in the appearance of tooth-colored restorative resins and is a desirable characteristic that allows restorative materials to better mimic the appearance of the enamel [160–162]
4. A smooth and well-polished surface improves the flexural strength of the restorations and decreases abrasion of the opposing teeth [163, 164]
5. The quality of intraoral aesthetic finishing depends on the restorative materials used, finishing techniques, finishing tools and materials selected, and skill of the operator
6. The quality of polishing of the restoration surfaces is vital for long-term health, function, and aesthetics of the oral tissue

multibite pattern, to enhance the patient's physiologic resistive and adaptive capacity of their masticatory system).

The Force Finishing protocol has three fundamental steps:

- *Force finishing*: Digitally measures the fundamental occlusal components, correlate digital tooth contact location and tooth contact size using conventional articulating paper, and selectively optimize the necessary occlusal components using minimally invasive additive (composite resin) or reductive tooth contouring technique.
- *Aesthetic finishing*: After Force Finishing procedures, enamel and restorative surfaces which were adjusted for force harmony are polished meticulously with the surfaces smooth and glossy to ensure aesthetic polishing facts (Table 8.8) and maintain long-term health, aesthetic, and function.
- *Finishing evaluation*: This is last step of force finishing to document and evaluate the desired end result. Each step of force, aesthetic, and finishing evaluation requires particular tools and materials as shown in the pictures (Fig. 8.10a–d).

8.13 Clinical Cases

Force Finishing can be applied in every field of dentistry where dental occlusion is involved. Clinicians who perform orthodontic treatment, who regularly fabricate full mouth reconstructions, perform smile makeovers, place multiple restorations at one time, fabricate implant-supported prostheses, and treat temporomandibular disorders with occlusal adjustment or modification procedures would obtain significant benefits form employing Force Finishing in clinical practice. As mentioned earlier, in clinical practice, there are three treatment categories routinely employed in occlusal treatment: occlusal maintenance, occlusal modification, and occlusal reconstruction. To aid the reader in understanding the simplicity of, and the clinical benefits of using Force Finishing in daily practice, few clinical cases with Occlusal

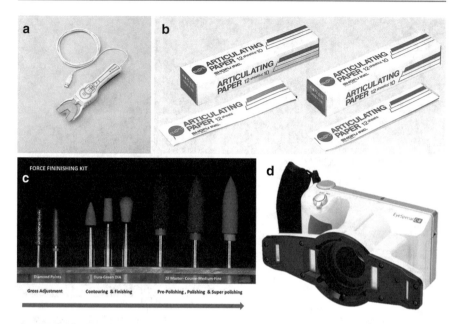

Fig. 8.10 (**a**) Force Finishing Materials and Tools—T-Scan for dental occlusion pattern and force scanning *(Photos Courtesy of Tekscan™, Inc.).* (**b**) Force Finishing Materials and Tools—Manual articulating paper to mark the contact location on the tooth (***Picture Courtesy** Shofu,Inc, Kyoto, Japan).* (**c**) Force Finishing Materials and Tools: Force Finishing Kit is the items selected by the author to be used for different steps of bite adjustment. Gross adjustment (Diamond points), contouring and finishing (Dura-Green DIA) and for pre-polishing and super polishing steps (Zil Master—course, medium, and fine) (***Picture Courtesy** Shofu,Inc, Kyoto, Japan).* (**d**) Force Finishing Materials and Tools—Digital Smart Camera for before and after photographic case documentation *(Picture courtesy Shofu, Inc, Kyoto, Japan)*

Force Disorders (OFD) are explained where treatment was done by employing Force Finishing and necessary restorative procedures (*Clinical pictures and graphic diagrams are Courtesy Vedic Smile, Nepal and reprinted with permission*).

Case 1 shows the *Management of Non-Carious Tooth Lesions (NCLs) using simple Injectable Composite Resin Restorations and Preventive Force Finishing Protocol* (Fig. 8.11).

Vedic Smile and Minimal Invasive protocol was followed and a thorough clinical examination was performed, necessary dental imaging was taken, and intraoral clinical pictures were taken. Multiple signs and symptoms of Occlusal Force Disorders (OFD) (teeth erosion, abrasion, attrition, and tongue thrusting and slight anterior open bite) was diagnosed. An occlusal force analysis using Digital Force Scanner (T-Scan) was performed next. The patient denied comprehensive Force Finishing therapy necessary (like mandibular deprogramming, selective reduction of posterior teeth contact interferences during excursive movement, creating canine guidance, reducing disocclusion time, and restoring necessary attrited teeth using non-prep adhesive restorations) to prevent his ongoing OFD process. Hence the

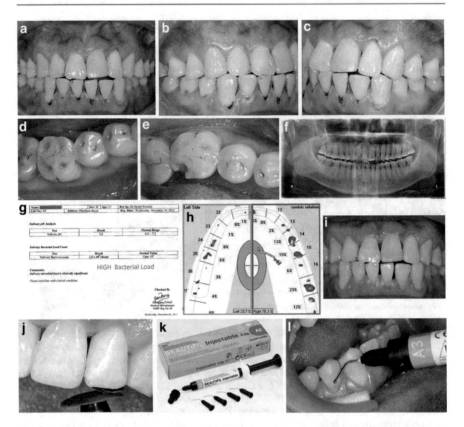

Fig. 8.11 (**a–e**) Retracted intraoral views: note poor oral hygiene, anterior open bite, cervical abrasion, occlusal attrition, and erosion of the teeth. (**f**) OPG X-ray . Note the flat cusps and minimal enamel present on the posterior teeth, both visible in the radiograph. (**g**) Salivary pH and bacterial load analysis, note bacterial load before periodontal therapy (1.5×10^9 cfu/ml). (**h**) Occlusal force scanning using T-Scan. Note Center of Force (COF) icon was shifted towards the right side indicating more force on the right half of the arch (left side 23.7% vs. right side 76.3%). Moreover, tooth no 15 and 17 were taking high occlusal pressures. (**i**) After simple periodontal therapy, note the multiple diastemas in lower anterior region and black triangles on upper front region were visible after removing dental calculus. (**j**) Cosmetic contouring of tooth no 22 using Super snap Black disc. This was done just because the patient did not want to increase the length of upper two central incisors to harmonize the smile. (**k**) Restoration material: Beautifil Injectable (*Image Courtesy of Shofu., Inc . Kyoto, Japan*). (**l**) Restoration of the lesions. (**m, n**) Restoration of occlusion cervical lesions—before and after. (**o, p**) Restoration of occlusal erosion—before and after. (**q, r**) Restoration of occlusion erosion and chipped out—before and after. (**s, t**) Restoration of diastemas and black triangles—before and after. (**u**) Salivary pH and bacterial load analysis, note bacterial load after periodontal therapy (9×10^6 cfu/ml). (**v**) Force Finishing for habitual bite balance, note the before and after picture of occlusal force balance. Now Center of Force (COF) icon is almost in the middle. Occlusal force load is balanced with left side 52.0% and right side 48% and overload of tooth no 15 and 17 were reduced

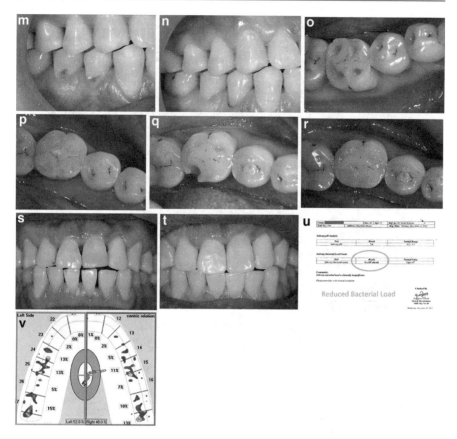

Fig. 8.11 (continued)

treatment performed was in accordance with the patient's desire using the simple approach of composite resin restorations and preventive force finishing protocol (occlusal force balance during the habitual bite of the patient), and night guard was given to protect night grinding and clenching habits of the patients.

Case 2 shows the *Oral Rehabilitation with Minimally Invasive Restorations and Preventive Force Finishing* (Fig. 8.12).

Case of a 62-years-old male with multiple signs and symptoms of Occlusal Force Disorders (OFD) (teeth erosion, abrasion, attrition, gingival recession, and notable occlusal forces disharmony). Digital occlusion analysis showed the overloading of occlusal force on tooth no 46, correlated with the thickening of PDL in radiology. Minimally invasive, quick and cost-effective treatment was performed. After routine oral hygiene prophylaxis and restorative treatment (restoration of abfraction, abrasion and erosion lesions using composite resin, and restoration of lost vertical

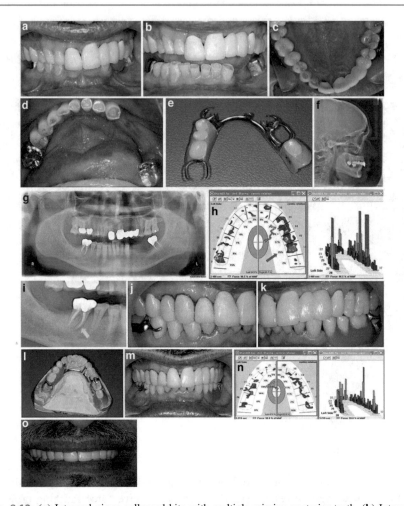

Fig. 8.12 (a) Intraoral view: collapsed bite with multiple missing posterior teeth. (b) Intraoral view: note multiple signs of Occlusal Force Disorders (attrition, erosion, abrasion, gingival recession). (c) Intraoral occlusal view: note enamel erosion on tooth no 12, 13, 14, and 26. (d) Intraoral occlusal view lower arch: note attrition of lower anterior due to reduced posterior support and bite imbalance. (e) A fully attrited cast partial denture that the patient was wearing. (f) CEPH X-ray collapsed bite. (g) OPG X-ray—note missing teeth, prominent mandibular angle, lost enamel in anterior region. (h) Occlusal Force Scan using T-Scan: Note the right side of the arch had 65.7% of occlusal load with high concentration of load (25%) on the tooth no 16 and occluding partner tooth no 46. The Center of Force icon was outside the inner circle showing occlusal force disharmony. (i) Digital occlusion analysis clearly showed the overloading of occlusal force (25%) on tooth no 46 which can be correlated with the thickening of PDL in radiology. (j–l) Restoration of abfraction, abrasion, and erosion lesions were completed using Beautifil II Composite resin from *Shofu, Inc, Kyoto Japan* . And restoration of lost vertical dimension of occlusion (VDO) was carried out by changing old metal crowns, restoring with composite overlay and fabrication of new lower cast partial denture as per new VDO. (m) After reconstruction of the compromised teeth and establishment of new VDO. (n) Occlusal force scan after Preventive Force Finishing. Note right and left side arch force balance, the high concentration of load on tooth no 16/46 was reduced. The Center of Force (COF) is now in the middle of the circle indicating proper force balance. (o) Smile after full mouth rehabilitation completed with minimally invasive approach

dimension of occlusion by changing old crows, restoring with composite overlay and fabrication of a new cast partial denture), the bite force adjustment using Force Finishing protocol was carried out with noticeable changes on the occlusal force balance.

8.14   Summary

Table 8.9 summarizes the different terminologies used and explained in this chapter. In the performance of clinical dental procedures, ranging from single restorations to complex full mouth reconstruction involving dental implants, the occlusal force components of the final case are often neglected and misunderstood. Therefore, the physical strength of the tooth-colored restorative materials is still an important topic in dentistry. Hence, the physical strength of the restorative materials chosen is often much stronger than the natural teeth because the clinician hopes the materials selected will overcome potential fracture of the restorations. Restorative clinicians must understand that overcoming the restoration fracture through material choice ignores the underlying occlusal force factors, shifting the effects of the occlusal force overload from the restoration, to other areas like the periodontium, the masticatory muscles, and the temporomandibular joints. Moreover, in the field of orthodontics, where clinicians routinely change the patient's occlusion during their treatment procedures, and there is no priority given for Force Finishing at the end of the treatment completion, yet orthodontic cases frequently encounter treatment replace, which is a direct response to masticatory force disharmony. Hence, to achieve the maximum therapeutic effect from any treatment, it is necessary to understand and harmonize the force components involved in a patient's masticatory system. And whatever the theory or concept of occlusal scheme selected during the treatment procedure, the role of Force Finishing is paramount to achieving long-term optimum results in terms of health, function, aesthetics, and high patient satisfaction with minimal biological cost.

8.15   Disclaimer

No conflict of interest has been declared by the author.

Table 8.9 Key terms

Key terms	Description
Vedic smile dentistry	A holistic dental care and treatment approach, which is based on the Vedic philosophy of consciousness and natural harmony
Dental occlusion	It is the relationship between the *maxillary* and *mandibular* teeth when they approach each other and generate occlusal forces within stomatognathic system)
Static occlusion	It refers to contact between the maxillary and mandibular teeth when the jaw is closed and stationary
Dynamic occlusion	It refers to occlusal contacts made when the jaw is moving
Centric occlusion (CO) or maximum Intercuspation(MIC)	Static occlusion where a position of mandible is in maximum intercuspation of the maxillary and mandibular teeth. CO/MIC is the functional relationship of the teeth and is influenced by "tooth shape" as well as neuromuscular "memory."
Centric relation (CO)	A position of the mandible dictated by the shape of the TMJ and mandibular condyles (this is maxillomandibular orientation, and is the only reproducible position of the mandibular and is used for complex occlusal rehabilitation)
Habitual occlusion or bite	The consistent relationship of maxillary and mandibular teeth in maximum intercuspation (it is the true centric occlusion)
Deflective occlusal contact	The initial tooth contact that diverts the mandible from a normal path of closure to centric jaw relation, moving the condyle to an eccentric position in habitual occlusion (also known as occlusal premature contact)
Occlusal interference contact	A tooth contact that concentrates adverse force on a single tooth and prevents other teeth from participating in an optimal occlusal scheme
Occlusal force disorders	The disorders of teeth masticatory muscles, temporomandibular joints, and airway, resultant from the presence of excess occlusal force that is greater than the individual's physiological resistive and adaptive capacity
Occlusal harmony	The physiologic and functional balance of the occlusion
Force finishing	A clinical procedure employed to optimize the occlusal force components of the masticatory system, using objective measurements of occlusal force and timing
Preventing force finishing	A procedure to optimize the occlusal force components of the masticatory system, to protect and maintain a physiologically accepted original occlusal scheme, while preventing existing restorations from future failure
Therapeutic force finishing	A procedure to customize the occlusal force components in the treatment of the specific signs and symptoms of occlusal force disorder (OFD) conditions
TMJA harmony	The physiologic and functional harmony of the entire stomatognathic systems; the teeth, muscles, temporomandibular joints, and airway
Digital occlusion	It refers to the computer-guided assessment of dental occlusion relationship. And the science of digital occlusion is the investigation and interpretation of the collected data

References

1. Koirala S. Smile design wheel—a simplified protocols of smile design. JNDA. 2008;9:1–6. 1[1]
2. Koirala S. Force finishing in dental medicine: a simplified approach to Occlusal Harmony. Handbook of Research on Computerized Occlusal Analysis Technology Application in Dental Medicine. Page 905–972, IGI Global Publication, 2015.
3. Ramfjord SP, Ash MM. Occlusion. 3rd ed. Philadelphia, PA: WB Saunders; 1983.
4. Dawson PE. Evaluation, diagnosis, and treatment of occlusal problems. 2nd ed. St. Louis: Mosby; 1989. p. 14–7.
5. Okeson J. Management of temporomandibular disorders and occlusion. 5th ed. St. Louis, MO: CV Mosby and co; 2003.
6. Moffett F Jr, Johnson L, McCabe J, et al. Articular remolding in the adult human temporomandibular joint. Am J Anat. 1964;115:119–30.
7. Dawson PE. Functional occlusion: from TMJ to smile design, vol. 1. St. Louis: Mosby, Inc; 2007.
8. McNeil C. Science and practice of occlusion. Carol Stream, IL: Quintessence Publishing; 1997.
9. Glickman MO. I. Clinical Periodontics. 5th ed. Philadelphia, PA: Saunders and Co.; 1979.
10. McLean DW. Physiologic vs pathologic occlusion. 17. J Am Dent Assoc. 1938;25: 1583–94.
11. Woda A, Vigneron P, Kay D. Non-functional and functional occlusal contacts: a review of the literature. J Prosthet Dent. 1979;42:335–41.
12. D'Amico A. The canine teeth: normal functional relation of the natural teeth of man. J S Calif Dent Assoc. 1958;26:6–23.
13. Gysi A. Masticating efficiency in natural and artificial teeth. Dent Dig. 1915;21:74–8.
14. Kaplan RL. Concepts of occlusion. Gnathology as a basis for a concept of occlusion. Dent Clin N Am. 1963;7:577–90.
15. Lucia VO. Modern gnathological concepts up dated. Chicago: Quintessence; 1983.
16. McAdam DB. Tooth loading and cuspal guidance in canine and group function occlusions. J Prosthet Dent. 1976;35:283–90.
17. Reynolds JM. The organization of occlusion for natural teeth. J Prosthet Dent. 1971;26:56–67.
18. Schwartz H. Occlusal variations for reconstructing the natural dentition. J Prosthet Dent. 1986;55:101–5.
19. Stuart CH, Stallard CE. Concepts of occlusion what kind of occlusion should recusped teeth be given? Dent Clin N Am. 1963;7:591–600.
20. Alexander PC. Analysis of the cuspid protected occlusion. J Prosthet Dent. 1963;13:309–17.
21. Beyron H. Occlusal relation and mastication in Australian aborigines. Acta Odontol Scand. 1964;22:597–60.
22. MacMillan HW. Unilateral vs bilateral balanced occlusion. J Am Dent Assoc. 1930;17:1207–20.
23. Mann AW, Pankey LD. Concepts of occlusion. The PM philosophy of occlusal rehabilitation. Dent Clin N Am. 1963;7:621–36.
24. Schuyler CH. Factors contributing to traumatic occlusion. J Prosthet Dent. 1961;11:708–16.
25. Rinchuse DJ, Kandasamy S, Sciote J. A contemporary and evidence-based view of canine protected occlusion. An evaluation of eccentric occlusal contacts in orthodontically treated subjects. Am J Orthod. 1982;82:251–6.
26. Begg PR. Stone Age man's dentition. Am J Orthod. 1954;40:298–312.
27. DeShields RW. Gnathological considerations of a controversial nature. Dent Surv. 1978;54:12–8.
28. Isaacson D. A biologic concept of occlusion. J Prevent Dent. 1976;3:12–6.

29. Thornton LJ. Anterior guidance: group function/ canine guidance. A literature review. J Prosthet Dent. 1990;64:479–81.
30. Anderson DM. Dorland's illustrated medical dictionary. 28th ed. Philadelphia, PA: WB Saunders; 1988.
31. Ahlgren J. Mechanism of mastication. Acta Odontol Scand. 1966;24(Suppl.44)
32. Anderson FJ, Picton DCA. Tooth contact during chewing. J Dent Res. 1957;36(1):21–6.
33. Adams SH, Zander HA. Functional tooth contacts in lateral and centric relation. J Am Dent Assoc. 1964;69:465–743.
34. Gibbs CH, Mahan PE, Lundeen HC, Brehnan K, Walsh EK, Sinkewiz SL, Ginsberg SB. Occlusal forces during chewing – influences of biting strength and food consistency. Prosthet Dent. 1981;46:561–7.
35. Gibbs CH, Mahan PE, Lundeen HC, Brehnan K, Walsh EK, Holbrook WB. Occlusal forces during chewing and swallowing as measured by sound transmission. J Prosthet Dent. 1981;46(4):443–9.
36. Gibbs CH, Mahan PE, Lundeen HC. Jaw movements and forces during chewing and swallowing and their clinical significance. In: Lundeen HC, Gibbs CH, editors. Advances in occlusion. Boston: John Wright; 1982. p. 23.
37. Nishigawa K, Bando E, Nakano M. Quantitative study of bite force during sleep associated bruxism. J Oral Rehabil. 2001;28(5):485–91.
38. Shimada A, Tanaka M, Yamashita R, Noguchi K, Torisu T, Yamabe Y, Fujii H, Murata H. Automatic regulation of occlusal force because of hardness-change of the bite object. J Oral Rehabil. 2008;35(1):12–9. Epub 2007 Nov 29
39. Dawson PE. Want a thriving practice? Concentrate on clinical excellence. Dent Econ. 1992;82(10):78–9.
40. van der Bilt A, Tekamp A, van der Glas H, Abbink J. Bite force and electromyograpy during maximum unilateral and bilateral clenching. Eur J Oral Sci. 2008;116(3):217–22.
41. Cleall JF. Study of form and function. Am J Orthod. 1965;51(8):566–94.
42. Jenkins GN. The physiology and biochemistry of the mouth. 4th ed. Oxford: Blackwell Scientific Publications; 1974.
43. Alex G, Polimeni A. Comprehensive dentistry: the key to predictable smile design. AACD Monogr. 2006:15–20.
44. Miller L. Symbiosis of esthetics and occlusion: thoughts and opinions of a master of esthetic dentistry. J Esthet Dent. 1999;11(3):155–65.
45. Spear FM. The business of occlusion. J Am Dent Assoc. 2006;137(5):666–7.
46. Baldini A, Nota A, Cozza P. The association between occlusion time and temporomandibular disorders. J Electromyogr Kinesiol. 2015;25(1):151–4.
47. Clark GT, Tsukiyama Y, Baba K, Simmons M. The validity and utility of disease detection methods and of occlusal therapy for temporomandibular disorders. Oral Surg Oral Med Oral Pathol Oral Radiol Endod. 1997;83(1):101–6. [Internet]
48. Cooper BC, Kleinberg I. Relationship of temporomandibular disorders to muscle tension type headaches and a neuromuscular orthosis approach to treatment. Cranio J Craniomandib Pract. 2009;27(2):101–8.
49. Dawson PE. A classification system for occlusions that relates maximal intercuspation to the position and condition of the temporomandibular joints. J Prosthet Dent. 1996;75(1):60–6.
50. Ferreira LA, Grossmann E, Januzzi E, de Paula MVQ, Carvalho ACP. Diagnosis of temporomandibular joint disorders: indication of imaging exams. Braz J Otorhinolaryngol. 2016;82(3):341–52.
51. McNamara JA. Orthodontic treatment and temporomandibular disorders. Oral Surg Oral Med Oral Pathol Oral Radiol Endod. 1997;83(1):107–17.
52. McNeill C. Management of temporomandibular disorders: concepts and controversies. J Prosthet Dent. 1997;77(5):510–22.
53. Wieckiewicz M, Boening K, Wiland P, Shiau Y-Y, Paradowska-Stolarz A. Reported concepts for the treatment modalities and pain management of temporomandibular disorders. J Headache Pain. [Internet. 2015;16(1):106.

54. Yamada K, Hanada K, Fukui T, Satou Y, Ochi K, Hayashi T, et al. Condylar bony change and self-reported parafunctional habits in prospective orthognathic surgery patients with temporomandibular disorders. Oral Surg Oral Med Oral Pathol Radiol Endod. 2001;92(3):265–71.
55. Mohl ND, Zarb GA, Carlsson GE, Rugh JDA. Textbook of occlusion. Chicago: Quintessence Publishing; 1988.
56. Schuyler CH. Fundamental principles in the correction of occlusal disharmony, natural and artificial. JADA. 1935;22:1193–202.
57. Stuart CH, Stallard CE. Principles involved in restoring occlusion to natural teeth. J Prosthet Dent. 1960;10:304–13.
58. da Silva Martins MJ, Caramelo FJ, Ramalho da Fonseca JA, Gomes Nicolau PM. In vitro study on the sensibility and reproducibility of the new T-scan® III HD system. Revista Portuguesa de Estomatologia, Medicina Dentária e Cirurgia Maxilofacial. 2014;55:14–22.
59. Hannukseal A. The effect of moderate and severe atrophy on the facial skeletal. Eur J Orthod. 1981;3(3):187–93.
60. Linder-Aronson S. Adenoids: their effect on mode of breathing and nasal airflow and their relationship to characteristics of the facial skeletal and the dentition. Acta Otolaryngol. 1970;265(supplement):1–32.
61. Sassuni V, Shnorhokain H, Beery Q, Zullo T, Friday GA. Influence of perennial allergic rhinitis (PAR) on facial type. L. J Allergy Clin Immunol. 1982;69(149):29–64.
62. Trask GM, Shipiro GC, Shapiro PA. The effects of perennial allergic rhinitis on dental and skeletal development: a comparison of sibling pairs. J Am Dent Assoc. 1987;33:151–80.
63. Woodside DG, Linder- Arnonson S. The channelization of upper and lower anterior face heights compared to population standards in mates between ages six to twenty tears. Eur J Orthod. 1979;1(1):24–40.
64. Hannam AG, De CR, Scott JD, Wood WW. The relationship between dental occlusion, muscles activity and associated jaw movement in man. Arch Oral Biol. 1977;22:25–32.
65. Rodrigues AF, Fraga MR, Vitral RWF. Computed tomography evaluation of the temporomandibular joint in class II division 1 and class III malocclusion patients: condylar symmetry and condyle fossa relationship. Am J Orthod Dentofac Orthop. 2009;136:199–206.
66. Weinberg LA, Lager LA. Clinical report on the etiology and diagnosis of TMJ dysfunction-pain syndrome. J Prosthet Dent. 1980;44(6):642–53.
67. Weinberg LA. The etiology, diagnosis, and treatment of TMJ dysfunction-pain syndrome. Part I: Etiology. J Prosthet Dent. 1979;42(6):654–64.
68. Weinberg LA. The role of stress, occlusion, and condyle position in TMJ dysfunction-pain. J Prosthet Dent. 1983;49(4):532–45.
69. Celić R, Jerolimov V, Pandurić J. A study of the influence of occlusal factors and parafunctional habits on the prevalence of signs and symptoms of TMD. Int J Prosthodont. 2002;15(1):43–8.
70. Crawford SD. Condylar axis position as determined by the occlusion and measured by the CPI instrument, and signs and symptoms of temporomandibular dysfunction. Angle Orthod. 1999;69(2):103–14.
71. Bonilla-Aragon H, Tallents RH, Katzberg RW, Kyrkanides S, Moss ME. Condyle position as a predictor of temporomandibular joint internal derangement. J Prosthet Dent. 1999;82(2):205–8.
72. Areso MP, Giralt MT, Sainz B, Prieto M, Garcia-Vallejo P, Gomez FM. Occlusal disharmonies modulate central catecholaminergic activity in the rat. J Dent Res. 1999;78(6):1204–13.
73. Budtz-Jørgensen E. Occlusal dysfunction and stress. An experimental study in macaque monkeys. J Oral Rehabil. 1981;8(1):1–9.
74. Kirveskari P, Jamsä T. Health risk from occlusal interferences in females. Eur J Orthod. 2009;31(5):490–5.
75. Kirveskari P, Le Bell Y, Salonen M, Forssell H, Grans L. Effect of elimination of occlusal interferences on signs and symptoms of craniomandibular disorder in young adults. J Oral Rehabil. 1989;16(1):21–6.

76. Kubo KY, Yamada Y, Iinuma M, Iwaku F, Tamura Y, Watanabe K, et al. Occlusal dishar-
    mony induces spatial memory impairment and hippocampal neuron degeneration via stress
    in SAMP8 mice. Neurosci Lett. 2007;414(2):188–91.
77. Le Bell Y. Are occlusal treatments still possible and appropriate methods in clinical dentistry?
    J Craniomand Func. 2014;6(4):317–32.
78. Onozuka M, Fujita M, Watanabe K, Hirano Y, Niwa M, Nishiyama K, et al. Age-related
    changes in brain regional activity during chewing: a functional magnetic resonance imaging
    study. J Dent Res. 2003;82(8):657–60.
79. Onozuka M, Fujita M, Watanabe K, Hirano Y, Niwa M, Nishiyama K, Saito S. Mapping brain
    region activity during chewing: a functional magnetic resonance imaging study. J Dent Res.
    2002;81(11):743–6.
80. Randow K, Carlsson K, Edlund J, Oberg T. The effect of an occlusal interference on the
    masticatory system. An experimental investigation. Odontol Revy. 1976;27(4):245–56.
81. Yoshihara T, Matsumoto Y, Ogura T. Occlusal disharmony affects plasma corticosterone and
    hypothalamic noradrenaline release in rats. J Dent Res. 2001;80(12):2089–92.
82. Jankelson R. Neuromuscular dental diagnosis and treatment: Ishiyaku Euroamerica; 1990.
83. McHorris WH. Focus on anterior guidance. J Gnatol. 1989;8:3–13.
84. Shimazaki T, Otsuka T, Akimoto S, Kubo KY, Sato S, Sasaguri K. Comparison of brain acti-
    vation via tooth stimulation. J Dent Res. 2012;91(8):759–63.
85. Slavicek R. Functional determinants of the masticatory system. Dentistry (German).
    1985;29(10):663–4.
86. Greven M, Otsuka T, Zutz L, Weber B, Elger C, Sato S. The amount of TMJ displacement
    correlates with brain activity. Cranio. 2011;29(4):291–6.
87. Otsuka T, Sasaguri K, Watanabe K, Hirano Y, Niwa M, Kubo K, et al. Influence of the TMJ
    position on limbic system activation – an fMRI study. J Craniomand Func. 2011;3(1):29–39.
88. Otsuka T, Watanabe K, Hirano Y, Kubo K, Miyake S, Sato S, et al. Effects of mandibu-
    lar deviation on brain activation during clenching: an fMRI preliminary study. Cranio.
    2009;27(2):88–93.
89. Tamaki K, Hori N, Fujiwara M, Yoshino T, Toyoda M, Sato S. A pilot study on masticatory
    muscle activities during grinding movements in occlusion with different guiding areas on
    working side. Bull Kanagawa Dental Coll. 2001;29:26–7.
90. Issa TS, Huijbregts PA. Physical therapy diagnosis and management of a patient with chronic
    daily headache: a case report. J Man Manip Ther. 2006;14(4):E88–123.
91. Scrivani SJ, DAS K, Kaban LB. Temporomandibular disorders. N Engl J Med. 2008:2693–705.
92. Gross M. The science and art of occlusion and oral rehabilitation, vol. 205: Quintessence
    Publishing Co, Ltd. p. 265–74.
93. Buescher J. Temporomandibular joint disorders. Am Fam Physician [Internet]. Elsevier; 2007
    [cited 2016 Dec 15]. pp. 1477–1482.
94. Yuasa H, Kino K, Kubota E, Kakudo K, Sugisaki M, Nishiyama A, et al. Primary treatment
    of temporomandibular disorders: The Japanese Society for the Temporomandibular Joint
    Evidence-Based Clinical Practice Guidelines. 2013.
95. Carey JP, Craig M, Kerstein RB, Radke J. Determining a relationship between applied occlu-
    sal load and articulation paper mark area. Open Dent J. 2007;1:1–7.
96. Millstein P, Maya A. An evaluation of occlusal contact marking indicators. Descriptive quan-
    titative methods. J Am Dent Assoc. 2001;132(9):1280–6.
97. Qadeer S, Kerstein R, Kim RJ, et al. Relationship between articulation paper mark size
    and percentage of force measured with computerized occlusal analysis. J Adv Prosthodont.
    2012;4(1):7–12.
98. Harper KA, Setchell DJ. The use of shimstock to assess occlusal contacts: a laboratory study.
    Int J Prosthodont. 2002;15(4):347–52.
99. Qadeer S, Kerstein RB, Yung-Kim RJ, Huh JB, Shin SW. Relationship between articulation
    paper mark size and percentage of force measured with computerized occlusal analysis. J
    Adv Prosthodont. 2012;4:7–12.

100. Saad MN, Weiner G, Ehrenberg D, Weiner S. Effects of load and indicator type upon occlusal contact markings. J Biomed Mater Res Part B. 2008;85(1):18–22.
101. Panigrahi D, Satpathy A, Patil A, Patel G. Occlusion and occlusal indicating materials. Int J Appl Dent Sci. 2015;1(4):23–6.
102. Gözler S. Courtesy of Dr Serdar Gözler. In: Erdemir U, Yildiz E, editors. Esthetic and functional management of diastema: a multidisciplinary approach [internet]. 1st ed. Istanbul: Springer; 2015. p. 35.
103. Iwase M, Ohashi M, Tachibana H, Toyoshima T, Nagumo M. Bite force, occlusal contact area and masticatory efficiency before and after orthognathic surgical correction of mandibular prognathism. Int J Oral Maxillofac Surg. 2006;35(12):1102–7.
104. Kürklü D, Yanikoglu N, Gözler S. Oklüzal Analiz Metodları ve T-scan. Atatürk Üniv Diş Hek Fak Derg. 2009;19(1):55–60.
105. Qadeer S, Yang L, Sarinnaphakorn L, Kerstein RB. Comparison of closure occlusal force parameters in post-orthodontic and non-orthodontic subjects using T-scan® III occlusal analysis. J Craniomandib Sleep Pract. 2016;26:1–7.
106. Ruge S, Quooss A, Kordass B. Variability of closing movements, dynamic occlusion, and occlusal contact patterns during mastication. Int J Comput Dent. 2011;14:119–27.
107. Suit SR, Gibbs CH, Benz ST. Study of gliding tooth contacts during mastication. J Periodontol. 1976;47(6):331–4. Internet
108. Maness WL Benzamin M, Podoloff R, Bobick A, Golden RF. Computerized occlusion analysis, a new technology. Quintessence Int. 1987;18(4):287–92.
109. Cerna M, Ferreira F, Zaror C, Navarro P, Sandoval P. Validity and reliability of the T-scan III for measuring force under laboratory conditions. J Oral Rehabil. 2015;42:544–51.
110. Ferreira F, Zaror C, Navarro P, Sandoval P. In vitro evaluation of T-scan® III through study of the sensels. Cranio. 2016;33(4):300–6.
111. Kerstein RB. The evolution of the T-scan I system from 1984, to the present day T-scan 10 system. In: Kerstein RB, editor. Handbook of research on clinical applications of computerized occlusal analysis in dental medicine. Hershey, PA: IGI Global; 2019. p. 1–54.
112. Kerstein RB, Chapman R, Klein M. A comparison of ICAGD (immediate complete anterior guidance development) to "mock ICAGD" for symptom reductions in chronic myofascial pain dysfunction patients. J Craniomandib Pract. 1997;15(1):21–37.
113. Kerstein RB, Lowe M, Harty M, Radke J. A force reproduction analysis of two recording sensors of a computerized occlusal analysis system. J Craniomandib Pract. 2006;24(1):15–24.
114. Koos B, Holler J, Schille C, Godt A. Time-dependent analysis and representation of force distribution and occlusion contact in the masticatory cycle. J Orofac Orthop. 2012;73: 204–14.
115. Koos B, Godt A, Schille C, Göz G. Precision of an instrumentation-based method of analyzing occlusion and its resulting distribution of forces in the dental arch. J Orofac Orthop. 2010;71(6):403–10.
116. Mitchem JA, Katona TR, Moser EAS. Does the presence of an occlusal indicator product affect the contact forces between full dentitions? J Oral Rehabil. 2017;44:791–9.
117. Cohen-Levy J, Cohen N. Computerized analysis of occlusal contacts after lingual orthodontic treatment in adults. Int Orthod. 2011;9(4):410–31.
118. Kerstein RB, Radke J. Average chewing pattern improvements following disclusion time reduction. Cranio. 2017;35:135–51.
119. Kerstein RB, Radke J. Masseter and temporalis excursive hyperactivity decreased by measured anterior guidance development. J Craniomandib Pract. 2012;30(4):243–54.
120. Kerstein RB. Disclusion time measurement studies: stability of disclusion time. A 1 year follow-up study. J Prosthet Dent. 1994;72(2):164–8.
121. Kerstein RB. Treatment of myofascial pain dysfunction syndrome with occlusal therapy to reduce lengthy disclusion time—a recall study. J Craniomandib Pract. 1995;13(2):105–15. 27–40
122. Kerstein RB, Radke J. The effect of Disclusion time reduction on maximal clench muscle activity level. J Craniomandib Pract. 2006;24(3):156–65.

123. Koirala S. MiCD—customized case finishing concept and clinical protocol. MiCD Clin J. 2011;1(1):32–42.
124. Qadeer S, Yang L, Sarinnaphakorn L, Kerstein RB. Comparison of closure occlusal force parameters in post-orthodontic and non-orthodontic subjects using T-scan(R) III DMD occlusal analysis. Cranio [Internet]. 2016;9634:1–7.
125. Qadeer S, Abbas AA, Sarinnaphakorn L, Kerstein RB. Comparison of excursive occlusal force parameters in post-orthodontic and non-orthodontic subjects using T-Scan® III. Cranio. 2016;36:11.
126. Thumati P, Manwani R, Mahant shetty M. The effect of reduced Disclusion time in the treatment of myofascial pain dysfunction syndrome using immediate complete anterior guidance development protocol monitored by digital analysis of occlusion. Cranio. 2014;32(4):289–99.
127. Thumati P, Sutter B, Kerstein RB, Yiannios N, Radke J. Changes in the Beck depression inventory - II scores of TMD subjects after measured occlusal treatment. Adv Dent Technol Tech. 2018;1(1):1–13.
128. Yiannios N, Kerstein RB, Radke J. Treatment of frictional dental hypersensitivity (FDH) with computer-guided occlusal adjustments. J Craniomandib Sleep Pract. 2016;35(6):1. -11-40
129. Yiannios N, Sutter B, Radke J, Kerstein RB. TMJ vibration changes following immediate complete anterior guidance development. Adv Dent Technol Tech. 2018;1(1):13–28.
130. Dees A, Kess K, Proff P, Schneider S. The use of the T-scan system in occlusal diagnosis. Zahn Mund Kieferheilkd Zentralbl. 1992;80(3):145–51.
131. Garrido García VC, García Cartagena A, González Sequeros O. Evaluation of occlusal contacts in maximum intercuspation using the T-Scan system. J Oral Rehabil. 1997;24(12):899–903.
132. Harvey WL, Hatch RA, Osborne JW. Computerized occlusal analysis: an evaluation of the sensors. J Prosthet Dent. 1991;65(1):89–92.
133. Hirano S, Okuma K, Hayakawa I. In vitro study on the accuracy and repeatability of the T-Scan II system. Kokubyo Gakkai Zasshi. 2002;69(3):194–201.
134. Maeda Y, Ohtani T, Okada M, Emura I, Sogo M, Mori T, Yoshida M, Nokubi T, Okuno Y. Clinical application of T-Scan system. Sensitivity and reproducibility and its application. Osaka Daigaku Shigaku Zasshi. 1989;34(2):378–84.
135. Okamoto K, Okamoto Y, Shinoda K, Tamura Y. Analysis of occlusal contacts of children by the T-Scan system. The reproducibility of the sensor. Shoni Shikagaku Zasshi. 1990;28(4):975–83.
136. Patyk A, Lotzmann U, Paula JM, Kobes LW. Is the T-scan system a relevant diagnostic method for occlusal control? Das Deutsche Zahnarzteblatt. 1989;98(8):686–8.
137. Ash MM, Nelson SJ. Wheeler's dental anatomy, physiology, and occlusion. 8th ed. St Louis: Saunders; 2003. p. 29–64.
138. Glickman I. Inflammation and trauma from occlusion. J Periodontol. 1963;34:5–15.
139. Goldman HM, Cohen WD. Periodontal therapy. St. Louis: Mosby; 1968.
140. Guichet NE. Occlusion: a teaching manual. Anaheim, CA: The Denar Corporation; 1977.
141. Howell AH, Manly RS. An electrical strain gauge for measuring oral forces. J Dent Res. 1948;27:705–12.
142. Kerstein RB. Reducing chronic masseter and temporalis muscular hyperactivity with computer-guided occlusal adjustments. Compend Contin Educ. 2010;31(7):530–43.
143. Korioth TWP, Hannam AG. Effect of bilateral asymmetric tooth clenching on load distribution at the mandibular condyle. J Prosthet Dent. 1990;64:62–78.
144. Kraua BS, Jordon RE, Abrahams L. Dental anatomy and occlusion. Baltimore: Waverly Press; 1973. p. 226.
145. Lee RL. Anterior guidance advances in occlusion. Boston: John Wright PSG; 1982. p. 51–80.
146. Standlee JP. Stress transfer to the mandible during anterior guidance and group function in centric movements. J Prosthet Dent. 1979;34:35–45.
147. Williamson EH, Eugene H. Willamson on occlusion and TMJ dysfunction. (part 2) (interviewed by Sidney Brandt.). J Clin Orthod. 15:39.
148. Williuams EH, Lundquist DO. Anterior guidance: its effect on the electromyographic activity of the temporal and masseter muscles. J Prosthet Dent. 1983;49:816–25.

149. Downs DH. An investigation into condylar position with leaf gauge and bimanual manipulation. J Gnathol. 1988;7:75–81.
150. Gelb ML, Gelb H. Gelb appliance: mandibular orthopedic repositioning therapy. Cranio Clin Int. 1991;1(2):81–98.
151. Quiryen M, Bollen CML. The influence of surface roughness and surface free energy on supra and sub gingival plaque formation in man. J Clin Periodontol. 1995;22(1):1–14.
152. Bollen CML, Lambrechts P, Quirynen M. Comparison of surface roughness of oral hard materials to the threshold surface roughness for bacterial plaque retention: a review of the literature. Dent Mater. 1997;13(4):258–69.
153. De Silva MFA, Davies RM, Stewart B, et al. Effect of whitening gels on the surface roughness of the restorative materials in situ. Dent Mater. 2006;22(10):919–24.
154. Kawai K, Urano M, Ebisu S. Effect of surface roughness of porcelain on adhesion of bacteria and their synthesizing glucans. J Prosthet Dent. 2000;83(6):664–7.
155. Martinez-Gomis J, Bizar J, Anglada JM, et al. Comparative evaluation of four systems on one ceramic surface. Int J Prosthodont. 2003;16(10):74–7.
156. Roeder LB, Tate WH, Powers JM. Effect of finishing and polishing procedures on the surface roughness of packable composites. Oper Dent. 2000;25(6):534–43.
157. Setcos JC, Tarim B, Suzuki S. Surface finish produced on resin composites by new polishing systems. Quintessence Int. 1999;30(3):169–73.
158. Yap AUJ, Yap SH, Teo CK, Ng JJ. Finishing/polishing of composite and compomer restorative: effectiveness of one-step systems. Oper Dent. 2004;29(3):275–9.
159. Brewer JD, Gariapo DA, Chipps EA, et al. Clinical discrimination between autoglaze and polished porcelain surfaces. J Prosthet Dent. 1990;64(60):631–4.
160. O'brien WJ, Johnston WM, Fanian F, Lambert S. The surface roughness and gloss of composites. J Dent Res. 1984;63:685–8.
161. Da Costa J, Ferracane J, Paravina RD, Mazur RF, Roeder L. The effect of different polishing systems on surface roughness and gloss of various resin composites. J Esthet Restor Dent. 2007;19:214–26.
162. Paravina RD, Roeder L, Lu H, Vogel K. Powers. Jm. Effect of finishing a polishing procedures on surface roughness, gloss and color of resin- based composites. Am J Dent. 2004;17:252–66.
163. Giordano RA, Cima M, Pober R. Effects of surface. Finish on the flexural strength of feldpathic and aluminous dental ceramics. Int J Prosthodont. 1995;8(4):311–7.
164. Chu FCS, Frankel N, Samales RJ. Surface roughness and flexural strength of self- glazed, polished and reglazed in-ceramic /vitadur alfa porcelain laminates. Int J Prosthodont. 2000;13(1):66–71.

Digitization in Management of Temporomandibular Disorders

9

Wael M. Talaat

9.1 Introduction

9.1.1 Temporomandibular Disorders (TMD)

These are a prevailing group of musculoskeletal and neuromuscular disorders that affect the muscular, soft tissue and osseous components of the Temporomandibular Joint. TMD have a multifactorial origin, where the predisposing, trigger, and perpetuating factors may include trauma, psychosocial, and physiopathological aspects. TMD have been reported as the most common origin of non-odontogenic oro-facial pain. In addition to pain, patients may present with joint sounds, limited or asymmetric mandibular movements, and different forms of disabilities which may severely affect the quality of life. The yearly cost for TMD treatment in the USA has been estimated to be $4 billion, not including imaging, thus TMD is regarded as a significant public health problem [1]. The management of TMD is often complicated, mainly due to the overlap between different medical specialties like dentistry, otology, neurology, orthopedic surgery, psychiatry, and others [2].

9.1.1.1 Classification of Temporomandibular Disorders
Clinicians and researchers benefit from the use of standardized, well-defined, and clinically relevant taxonomy for diseases to facilitate the transfer of information in both research and clinical practice. Among the pioneers in classifying TMD was Helkimo, who developed the Helkimo's clinical dysfunction index (Di) in 1974. Di is a functional assessment of the TMD-related signs including the TMJ functional impairment,

. M. Talaat (✉)
Department of Oral and Craniofacial Health Sciences, College of Dental Medicine, University of Sharjah, Sharjah, UAE

Department of Oral and Maxillofacial Surgery, Suez Canal University, Ismailia, Egypt

Research Institute of Medical and Health Sciences, University of Sharjah, Sharjah, UAE
e-mail: wtaha@sharjah.ac.ae

© Springer Nature Switzerland AG 2021
P. Jain, M. Gupta (eds.), *Digitization in Dentistry*,
https://doi.org/10.1007/978-3-030-65169-5_9

muscle tenderness, TMJ pain during palpation and mandibular movement, and range of mandibular mobility. Since Di is a purely clinical evaluation, it can be considered a useful tool to qualify patients for radiographic assessment and justify X-ray exposure [3]. Later, the International Headache Society (IHS) offered a classification for headache including 13 categories, among which the 11th was related to TMD.

The American Academy of Orofacial Pain provided a more detailed description of the 11th category of the IHS classification by introducing subcategories and their diagnostic criteria [4, 5]. The Research Diagnostic Criteria for Temporomandibular Disorders (RDC/TMD) has been the most widely accepted and commonly used classification for TMD since its publication in 1992 [6]. The strength of RDC/TMD lies in recognizing the psychosocial component and pain-related disabilities of TMD. The RDC/TMD has two evaluation Axis:

Axis I includes a clinical assessment of signs and symptoms augmented with radiographic evaluation, leading to the classification of three groups of TMD: Group I, muscular disorders (Group Ia, myofascial pain; Group Ib, myofascial pain with limited mouth opening); Group II, disk displacement (Group IIa, disk displacement with reduction; Group IIb, disk displacement without reduction with limited opening; group IIc, disk displacement without reduction without limited opening); and Group III, arthralgia, osteoarthritis, and osteoarthrosis (Group IIIa, arthralgia; Group IIIb, osteoarthritis; Group IIIc, osteoarthrosis).

Axis II comprises different instruments for the biobehavioral assessment, specifically the psychosocial status and pain-related disabilities as mentioned.

A new evidence-based protocol was published in 2014 to improve the sensitivity and specificity of the original RDC/TMD and add new comprehensive instruments for Axis I and Axis II to allow the diagnosis of simple and complex forms of TMD [7]. The modified protocol was called diagnostic criteria for temporomandibular disorders (DC/TMD) and included new Axis I instruments and assessment algorithms and new Axis II instruments. The new Axis I and II instruments proposed new terminology for several TMD diagnoses using more concise algorithms which are suitable for clinical application.

9.1.1.2 Prevalence of Temporomandibular Disorders

TMD are prevalent and divergent admixture of disorders affecting the osseous and soft tissue components of the TMJ. The reported prevalence of TMD differed greatly between different studies, not only due to the differences in populations but also due to the lack of standardization in the examination procedures, taxonomy, and diagnostic criteria. Patients might ignore the early signs of TMD or lose their way between different medical specialties before their diagnosis is confirmed. The prevalence of non-self-reported TMD which were discovered incidentally during the routine dental examination was found to be 10.8% in one study [8]. A questionnaire-based study in Brazil showed that 37.5% of the population had at least one TMD symptom [9], whereas epidemiologic surveys reported at least one TMD sign to be present in 40–75% of the population and at least one TMD symptom to be present in 33% of the population [10]. Normal joints were found only in 50% of boys and in 23–29% of girls in another study, whereas the rest of the study population showed partial to full disc displacement on magnetic resonance images (MRI) [11]. It has been confirmed that TMD are common disorders and have a negative impact on the quality of patients' life, thus a costly effect on the nation's economy.

9.2   Diagnosis of Temporomandibular Disorders

The diagnosis of TMD is a complicated process, mainly due to the multifactorial origin of TMD and the overlap of signs and symptoms between the different disorders. Many of the symptoms of TMD appear to arise from outside the TMJ, for example, ear pain, dizziness, neck pain, tinnitus, and headache. Accordingly, patients may lose their way between different medical specialties before reaching a proper TMD diagnosis. TMD has been declared to be within the scope of practice of dentistry, so dental graduates are considered the primary care providers for TMD [12]. It's the duty of each dentist to screen patients for TMD, even when no signs and symptoms are reported by the patient.

The diagnosis of TMD involves history taking, clinical examination, and imaging. In addition, biobehavioral and psychosocial assessments are essential components of the diagnosis process as indicated by the DC/TMD [7]. According to the DC/TMD, the following disorders represent the latest disease entities: myalgia, local myalgia, myofascial pain, myofascial pain with referral, four-disc displacement disorders, arthralgia, degenerative joint disorder, subluxation, and headache. Different diagnostic algorithms for most disorders were created that map the patient's history, clinical, and radiographic findings to a final diagnosis using a decision tree. The Axis I diagnostic criteria include specific clinical examination procedures and instruments to assess pain, joint noises, jaw locking, and headache. Axis II assessment instruments include pain intensity and disability, jaw function and para-function, and psychosocial distress [7].

9.2.1   The Conventional Diagnostic Approach

Although the treatment guidelines for TMD have been well established, however, TMD diagnosis is still considered a dilemma. Imaging is a crucial component of the diagnostic process. It has been noted that TMD prevalence was overestimated in studies that used questionnaires and clinical examination only, without confirming the primary diagnosis with imaging [8]. Several imaging modalities have been used to diagnose TMD, including panoramic radiography, linear and complex motion tomography, computed tomography (CT) to evaluate the osseous components, and magnetic resonance imaging to evaluate the soft tissue components of the joint [13].

The transcranial view, a two-dimensional projection, has been used in the past for TMJ evaluation; however, its use is currently limited due to the superimposition of nearby structures, resulting in inaccurate assessment of the pathologic changes. Panoramic radiography may be useful for initial screening for TMD and for detecting the gross osseous changes. However, several limitations are associated with the use of panoramic radiography like the inability to show the entire articular surface, superimposition of the zygoma, and the possible image distortion. Accordingly, panoramic radiography has been reported to have poor reliability and low sensitivity in the assessment of bony changes associated with TMD [14]. Linear and complex motion tomography have been utilized for TMJ assessment for years, with a reported sensitivity range of 53–90% in spotting bony changes associated with TMD and a specificity range of 73–95%. Nevertheless, the diagnostic accuracy of tomography is deficient, due to the inadequacy in detecting small osseous changes [15].

9.3 Digitization in the Diagnosis of Temporomandibular Disorders

9.3.1 Cone Beam Computed Tomography

Osteoarthritis of the TMJ is the most common TMD to be seen in the dental clinic. The reason is the association between osteoarthritis, severe pain, and disability. Osteoarthritis is linked to TMJ inflammation and degenerative changes in the different components of the TMJ [16]. In addition to history and clinical examination, different imaging modalities have been used to diagnose osteoarthritis definitely. Panoramic radiography and linear and complex tomography have serious limitations as discussed before. CT has been used successfully for the assessment of the bony changes associated with osteoarthritis. However, the use of CT in dentistry, in general, has been limited due to high cost, high level of radiation, and limited access to equipment in the dental clinics.

The introduction of cone beam computed tomography has led to a dramatic change in the process of TMD diagnosis. CBCT uses a cone-shaped source of radiation incorporating the entire field of view and enables quick data acquirement. Compared to CT, CBCT has been reported to have similar accuracy but with lower cost, lower doses of radiation, and easier access to equipment and accordingly is present in many dental clinics nowadays. In addition, CBCT allows for a shorter exposure time, sharper images, and less image distortion [17]. In a medium field of view, CBCT warrants 35% less dose of radiation compared to multidetector CT. CBCT allows the evaluation of every aspect of the bony components of the TMJ, unlike panoramic and sagittal radiography. Compared to CT, CBCT was reported to have similar specificity in assessing condylar osseous abnormalities (1.0); however, CBCT had higher diagnostic accuracy (0.9) compared to CT (0.86) and higher sensitivity (0.8) compared to CT (0.7) [18].

To evaluate the value of CBCT in the diagnosis of TMD, the association between the CBCT findings and the clinical TMD diagnosis was investigated.

In one study which evaluated patients diagnosed with osteoarthritis and closed lock, the following radiographic criteria were assessed in sagittal, coronal, and axial planes; flattening of the articular surfaces, osteophyte formation, Ely's cyst (subcortical cyst), condylar surface irregularities, and joint space measurements. This study showed that condylar superior surface irregularities were detected by CBCT in 80% of joints with osteoarthritis and in 11.54% of joints with closed lock, whereas osteophytes were found in 40% of joints with osteoarthritis and in 3.85% of joints with closed lock. CBCT also showed the flattening of the condylar surfaces in 30% of osteoarthritic joints and in 7.69% of closed lock joints, whereas Ely's cysts were found in 10% of osteoarthritic joints and in 3.85% of closed lock joints. Joint space measurements done by CBCT showed that normal patients have significantly more joint space (5.64 ± 1.88) compared to patients with osteoarthritic joints (4.57 ± 1.97) (Fig. 9.1). This study concluded that CBCT diagnosis was significantly associated with the clinical findings in cases with osteoarthritis and closed lock [19].

Another study also found a strong correlation between the condyle and glenoid fossa CBCT findings and the score and degree of Helkimo's clinical dysfunction index [20]. Interestingly, the use of CBCT led to a change in the primary TMD diagnosis in 26.08% of cases in one study [8] and in 65% of cases in another study [21]. CBCT also led to changes in management decisions in 40% of cases in the latter study.

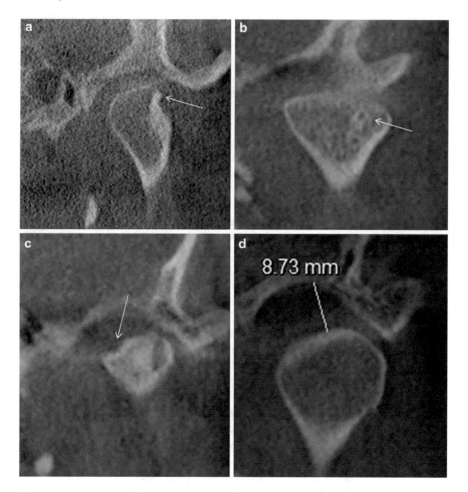

Fig. 9.1 Radiographic criteria detected on CBCT during the process of diagnosis of TMD: (**a**) osteophyte, (**b**) subcortical cyst (Ely's cyst), (**c**) condylar surface irregularities, and (**d**) joint space measurement

9.3.2   Analysis of Occlusion and Occlusal Forces

The question of whether dental occlusion is a contributing factor for TMD or not has been debatable for years. There is still no clear answer to this controversy; however, with the introduction of more objective evidence-based approaches for the diagnosis of TMD and with the use of modern digital analysis technologies which are able to quantify occlusal forces, we might come closer to an answer for this question soon. In one study, 11 common occlusal features were analyzed as possible risk factors for TMD. In this study, five TMD classes were analyzed: disc displacement with reduction, disc displacement without reduction, myalgia, primary osteoarthrosis, and secondary osteoarthrosis. This study concluded that the contribution of occlusion to the different TMD categories could not be proven; however, out of the 11 occlusal features, the following showed a high risk: anterior open bite, unilateral maxillary lingual crossbite, overjets greater than 6–7 mm, more than 5–6 missing posterior teeth, and retruded contact position to intercuspal position greater than 2 mm. The authors of this study stated that occlusion should not be regarded as an etiologic factor for TMD; nevertheless, anterior open bite in osteoarthrosis cases can be regarded as a result rather than a cause for TMD [22].

On the other hand, studies which support the effects of occlusion on TMD describe the consequences of premature contacts which lead to condyle displacement, resulting in friction and increased pressure inside the joint. This will result in pathologic intra-articular changes if the adaptation capacity of the joint is exceeded [23, 24]. The modern digital occlusal analysis technologies provide detailed information about occlusion time, the center of occlusal forces, and the arrangement of occlusal forces on both sides. An example of this technology is the T-Scan computerized occlusal analysis system (Tekscan Inc., South Boston, MA, USA). T-Scan, which is composed of a digital pressure mapping sensor, a headpiece, and software, provides a comprehensive occlusal analysis which overcomes many of the limitations of the traditional occlusal analysis practices (Fig. 9.2). The system provides information on the level and timing of force on each tooth, quadrant and side, the stability of the bite, the center of force target and trajectory, and contact time sequencing and enables the comparison between the pre- and posttreatment records. The system also enables the assessment of the dynamics of chewing movements and muscles' stress on teeth. Using T-scan, one study was able to correlate TMD symptoms with group function occlusion, whereas the canine-guided occlusion was significantly associated with normal joints [25].

It is well-known that canine-guided occlusion is favorable for the TMJ due to the disclosure of posterior teeth during lateral excursions, better tolerance to horizontal forces, and less muscular activity during movements. In the same study, balancing side interferences were found to have a significant correlation to TMD compared with poor correlations with working side and protrusive interferences. Balancing side interferences were shown to be associated with high muscular activity and destructive forces using electromyography [26]. T-scan showed that the occlusion and disocclusion times for TMD patients were longer than control, leading to an increase in muscular activity and an increase in stresses on joint components [25].

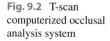
Fig. 9.2 T-scan computerized occlusal analysis system

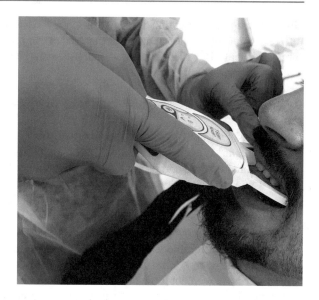

In another study, T-scan has proved that in intracapsular disorders, there is a change in condylar position from the normal centric relation position associated with an increase in the percentage of force due to occlusal interferences [27].

9.3.3 Real-Time Jaw Movement Tracking

Measuring the 3D in vivo kinematics of the mandible during different movements would potentially enhance the diagnostic process of TMD. Attempts to achieve this goal started with the use of two mechanical face bows [28] and progressed to the use of more compact and refined systems [29–31]. Stereophotogrammetric systems were developed for this purpose and were depending on skin marks; however, these systems had limitations due to the artifacts associated with the skin movements relative to the underlying bones. Transoral devices were developed to overcome these limitations, but these devices had also their own limitations, as they were interfering with the natural movements of the mandible [32].

Subsequently, a fluoroscopic 3D imaging modality enabled the registration of TMJ rigid-body kinematics in three dimensions. This system depended on recording the data obtained from the CT images on single-plane fluoroscopic images. The system was then modified to use CBCT data instead of CT as the former is more widely used in dental practice. The system was capable of recording the midpoint of the interincisal edge during opening and closing, protrusion and retrusion, chewing, and lateral gliding movements. Thus, this system was able to quantify the different complicated movement patterns of the TMJ and provided a complete analysis of the mandibular motion using different reference points [33]. Such systems allow for better understanding of the biokinetics of the TMJ and the etiology of TMD and would facilitate the refinement of management approaches as well. The

CBCT-based jaw motion tracking systems allow measuring the movement paths of different points of interest in different planes and can be exported to other software for further analysis, patient education, and treatment planning.

9.3.4 Real-Time Magnetic Resonance Imaging (MRI) of the TMJ

When the diagnosis of TMJ soft tissue-related disorders are considered, MRI is definitely regarded as the gold standard [34]. The location of the disc in opened and closed mouth positions and its configuration are required for a definite diagnosis of certain TMD classes. However, the traditional MRI assesses the soft tissue components of the TMJ only at static positions. Recently, high-speed real-time MRI was introduced in order to augment the diagnosis of TMD with dynamic information concerned with the movement of the TMJ [35].

Researchers were able to transform the single-slice real-time MRI records to movie recordings in several layers with improved contrast and superior image quality during movement [36]. The protocol used in this study involved triple-slice recordings for both joints, followed by dual-slice recordings and quadruple-slice recordings on an average slice thickness of 6–8 mm. The method used achieved thorough volume coverage of the entire jaw enabling precise dynamic characterization for both joints. Another approach combined fast low-angle exposures MRI sequences with radial data sampling and view sharing of consecutive acquisitions. The resulting reconstructions allowed for dynamic images visualizing the movements of the TMJ which were free from motion artifacts [37]. Such technologies are extremely beneficial for the diagnosis of TMD, especially internal derangements, due to the merit achieved by visualizing the TMJ disc during the movements of the jaw.

9.3.5 Artificial Intelligence (AI)

Many of the recent advances in the healthcare sector have been influenced by AI. AI is geared toward improving the accuracy of the diagnosis of different diseases, saving the patient's and medical practitioner's time, and improving work efficiency in general. In dentistry, AI has been used to develop programs that can assist in the diagnosis of diseases, identification of pathologies, detection of radiographic landmarks, and segmentation of radiographic structures. To achieve such goals, several programming approaches were utilized, including machine learning techniques and computer vision algorithms [38–40]. From this perspective, neural networks were developed to provide highly efficient and sound mathematic models that are able to classify, predict, and recognize patterns in different fields including medicine. Neural networks assist medical practitioners in the process of decision-making for the diagnosis of different disease and treatment planning [41].

In the field of oral and maxillofacial surgery, neural networks have been used to identify patients with risk of oral cancer [42], to assist in treatment planning for lower third molars [43], and to detect cervical lymph node metastasis of squamous cell carcinoma [44]. As pertaining to TMD, an artificial neural network was trained to diagnose disc displacement with acceptable sensitivity and specificity using frontal chewing patterns of normal subjects and of TMD patients. The neural network training module in this study used data related to clinical symptoms and diagnoses of 161 patients, whereas 58 patients were used for testing. This study reported a low accuracy in the diagnosis of disc displacement without reduction compared to a high accuracy achieved in the diagnosis of disc displacement with reduction. The authors contributed this discrepancy to the variability of the symptoms associated with disc displacement without reduction [45].

Another neural network application was used in a study to diagnose TMJ osteo-arthritis through a minimally invasive approach. This study analyzed the serum and salivary levels of 17 different biomarkers associated with osteoarthritis and then assessed the correlations between the morphological changes in different surfaces of the condyle with the biomarkers through a neural network. The neural network was trained using data from 154 condyles with osteoarthritis and 105 controls and then tested using 34 condyles. The network was trained to calculate the condyles' geometric characteristics and dysmorphology and to detect different degrees of deformations in the osteoarthritic condyles. In this study, AI was used to stage the condylar morphology in TMJ osteoarthritis into six stages ranging from normal to severely degenerated condyles. Although the deep learning design used in this study analyzed complex condylar morphologies, significant agreements were found between clinician experts' classifications and the neural network classifications. The study recommended the use of larger datasets in future studies to overcome any discrepancies in clinician experts' visual perception and any inaccuracies in the computation of features in the neural networks. The study concluded that the used neural network provided a high degree of accuracy in classifying the stages of osteoarthritis of the TMJ depending on the condylar morphologies [46].

Another example of the application of the neural network deep learning approach in the field of TMJ used the "Data Storage for Computation and Integration" web-based system to remotely compute a neural network classifier for the diagnosis of TMJ osteoarthritis. This study focused on improving the accuracy of the radio-graphic interpretations of TMJ osteoarthritis and refining the classifications of osteoarthritis which depend on data from biological markers and clinical variables. The approach used in this study was to detect the hidden patterns which are present in the big data obtained during the diagnostic process using machine learning algo-rithms to improve the diagnostic decision-making. The study used radiographic, clinical, and biological data obtained from patients with TMJ osteoarthritis. Two clinician experts classified subjects into five subgroups of osteoarthritis with vari-able degrees of degeneration and compared their classifications to the results obtained from the neural network. The neural network utilized a slicer plug-in (shape variation analyzer) to evaluate average morphologies and classify morpho-logical changes. The results of this study defined eight groups of morphological variability in the condyles after excluding bone proliferations and overgrowth as they do not seem to follow a pattern. The authors recommended using larger databases in future research to accurately train the neural networks to recognize different patterns of TMJ degeneration and thus improve the precision of the classifications [47].

AI is expected to improve the performance of medical practitioners in the near future and thus improve productivity by eliminating subjective interpretations and allowing for smart clinical decisions. Recently, many algorithms have been tested and showed excellent results in mining medical data.

9.4   Treatment of Temporomandibular Disorders

The success of TMD treatment depends on the choice of the correct treatment approach at the correct time. TMD are progressive disorders, which may deteriorate to more advanced forms over time if not treated. With the advances in the diagnostic approaches for TMD and the development of universally accepted guidelines for treatment, it was expected that the high prevalence of advanced forms will decrease. However, TMD treatment still suffers from the lack of training in undergraduate dental education, the inconsistency in the offered treatment modalities between different medical and dental specialties, and the scarcity of the recommended multidisciplinary approach which is essential for the success of treatment. The refinement of the treatment modalities using the recent advancement in technology is expected to improve the treatment outcomes and reduce the high prevalence of TMD.

9.4.1   The Conventional Treatment Approach for Temporomandibular Disorders

Conservative treatment has been recommended as the starting point in the management of TMD, which may include rest, soft diet, drug therapy, physiotherapy, and several types of occlusal guards. The goals of TMD treatment are to reduce pain and restore normal function. Contradicting results in the success rates of nonsurgical treatment have been reported in the literature, ranging from 36% [48] to 88% [49]. Patients refractory to conservative treatments are usually candidates for more invasive forms of treatment.

In the past, open joint surgeries were dominating the treatment approaches for patients not responding to conservative treatment. Currently, open joint surgeries are only recommended if minimally invasive surgeries fail. Procedures like synovectomy, discectomy, eminoplasty, eminectomy, and disc plication were utilized to manage advanced TMD cases and were reported to be successful in reducing pain and improving function, but a high rate of complications was reported as well [50, 51]. If no improvement was achieved following minimally invasive surgeries and open joint surgeries, then total joint replacements are recommended. The minimally invasive procedures, like arthroscopy and arthrocentesis, are nowadays the treatment modalities of choice for managing TMD cases not responding to conservative treatment. The use of the arthroscope in the TMJ was first described by Onishi in 1975 [52].

Since then, a lot of progress has been achieved in the field of TMJ arthroscopy [53, 54]. Arthroscopic lysis and lavage were shown to be effective in treating osteoarthritis and disc displacement without reduction of the TMJ by releasing the fibrous adhesions inside the joint, washing out the inflammatory mediators and preventing the suction effect of the TMJ disk to the fossa [54]. Operative arthroscopy is a different technique which allows instrumentation to carry out strategies more advanced than lysis and lavage as debridement, miotomy, disc reduction, and disc fixation [55]. In 1987, Murakami et al. applied the same concepts of lysis and lavage without the visualization in arthrocentesis of the TMJ [56]. The double-puncture arthrocentesis technique as used today was first described by Nitzan et al. [57], while later several proposals for single-puncture arthrocentesis were introduced [58–60].

9.5   Digitization in the Treatment of Temporomandibular Disorders

9.5.1   Computer-Assisted Arthroscopy of the TMJ

Refinement of the technique of TMJ arthroscopy is an ongoing process [61]. Among the technological advances in this field was the introduction of a system that facilitated the navigation of the arthroscope between the different anatomical structures. The system allowed the visualization of digital data and videos simultaneously on independent channels. The digital data can be obtained from CT scans, MRI, and radiographic records. The system then allowed the superimposition of projected computer graphics on online pictures to define the anatomical structures more clearly on video monitors. This was done through the consolidation of the digital data sets with real-time position data through different tracking technologies. This system facilitated accurate navigation of the arthroscope inside the TMJ between the anatomical structures during the different surgical procedures in a composite-reality environment.

The system also allowed the recording of the 3D data of the surgical procedure. The system used an optoelectronic tracking technology with an orthotopic matching technology allowing the registration of any movement of the equipment attached to the tracking devices. Accordingly, the puncturing locations and the working channels were identified using the preoperative CT data, and the surgical access path was followed in a real-time superimposition in the live video image on a head display or monitor. A safe pathway for the arthroscope was thus displayed using virtual rectangles superimposed on the real patient and leading the surgeon to the correct puncture point and target anatomical structure. This study concluded that computer-assisted arthroscopy can reduce the possible complications associated with the surgery and reduce the operative time as well. In addition, it allows a remote expert to observe the surgical procedure and even interfere in the intraoperative decision-making process. The authors recommended that further studies should concentrate on integrating MRI records with computer-assisted technology to allow for the interpretation of soft tissues of the joint [62].

Another study evaluated a TMJ computer-assisted surgical navigation system for the treatment of ankylosis. The authors of this study performed computer-assisted gap arthroplasty in one group of patients and compared the results to another group where the procedure was done without a computer-assisted approach. CT was used postoperatively to assess the accuracy of gap arthroplasty in both groups. The results of the study showed that using a computer-assisted approach the authors were able to achieve a more extensive removal of the ankylosed bone while ensuring a proper safety distance [63].

A technical report, published in 2017, introduced a surgical template for TMJ access during minimally invasive surgeries. The template was based on the use of CBCT and computer-aided design/computer-aided manufacturing (CAD/CAM). The workflow in this report was composed of obtaining CBCT, CT, or MRI data, followed by optical scanning of the face, and then the conversion of DICOM data to surface data which was aligned to the optical scan data using an algorithm. This workflow allowed for the designing of a printable biocompatible template with two working channels for the scope and manipulation instruments that were aligned to the anatomy of the patient. The template was used to direct the surgeon to the correct puncture points and direct the arthroscope to the correct working site inside the TMJ. The puncture point on the template was supposed to be chosen so that it allows all planned movements during the surgical procedure. The advantages of this approach have been identified as making the minimally invasive surgeries easier and safer for the inexperienced surgeons and allowing the identification of the correct puncturing point, which might be tricky even for the experienced surgeon. The procedure has been described as being affordable; however, planning was time-consuming, which is expected to improve with further training [64].

9.5.2 Customized Design: Total TMJ Prosthesis

The indications for total TMJ prosthesis include end-stage osteoarthritis of the TMJ, comminuted condylar fractures, tumors, and idiopathic resorption of the joint. The two main total joint prosthesis systems available at the market are Zimmer Biomet (Biomet Microfixation, Jacksonville, FL, USA) [65] and TMJ Concepts (TMJ Concepts Inc., Camarillo, CA, USA) [66]. Despite the fact that the available stock prostheses have been reported to be highly efficient, they are not essentially suitable for every case, partially due to the unmatching TMJ anatomy and partially due to the high cost. This was the drive for the development of customized TMJ prosthesis using 3D printing and CAD/CAM technologies.

This approach was used in a study to evaluate the safety and efficacy of a customized TMJ prosthesis for a Chinese population. The study was conducted on patients with unilateral end-stage osteoarthritis. The procedure started by taking a CT scan and creating a 3D craniomaxillofacial model using DICOM files. Using the software, the lower part of the eminence and the whole condyle were cut, followed by designing the prosthesis using another software. The designed prosthesis had

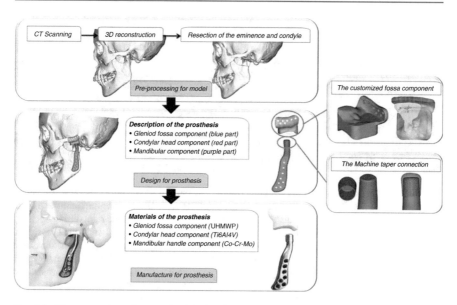

Fig. 9.3 The processing of customized design TMJ prosthesis, showing the preprocessing of the model, the design of the prosthesis, and the materials used. UHMWP ultrahigh-molecular-weight polyethylene; Ti6Al4V titanium alloy; Co–Cr–Mo cobalt–chromium–molybdenum alloy [67]

three components; a glenoid fossa, a condylar head, and the mandibular handle component, which was fixed on the ramus of the mandible (Fig. 9.3).

The design of the prosthesis was tailored to fit the Chinese TMJ anatomy, whereas the manufacturing of the three components was done using a five-axis milling device for the fossa and condylar head and a 3D printing machine for the mandibular handle component. Under general anesthesia, a modified preauricular approach was performed in all patients followed by cutting the entire condyle and lower part of the articular eminence. The three components of the prosthesis were then fixed using titanium screws. The postoperative radiographic assessment showed that there was no loosening, displacement, or break down of the prosthesis during the entire 12-month follow-up period. The study confirmed the safety of the system by evaluating the surgical complications, occlusion, and laboratory tests like liver and kidney functions and blood, urine, and stool tests. In addition, the study has also proved the efficacy of the prosthesis by assessing several subjective and objective evaluation criteria. Accordingly, 3D printing technology has allowed the production of sophisticated customized TMJ prosthesis from CAD/CAM data, which has proven to be a safe and efficient joint prosthesis [67].

9.6 Clinical Applications

The positive impact of digitization was clearly evident in the diagnosis and management of a rare TMJ case. Figure 9.4 describes the treatment of a rare malignant TMJ lesion with the use of computer technology to assess the relation of the tumor to the

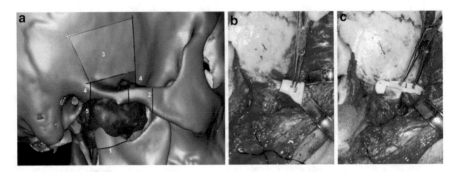

Fig. 9.4 Digital design of the surgical osteotomy and the use of digitally designed osteotomy templates. Patient with pain and swelling in the right pre-auricular region, limitation of mouth opening, crepitation of the right joint, and deviation of the mouth towards the right during opening. CT revealed a calcified mass arising from the right TMJ which eroded the right skull base and extended to the infra-temporal fossa and the middle cranial fossa. The lesion measured 45 mm × 36 mm × 32 mm. MRI showed the outspread of the lesion to the subdural space; however, the dura was intact. The lesion was highly suggestive of synovial chondromatosis. The lesion was critically close to important vital structures showing 5 mm to the internal carotid, 5 mm to the jugular vein, and very close proximity to the spinous foramen and the middle meningeal artery. The proposed surgical resection of the lesion was designed digitally through the use of the CT scan data for the 3D reconstruction and segmentation of the lesion. The design of the surgical osteotomy was conducted on the 3D reconstruction, and templates were fabricated to demarcate the outline of the osteotomy. Through pre-auricular and submandibular approaches, and by the use of the digital osteotomy template, the lesion was resected as a whole while preserving the facial nerve, the dura, and the other nearby vital structures. Biopsy revealed a synovial chondrosarcoma secondary to synovial chondromatosis, a very rare cartilaginous malignancy affecting large joints. There was no tumor infiltration to the surrounding soft tissues, thus immediate reconstruction was performed. The patient recovered following the surgery with neither facial asymmetry nor paralysis, and with improved mouth opening. The radiographic assessment after 1 year showed an acceptable remodeling of the joint. (**a**) Digitally designed outline for the resection; 1, outline for condylar osteotomy; 2, outline for temporary zygomatic arch osteotomy; 3, outline for temporary cranial osteotomy; 4, anterior and posterior limits of the designed osteotomy; 5, outline for the anticipated resection of tissues between the TMJ capsule and the lesion. (**b, c**) The use of the digitally designed templates during the surgical osteotomies [68]

important nearby vital structures and design the osteotomy in a safe manner. The precision of the digital design and resection allowed the execution of the surgery without complications [68].

9.7 Conclusions

In conclusion, the management of TMD has benefited from digitization, likewise the other fields of dentistry. Although this chapter is not inclusive of all the clinical and research applications of digitization in the field of TMD; however, the chapter provides an overview of the applications with remarkable influence in the field. The diagnosis of TMD is a challenge, and digitization will aid in achieving more precise interpretations by eliminating human errors. In addition, digitization will assist the treatment planning and decision-making processes in managing TMD. Digitization will soon help in the preclinical training of surgeons specialized in TMD and will even allow the remote supervision of the surgical procedures. The designing of tailored patient-specific management approaches for TMD patients is an important achievement in managing advanced forms of TMD. Furthermore, the current developments will encourage future research in different aspects of TMD management, with the ultimate goal of facilitating and standardizing the diagnosis and improving the treatment outcomes.

References

1. National Institute of Dental and Craniofacial Research. https://www.nidcr.nih.gov/research/data-statistics/facial-pain/ (accessed 25/11/2019).
2. Di Paolo C, Costanzo GD, Panti F, Rampello A, Falisi G, Pilloni A, Cascone P, Iannetti G. Epidemiological analysis on 2375 patients with TMJ disorders: basic statistical aspects. Ann Stomatol. 2013;4(1):161–9.
3. Helkimo M. Studies on function and dysfunction of the masticatory system. II. Index for anamnestic and clinical dysfunction and occlusal state. Sven Tandlak Tidskr. 1974;67:101–21.
4. Oleson J, for The International Headache Society. Classification and diagnostic criteria for headache disorders, cranial neuralgias and facial pain. Cephalalgia. 1988;8(suppl 7):1–97.
5. McNeill C, editor. Temporomandibular disorders: guidelines for classification, assessment, and management. 2nd ed. Chicago: Quintessence Publishing; 1993. p. 39–60.
6. Dworkin SF, LeResche L. Research diagnostic criteria for temporomandibular disorders: review criteria, examinations and specifications, critique. J Craniomandib Disord. 1992;6:301–55.
7. Schiffman E, Ohrbach R, Truelove E, Look J, Anderson G, Goulet JP, et al. Diagnostic criteria for temporomandibular disorders (DC/TMD) for clinical and research applications: recommendations of the international RDC/TMD consortium network and orofacial pain special interest group. J Oral Facial Pain Headache. 2014;28(1):6–27.
8. Talaat WM, Adel OI, Al Bayatti S. Prevalence of temporomandibular disorders discovered incidentally during routine dental examination using the research diagnostic criteria for temporomandibular disorders. Oral Surg Oral Med Oral Pathol Oral Radiol. 2018;125(3):250–9.
9. Gonçalves DA, Speciali JG, Jales LC, Camparis CM, Bigal ME. Temporomandibular symptoms, migraine and chronic daily headaches in the population. Neurology. 2009;73:645–6.
10. Leeuw R. Dor Orofacial: Guia de Avaliação, Diagnóstico e Tratamento. 4th ed. Quintessence: São Paulo, Brazil; 2010.
11. Nebbe B, Major PW. Prevalence of TMJ disc displacement in a pre-orthodontic adolescent sample. Angle Orthod. 2000;70:454–63.
12. Simmons HC 3rd. Why are dentists not trained to screen and diagnose temporomandibular disorders in dental school? Cranio. 2016;34:76–8.
13. Brooks SL, Brand JW, Gibbs SJ, Hollender L, Lurie AG, Omnell KA, Westesson PL, White SC. Imaging of the temporomandibular joint: a position paper of the American Academy of Oral and Maxillofacial Radiology. Oral Surg Oral Med Oral Pathol Oral Radiol Endod. 1997;83:609–18.
14. Ahmad M, Hollender L, Anderson Q, Kartha K, Ohrbach R, Truelove EL, John MT, Schiffman EL. Research diagnostic criteria for temporomandibular disorders (RDC / TMD): development of image analysis criteria and examiner reliability for image analysis. Oral Surg Oral Med Oral Pathol Oral Radiol Endod. 2009;107:844–60.
15. Flygare L, Rohlin M, Akerman S. Microscopy and tomography of erosive changes in the temporomandibular joint. An autopsy study. Acta Odontol Scand. 1995;53:297–303.

16. Zarb GA, Carlsson GE. Temporomandibular disorders: osteoarthritis. J Orofac Pain. 1999; 13(295):306.
17. Barghan S, Tetradis S, Mallya SM. Application of cone beam computed tomography for assessment of the temporomandibular joints. Aust Dent J. 2012;57:109–18.
18. Honda K, Larheim TA, Maruhashi K, Matsumoto K, Iwai K. Osseous abnormalities of the mandibular condyle: diagnostic reliability of cone beam computed tomography compared with helical computed tomography based on an autopsy material. Dentomaxillofac Radiol. 2006;35:152–7.
19. Talaat W, Al Bayatti S, Al Kawas S. CBCT analysis of bony changes associated with temporo-mandibular disorders. Cranio. 2016;34:88–94.
20. Su N, Liu Y, Yang X, Luo Z, Shi Z. Correlation between bony changes measured with cone beam computed tomography and clinical dysfunction index in patients with temporomandibu-lar joint osteoarthritis. J Craniomaxillofac Surg. 2014;42(7):1402–7.
21. de Boer EW, Dijkstra PU, Stegenga B, de Bont LG, Spijkervet FK. Value of cone-beam com-puted tomography in the process of diagnosis and management of disorders of the temporo-mandibular joint. Br J Oral Maxillofac Surg. 2014;52(3):241–6.
22. Pullinger AG, Seligman DA, Gornbein JA. A multiple regression analysis of risk and relative odds of temporomandibular disorders as a function of common occlusal features. J Dent Res. 1993;72(6):968–79.
23. Wang C, Yin X. Occlusal risk factors associated with temporomandibular disorders in young adults with normal occlusions. Oral Surg Oral Med Oral Pathol Oral Radiol. 2012;114(4): 419–23.
24. Kerstein RB, Radke J. Masseter and temporalis excursive hyperactivity decreased by measured anterior guidance development. Cranio. 2012;30(4):243–54.
25. Haralur SB. Digital evaluation of functional occlusion parameters and their association with temporomandibular disorders. J Clin Diagn Res. 2013;7(8):1772–5.
26. Williamson EH, Lundquist DO. Anterior guidance: its effect on electromyographic activity of the temporal and masseter muscles. J Prosthet Dent. 1983;49(6):816–23.
27. Ciavarella D, Parziale V, Mastrovincenzo M, Palazzo A, Sabatucci A, Suriano MM, Bossù M, Cazzolla AP, Lo Muzio L, Chimenti C. Condylar position indicator and T-scan system II in clinical evaluation of temporomandibular intracapsular disease. J Craniomaxillofac Surg. 2012;40(5):449–55.
28. Gibbs CH, Messerman T, Reswick JB, Derda HJ. Functional movements of the mandible. J Prosthet Dent. 1971;26:604–20.
29. Airoldi RL, Gallo LM, Palla S. Precision of the jaw tracking system JAWS-3D. J Orofac Pain. 1994;8:155–64.
30. Ferrario VF, Sforza C, Miani A, Serrao G. Kinesiographic three dimensional evaluation of mandibular border movements: a statistical study in a normal young nonpatient group. J Prosthet Dent. 1992;68:672–6.
31. Naeije M, Van der Weijden JJ, Megens CC. Okas-3D: optoelectronic jaw movement recording system with six degrees of freedom. Med Biol Eng Comput. 1995;33:683–8.
32. Chen C-C, Chen Y-J, Chen S-C, Lin H-S, Lu T-W. Evaluation of soft tissue artifacts when using anatomical and technical markers to measure mandibular motion. J Dental Sci. 2011;6:95–101.
33. Chen CC, Lin CC, Chen YJ, Hong SW, Lu TW. A method for measuring three-dimensional mandibular kinematics in vivo using single-plane fluoroscopy. Dentomaxillofac Radiol. 2013;42(1):95958184.
34. Behr M, Held P, Leibrock A, Fellner C, Handel G. Diagnostic potential of pseudo-dynamic MRI (CINE mode) for evaluation of internal derangement of the TMJ. Eur J Radiol. 1996;23: 212–5.
35. Frahm J, Schätz S, Untenberger M, Zhang S, Voit D, Merboldt KD, Sohns JM, Lotz J, Uecker M. On the temporal fidelity of nonlinear inverse reconstructions for real-time MRI—the motion challenge. Open Med Imaging J. 2014;8:1–5.
36. Krohn S, Joseph AA, Voit D, Michaelis T, Merboldt KD, Buergers R, Frahm J. Multi-slice real-time MRI of temporomandibular joint dynamics. Dentomaxillofac Radiol. 2018;20:20180162.

37. Zhang S, Block KT, Frahm J. Magnetic resonance imaging in real time: advances using radial FLASH. J Magn Reson Imaging. 2010;31:101–9.
38. Wang S, Li H, Li J, Zhang Y, Zou B. Automatic analysis of lateral cephalograms based on multiresolution decision tree regression voting. J Healthc Eng. 2018;2018:1–15.
39. Jiang F, Jiang Y, Zhi H, Dong Y, Li H, Ma S, et al. Artificial intelligence in healthcare: past, present and future. Stroke Vasc Neurol. 2017;2:230–43.
40. Fazal MI, Patel ME, Tye J, Gupta Y. The past, present and future role of artificial intelligence in imaging. Eur J Radiol. 2018;105:246–50.
41. Dayhoff JE, DeLeo JM. Artificial neural networks: opening the black box. Cancer. 2001;91:1615–35.
42. Speight PM, Elliott AE, Jullien JA, Downer MC, Zakzrewska JM. The use of artificial intelligence to identify people at risk of oral cancer and precancer. Br Dent J. 1995;179:382–7.
43. Brickley MR, Shepherd JP, Armstrong RA. Neural networks: a new technique for development of decision support systems in dentistry. J Dent. 1998;26:305–9.
44. Kann BH, Aneja S, Loganadane GV, Kelly JR, Smith SM, et al. Pretreatment identification of head and neck cancer nodal metastasis and extranodal extension using deep learning neural networks. Sci Rep. 2018;8:14036.
45. Radke JC, Ketcham R, Glassman B, Kull R. Artificial neural network learns to differentiate normal TMJs and nonreducing displaced disks after training on incisor-point chewing movements. Cranio. 2003;21(4):259–64.
46. Shoukri B, Prieto JC, Ruellas A, Yatabe M, Sugai J, Styner M, et al. Minimally invasive approach for diagnosing TMJ osteoarthritis. J Dent Res. 2019;98(10):1103–11.
47. de Dumast P, Mirabel C, Cevidanes L, Ruellas A, Yatabe M, Ioshida M, et al. A web-based system for neural network based classification in temporomandibular joint osteoarthritis. Comput Med Imaging Graph. 2018;67:45–54.
48. Moloney F, Howard JA. Internal derangements of the temporomandibular joint. III. Anterior repositioning splint therapy. Aust Dent J. 1986;31(1):30–9.
49. Randolph CS, Greene CS, Moretti R, et al. Conservative management of temporomandibular disorders: a post-treatment comparison between patients from a university clinic and from private practice. Am J Orthod Dentofac Orthop. 1990;98(1):77–82.
50. Bjørnland T, Larheim TA. Synovectomy and diskectomy of the temporomandibular joint in patients with chronic arthritic disease compared with diskectomies in patients with internal derangement. A 3-year follow-up study. Eur J Oral Sci. 1995;103:2–7.
51. Bjørnland T, Larheim TA, Haanaes HR. Surgical treatment of temporomandibular joints in patients with chronic arthritic disease: preoperative findings and one-year follow-up. Cranio. 1992;10:205–10.
52. Onishi M. Arthroscopy of the temporomandibular joint. Kokubyo Gakkai Zasshi. 1975;42:207–13.
53. Holmlund A, Hellsing G. Arthroscopy of the temporomandibular joint: an autopsy study. Int J Oral Maxillofac Surg. 1985;14:169–75.
54. Sanders B. Arthroscopic surgery of the temporomandibular joint: treatment of internal derangement with persistent closed lock. Oral Surg Oral Med Oral Pathol. 1986;62:361–72.
55. González-García R. The current role and the future of minimally invasive temporomandibular joint surgery. Oral Maxillofac Surg Clin North Am. 2015;27(1):69–84.
56. Murakami K, Iizuka T, Matsuki M, et al. Recapturing the persistent anteriorly displaced disk by mandibular manipulation after pumping and hydraulic pressure to the upper joint cavity of the temporomandibular joint. Cranio. 1987;5:17–24.
57. Nitzan DW, Franklin Dolwick MF, Martinez GA. Temporomandibular joint arthrocentesis: a simplified treatment for severe, limited mouth opening. J Oral Maxillofac Surg. 1991;49:1163–7.
58. Rehman KU, Hall T. Single needle arthrocentesis. Br J Oral Maxillofac Surg. 2009;47:403–4.
59. Guarda-Nardini L, Manfredini D, Ferronato G. Arthrocentesis of the temporomandibular joint: a proposal for a single-needle technique. Oral Surg Oral Med Oral Pathol Oral Radiol Endod. 2008;106:483–6.

60. Talaat W, Ghoneim M, Elsholkamy M. Single-needle arthrocentesis (Shepard cannula) vs. double-needle arthrocentesis for treating disc displacement without reduction. Cranio. 2016;34(5):296–302.
61. Talaat WM, McGraw TA, Klitzman B. Relationship between the canthal-tragus distance and the puncture point in temporomandibular joint arthroscopy. Int J Oral Maxillofac Surg. 2010;39:57–60.
62. Wagner A, Undt G, Watzinger F, Wanschitz F, Schicho K, Yerit K, et al. Principles of computer-assisted arthroscopy of the temporomandibular joint with optoelectronic tracking technology. Oral Surg Oral Med Oral Pathol Oral Radiol Endod. 2001;92(1):30–7.
63. He Y, Huang T, Zhang Y, An J, He L. Application of a computer-assisted surgical navigation system in temporomandibular joint ankylosis surgery: a retrospective study. Int J Oral Maxillofac Surg. 2017;46(2):189–97.
64. Krause M, Dörfler HM, Kruber D, Hümpfner-Hierl H, Hierl T. Template-based temporomandibular joint puncturing and access in minimally invasive TMJ surgery (MITMJS)—a technical note and first clinical results. Head Face Med. 2019;15(1):10.
65. Westermark A. Total reconstruction of the temporomandibular joint. Up to 8 years of follow-up of patients treated with Biomet (®) total joint prosthesis. Int J Oral Maxillofac Surg. 2010;39(10):951–5.
66. Wolford LM, Mercuri LG, Schneiderman ED, Movahed R, Allen W. Twenty-year follow-up study on a patient-fitted temporomandibular joint prosthesis: the Techmedica/TMJ concepts device. J Oral Maxillofac Surg. 2015;73(5):952–60.
67. Zheng J, Chen X, Jiang W, Zhang SY, Chen MJ, Yang C. An innovative total temporomandibular joint prosthesis with customized design and 3D printing additive fabrication: a prospective clinical study. J Transl Med. 2019;17:4.
68. Ye ZX, Yang C, Chen MJ, Huang D, Abdelrehem A. Digital resection and reconstruction of TMJ synovial chondrosarcoma involving the skull base: report of a case. Int J Clin Exp Med. 2015;8(7):11589–193.

Digitization in Operative Dentistry

10

Mahantesh Yeli and Mohan Bhuvaneswaran

10.1 Introduction

There has been tremendous advancements and innovations in the field of material science, technology and adhesive dentistry which has brought about a sea of change in the way we practice dentistry today. Transformations from the traditional dentistry to digital dentistry are making far-reaching consequences to patient care and also affecting the landscape of digitization of operative dentistry [1]. The CAD/CAM concepts were introduced into dental applications by Dr. Francois Duret in Lyon France in the year 1973. He later developed and patented the CAD/CAM device in the year 1984. Digital impressions were first used in orthodontics, but the use of the first intraoral scanner in restorative dentistry was in the 1980s by a Swiss dentist, Dr. Werner Mormann, and an Italian electrical engineer, Marco Brandestini. They further developed the concept which was introduced in 1987 as CEREC (Sirona dental systems) as the first commercially available CAD/CAM system for dental restorations [2].

The chapter will give a brief introduction about caries detection methods, which have already been introduced to the reader at the beginning of the book, and then guide through the digital processing of a ceramic inlay talking about all the steps from tooth preparation, digital impression taking, data processing and manufacturing/milling to try in and cementation. Subtraction and additive methods of digital manufacturing will also be discussed at the end of the chapter in brief. It is beyond the scope of this book to explain each and every digital technique currently available in detail, but every attempt has been made to introduce the reader to them.

M. Yeli (✉)
Department of Operative Dentistry and Endodontics, SDM College of Dental Sciences, Dharwad, India

M. Bhuvaneswaran
Sri Ramachandra University, Chennai, India

MAHSA University, Petaling Jaya, Malaysia

© Springer Nature Switzerland AG 2021
P. Jain, M. Gupta (eds.), *Digitization in Dentistry*,
https://doi.org/10.1007/978-3-030-65169-5_10

10.2   Digital Caries Diagnosis and Assessment

The carious lesion is a dynamic process, which is affected by numerous factors and varied aetiology. These factors tend to move the equilibrium either towards remineralization or demineralization [3], and as there is greater understanding regarding the advancements and the evidence supporting the carious process, it becomes more imperative to look for preventive measures which preserve the function, aesthetics and structure of the tooth.

The inability to detect early lesions leads to deep enamel caries, resulting in poor outcomes of the remineralization process, so methods have to be devised to quantify early mineral loss and to initiate correct intervention [4]. The traditional caries detection systems facilitated a more qualitative aspect of the disease progress, such as colour and anatomical location [5], and modifying factors like oral hygiene, salivary flow and microorganisms. These assessments gave limited information for early detection of noncavitated lesions; hence, the newer novel diagnostic systems offer true quantification and detection of lesions in the initial stages.

These newer detection systems work on the physical signals that include electronic current, x-rays, lasers, visible light and ultrasound (Table 10.1). These systems should be able to initiate, receive and interpret the signals so that the caries detection systems perform effectively [6].

10.3   Electrical Current Measurement

10.3.1 Electronic Caries Monitor (ECM)

The ECM works on single fixed-frequency alternating current which measures the 'bulk resistance' of the tooth tissue. The ECM probe is applied on a particular site or surface level at 5-second measurement cycle (Fig. 10.1). The ECM works on the principle of increased porosity associated with caries which is responsible for the mechanism of action of ECM [7].

Table 10.1 Methods of different caries detection based on their underlying principles

Medium of energy source	Clinical applications
X-rays	• Digital subtraction radiography
	• Digital image enhancement
Visible light	• Fibre optic transillumination. (FOTI)
	• Diode laser fluorescence (DLF)
	• Digital imaging fibre optic transillumination (DiFOTI)
Laser light	Laser fluorescence measurement (DIAGNOdent)
Electrical current	Electrical conductance measurement (ECM)
Ultrasound	Ultrasonic caries detector

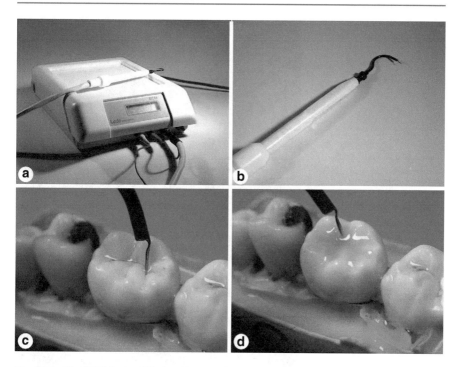

Fig. 10.1   The ECM device (Version 4) and its clinical application. (**a**) The ECM machine, (**b**) the ECM handpiece, (**c**) site-specific measurement technique, (**d**) surface-specific measurement technique. (*Reproduced with permission from Elsevier Publishing*) [6]

10.4   Radiographic Techniques

10.4.1 Digital Radiographs

A digital radiograph is a conventional radiograph which is digitized and comprises a number of pixels, each pixel carries a value of 0–255, with 0 being black and 255 being white [6] (Fig. 10.2) the values in between represent shades of grey. The digital radiographs offer potential of image enhancement by applying range of algorithms, so when these radiographs are assessed, their diagnostic value is as equivalent to that of conventional radiographs [8]. Other additional benefits include decrease in radiographic dose and replication and archiving of images. Detailed information about the digital radiographs is given in Chap. 3.

10.4.1.1   Subtraction Radiography
Digital radiographs have numerous advantages like image enhancement, processing and manipulation. The most important advancement in radiographic technologies is

Fig. 10.2 Radio
visiography

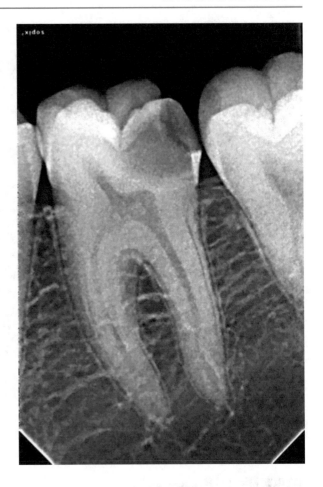

the development of subtraction radiography in the detection of caries and assessment of bone loss in periodontics. The principle is that two radiographs are compared using their pixel values and any difference in the values might be due to change in the object (Fig. 10.3).

10.4.1.2   DiFOTI

A new reliable method for detecting dental caries, where images of teeth are captured through visible-light is the fibre optic transillumination with CCD camera which are relayed to the computer for analysis with predetermined algorithms. The algorithms are developed to facilitate the location and diagnosis of carious lesions in real time which provides quantitative characterization for monitoring of lesions [9] (Fig. 10.4).

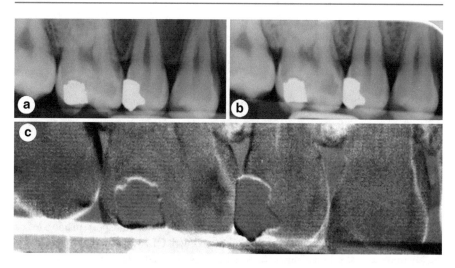

Fig. 10.3 (a) Radiograph showing proximal lesion on the mesial surface of the first molar, (b) follow-up radiograph taken 12 months later, (c) the areas of difference between the two films are shown as black, i.e. in this case, the proximal lesion has become more radiolucent and hence has progressed. *(Reproduced with permission from Elsevier Publishing)* [6]

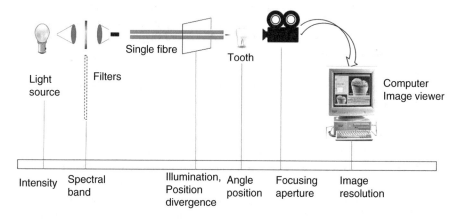

Fig. 10.4 DIFOTI working principle

10.5 Fluorescent Techniques

10.5.1 QLF (Quantitative Laser Fluorescence)

QLF is an optical diagnostic technique for the detection of early carious lesions in enamel. In 1998, Ferreira Zandona et al. used QLF technology for the very first time to assess caries on occlusal surfaces. Characteristic features of the technique are the detection, quantification and analysis of the lesion.

Table 10.2 Advantages and disadvantages of QLF

Advantages	Disadvantages
• Noninvasive diagnostic tool	• Not a confirmatory diagnostic tool
• User-friendly	• Not suitable for use on proximal lesions
• Reproducible and reliable method of quantifying mineral loss in enamel	• Plaque, calculus, and extrinsic stains obstruct detection of lesion
• Exhibits high sensitivity and specificity	• Fluorosis and developmental defects give a similar appearance as a white-spot lesion

10.5.1.1 Working Principle

QLF uses the natural fluorescence of teeth to differentiate between sound enamel and carious lesion. In a white-spot lesion, there is the disintegration of the crystalline structure resulting in more internal reflection sites. This results in the increased scattering of incident light which implies that the mean 'free path of photon transport' inside a lesion is shorter than in sound enamel. A lesion observed with QLF appears dark compared to highly luminescent sound enamel. Table 10.2 gives its benefits and drawbacks.

10.5.1.2 Uses

- Detection of early carious lesions in enamel in conjugation with ICDAS.
- Detection and differentiation of noncavitated root caries on root surfaces.
- Detection of early secondary caries adjacent to existing restorations.
- Detection of white-spot lesions after de-bracketing in orthodontic patients.
- Localization of enamel cracks and quantification of their severity.
- Assessment of severity of tooth wear and monitoring its changes in clinical situations.
- Measure the efficacy of treatment in patients, e.g. remineralization of a white-spot lesion.

10.5.1.3 DIAGNOdent

The DIAGNOdent is a device which utilizes fluorescence to detect caries. A red light is produced with the excitation of the laser at a wavelength of 655 nm which is designed to be delivered to pits and fissures and the smooth surfaces by one of the two intraoral tips. The tips emit the light and record the resultant fluorescence. The DIAGNOdent (Fig. 10.5) doesn't produce an image unlike the QLF, but displays a numerical value. Spitzer and Bosch (1975) suggested that when subjected to certain wavelengths, carious lesions emit more intense fluorescence than sound tissue due to organic compounds and proteinic chromophores in the affected tooth tissue. The DIAGNOdent produces a single-digit reading (0–99) and relies on the principle of validation that has high sensitivity for detecting early carious lesions [10].

10.6 Digital Restoration Workflow- the CAD/CAM Technique

This section will talk about the steps required for the fabrication of a CAD/CAM restoration, namely, the digital restoration workflow, beginning with the tooth preparation to digital impressions taking to data processing and manufacturing to finally try in and cementation.

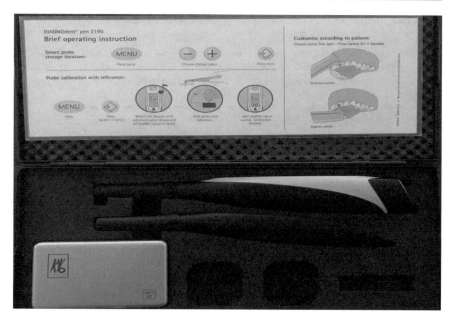

Fig. 10.5 DIAGNOdent

There are mainly three phases in the digital workflow:

1. The first phase is to record the geometry of the patient's intraoral status to a computer system using an intraoral camera. This is called as digital impression.
2. The second phase uses a software program to design and construct the volume proposal of the restoration.
3. The third phase involves the production of the restoration using a machining device [11].

10.6.1 Tooth Preparation for Digital Restorations/CAD/CAM Inlay or Onlay

The aesthetic inlay or onlay procedures using ceramic and composites began to be used in 1980s to counter the drawbacks of amalgam and direct composite restorations. The recent advances in adhesive dentistry coupled with material advancements in stacked, feldspathic porcelain were vital in addressing the deficiencies associated with direct composite like high wear, high shrinkage, low strength and technique sensitivity. The lab-fabricated ceramic and processed indirect composites had better physical properties, contacts and contours, and ideal proximal contacts and potential for better and efficient occlusal contacts; restorations and guidelines are based on the type of restorative material used for the particular type of restoration [12]. Tables 10.3 and 10.4 gives the indications, contraindications, advantages and drawbacks of

Table 10.3 Indications and Contraindications of CAD/CAM restorations

Indications	Contraindications
• Indirect tooth-coloured restorations are indicated in class 1 and class 2 (inlays and onlays) which are located in aesthetic areas as desired by the patient • Extensive carious lesions or large defects, (class 1 and class 2) with wide facio-lingual or mesiodistal caries and teeth which require cuspal coverage	• High occlusal forces, ceramic restorations which are subject to excessive occlusal stress for, e.g. bruxism or clenching habits • Isolation • Deep subgingival preparations, where margins are difficult to record in digital impressions and are difficult to evaluate and also for finishing and polishing

Table 10.4 Advantages and disadvantages of CAD/CAM restorations

Advantages	Disadvantages
• Improved physical properties • Varieties of materials and techniques • Wear resistance • Reduced polymerization shrinkage • Support of remaining tooth structure • More precise control of contact and contours • Biocompatibility and good tissue response	• Increased cost and time • Technique sensitivity • Difficult try in and delivery • Brittleness of ceramics • Wear of opposing dentition • Low potential for repair

using the technique. According to the author, there is not much demarcation between the digital CAD-CAM and conventional method of tooth preparation.

10.6.2 Principle of Inlay and Onlay

10.6.2.1 Outline Form

The outline form is generally governed by the extension of caries and existing restorations and is quite similar to the conventional metal inlay/onlay preparations, as the cavity preparation is dictated by the principles of adhesive dentistry employed; undercuts are avoided or blocked by resin-modified GIC and by preserving most of the enamel for adhesion.

Most of the undermined enamel or weakened enamel should be eliminated; the central groove reduction of 1.8 mm (occlusal surface) should follow the anatomy of the unprepared tooth surface. The outline should avoid occlusal contacts and have a clearance of 1.5 mm in all excursions to prevent ceramic fracture.

The box should be extended to allow for a minimum of 0.6 mm of proximal clearance for ease of impression making, margins are preferably kept supragingival for better recording and accuracy of a digital impression and also luting and finishing procedures. The width of the gingival seat should be approximately 1 mm. To prevent stress concentration all the internal line angles and point angles should be rounded and also to prevent voids during the cementation procedure.

10.6.2.2   Margin Design

Ceramic inlay margins are given a 90-degree butt joint; bevels are contraindicated as the margins need bulk of ceramic to prevent fracture. A heavy chamfer is recommended for ceramic onlay margins.

10.6.2.3   Occlusal Clearance

A clearance of approximately 1.5 mm is needed to prevent fracture in all excursions. This can be evaluated by using a dial caliper [13]. The principles of cavity preparation for aesthetic inlays differs from the gold restorations. In aesthetic inlay/onlay restorations, bevels and retention forms are not required, and resistance form is necessary for only large onlay restorations. An estimation of 5–15 degrees of flare is given on the cavity walls, and butt joint is given on the gingival seat/floor. All the internal line angles are rounded and a minimum of 2 mm isthmus width is given and depth of 1.5 mm (Fig. 10.6).

The functional and the nonfunctional cusps are given at least 1.5–2 mm of clearance so as to achieve bulk of material in these areas; if the margins of the onlay are visible on the buccal/facial side, then there can be further reduction of 1–2 mm with a minimum of 1 mm chamfer (Fig. 10.7).

When the occlusal aspect of the cavity is prepared, more amount of tooth structure should not be sacrificed while trying to eliminate undercuts; this is done so as to achieve conservative approach for cavity preparation. The bucco-palatal width of the lesion determines whether the cusp has to cap or not, cavo-surface margin of 50–75% on the cuspal inclines, and also when the cusp does not have sufficient dentin support underneath, the cusp gives a consensus to cap the cusp. This is done so as to reinforce the remaining tooth structure [13].

Intraoral digital scanners are line-of-sight cameras that record areas directly visible to the camera. Maximum amount of tooth structure is recorded when the camera lens is parallel to the tooth structure and the field of view is angulated perpendicular to the tooth surface, as it affords maximum surface of the tooth to be available to the camera.

Fig. 10.6 Inlay preparation

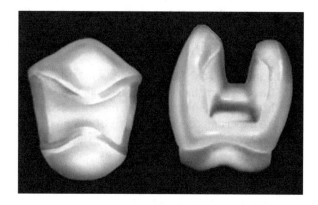

Fig. 10.7 Onlay
preparation

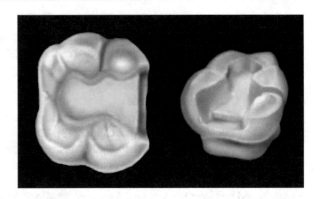

Fig. 10.7 Onlay preparation

10.6.3 Guidelines for Digital Impressions

The acquisition of an accurate negative copy of a prepared tooth or teeth and that of adjacent and opposing teeth are the ultimate goals of the impression process in restorative dentistry [14]. The CAD/CAM systems that are available in the market currently feed the data obtained from the digital scans of teeth directly into the milling machines capable of creating restorations out of ceramic or composite resin blocks without the need for a physical replica of the prepared, adjacent and opposing teeth. The marginal fit and the adaptation of the restoration is directly related to the accuracy of the recorded tooth preparation, these concepts hold true for both conventional and digital impressions.

Cavity preparation should be free of moisture, as the saliva, blood or soft tissues obscure the view. The digital camera only records those areas which are well isolated and visible; hence, a well-controlled scanning environment is essential for a perfectly fitting restoration.

Proper gingival displacement is essential so as to visualize the prepared margins for effective recording of the areas of the dentition. The digital scanners require only 150 microns of gingival displacement for sufficient visualization as compared to conventional impressions which require at least 1 mm of gingival retraction past the margins for recording, which is an advantage over conventional impressions.

The ultimate goal for the accurate recording of the digital impression is to have the 'real' or the 'actual' data than the 'calculated' or the 'extrapolated' data. In conventional impressions, the critical or non-critical areas in the impression are depended on the proper fit of the final restoration; if there is any discrepancy (voids, bubbles, undercuts), then the whole impression has to be repeated unlike in digital impressions where the virtual cast can be rotated and magnified on the computer monitor to search for the missing or distorted data. The advantage of a digital impression is that the missing area can be additionally scanned and can be added to the existing virtual cast than remaking the entire digital impression [11].

10.6.4 Intraoral Scanners

There are various types of intraoral scanners presently available in the market which use different methods to acquire the images. The scanners utilize lasers of different wavelengths and LEDs for scanning [15] (Figs. 10.8 and 10.9). For more detailed knowledge about them, the reader is referred to Chap. 11 in this book.

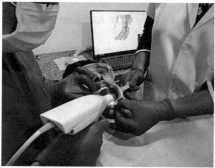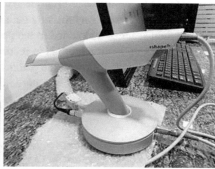

Fig. 10.8 Intraoral scanner

```
                          ┌──────────────────┐
                          │  Color/black and │
                          │      white       │
                          └──────────────────┘

┌──────────────────┐                          ┌──────────────────┐
│   Open/closed    │                          │ Corded/cordless  │
└──────────────────┘                          └──────────────────┘

┌──────────────────┐    ┌──────────────────┐  ┌──────────────────┐
│  Power/powder-   │    │     Scanner      │  │ Scanning speed:  │
│      free        │    │     system       │  │    fast/slow     │
└──────────────────┘    └──────────────────┘  └──────────────────┘

┌──────────────────┐                          ┌──────────────────┐
│ Single/multiple  │                          │    Top size:     │
│ image acquisition│                          │  small/thin or   │
└──────────────────┘                          │   large/thick    │
                                              └──────────────────┘

                          ┌──────────────────┐
                          │  STL/.OBJ/.PLY   │
                          │     (format)     │
                          └──────────────────┘
```

Fig. 10.9 Classification of different scanners

10.6.5 Digital Impression Workflow

Once the tooth preparation is completed, the margins are visualized and isolated from moisture. The preparation is coated with titanium dioxide powder which enhances the accuracy and speed of the scanning process.

The scanning is done over multiple passes over the preparation and adjacent teeth (as shown in the (Figs. 10.10 and 10.11) and the opposing teeth, and these data are sent over to the software program which will combine the scanned sections into one virtual single cast. Any missing data or areas desired to be included in the final cast are then scanned and added to the previous scan.

The most important feature is to record the occlusal contact relationships of the patients opposing dentition on the planned restoration. The maxillary and mandibular virtual casts are separately recorded for digital impressions, after which the patient is guided into maximum intercuspation and the digital scanning of the facial

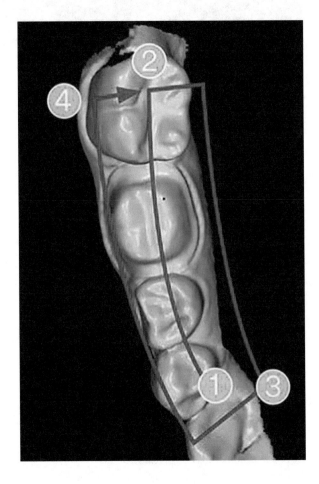

Fig. 10.10 Scanning recommended for quadrant wise scanning. *(Reproduced with Permission from Dr. Gary Kaye, The New York Center for Digital dentistry)* [1]

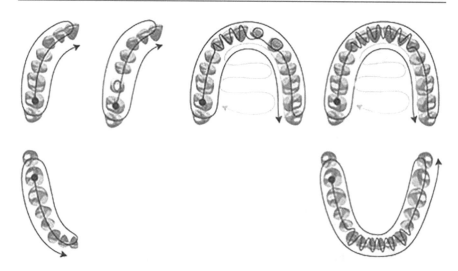

Fig. 10.11 Scan recommended for full arch scanning. *(Reproduced with Permission from Dr. Gary Kaye, The New York Center for Digital dentistry)* [1]

surfaces of the opposing teeth is done in a static position. The software uses the scan to match the facial surfaces of the opposing dentition to reproduce the patient's vertical dimension of the occlusion.

There has been no software developed to measure the protrusive and lateral functional movements available with current digital impressions systems yet in the market; studies have shown that there is no significant difference in the vertical dimension between the buccal scan mounting generated for the digital impressions and the master mounting [16].

Once the virtual casts have been recorded, the preparation can be visualized at a higher magnification on the monitor. This is done so as to critically evaluate whether the preparation margins have been recorded accurately before transferring the data to the lab/software. Another option is to quantitatively evaluate the occlusal clearance from the opposing cast, which is done to achieve adequate thickness for the proposed restoration (Fig. 10.12).

A stereolithography file (commonly referred to as .stl file) (Fig. 10.13) is commonly used to store the data derived from the digital impressions of the intraoral structures. Once the scanning process is completed, the data is electronically transmitted to the dental laboratory for processing.

There are two options in the laboratory:

- Firstly, the data file can be forwarded to the processing centre. Resin or polyurethane casts can be fabricated for the case, and on these articulated casts, the restoration can be fabricated with NiCr, gold or PFM.
- Secondly, the data file can be directly imported into the CAD/CAM software program for further designing and fabrication of the restoration [17] (Fig. 10.14).

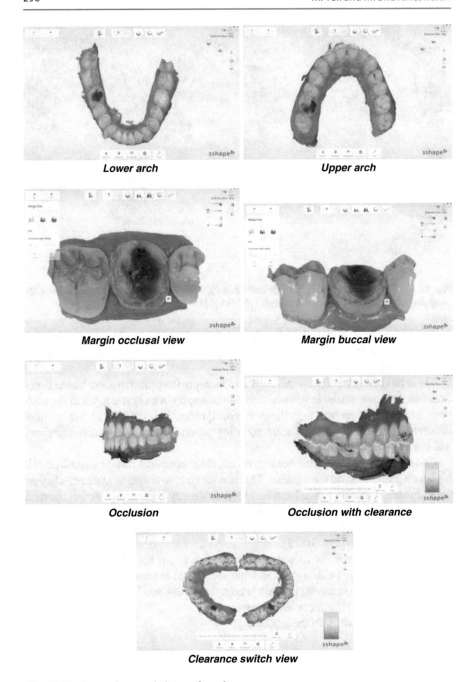

Lower arch

Upper arch

Margin occlusal view

Margin buccal view

Occlusion

Occlusion with clearance

Clearance switch view

Fig. 10.12 Intraoral scanned pictures for onlay

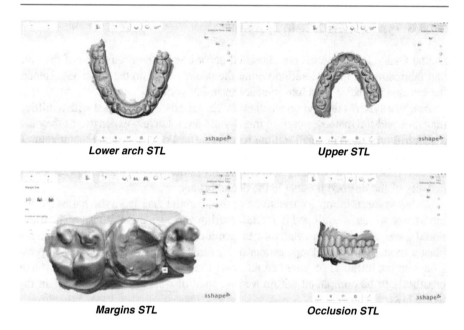

Fig. 10.13   Intraoral scanned images in STL format

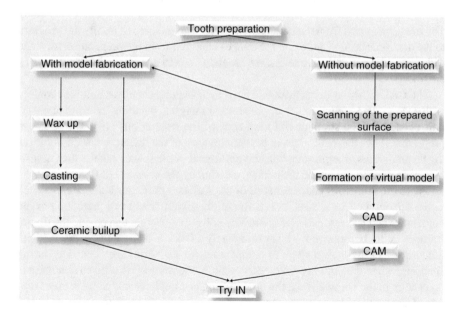

Fig. 10.14   Methods for using a digital impression data from an intraoral scanner according to the need for modelling

10.6.6 Types of CAD/CAM Systems

Dental CAD/CAM systems are classified according to the acquisition of the data and fabrication of the restoration within the dental office on the same day. Hence, the systems can be divided into in-office or in-lab systems.

In-office systems depend on whether the dental office is equipped with a milling machine, and the materials used in this system are relatively expensive as they use a mandrill type used in small milling machines (lava or Ivoclar) and manufactured exclusively for dental applications. The use is limited to manufacturing inlays and crowns and offers the advantage of being an all-in-one system that allows same-day delivery of the finished product in the dental office.

In-lab systems comprise transferring the scanned data from the patient to the laboratory which is equipped in manufacturing varieties of prostheses. The traditional Lava and Procera systems can produce zirconia crowns by scanning a plaster model with a desktop scanner or by directly acquiring the digital impression with the intraoral scanner and allowing the manufacture of the restoration or prosthesis to be completed within a short span of time at any laboratory in the world [18].

10.6.7 Data Processing of the Digital Impression

The image acquired from the data is transferred with the help of a software program to the data processing centre and the images captured from the preparation form the tridimensional network. These images are then used to design the inlays, onlays or prosthesis.

The CAD/CAM systems available have their own mechanisms and functioning, with each system having to detect preparation margins, planning the form and support needed for the strength and aesthetics of the restorations [19]. The software program follows the same steps in the construction of the restoration such as blocking the undercuts, margin selection and placement of die spacer, but the final adjustments are carried out by the technician, assisted by the software [20].

There are numerous characteristics of the software programs and materials such as the selection of the shades, evaluation of the digital model and prediction of the outcomes such as the CEREC system. The software program can enable the digital framework to be enlarged by approximately 20–25% compared to the original dimensions in the design stage to compensate for the shrinkage occurring during sintering, when the partially sintered zirconia-based material is used so that there is no change in the volume when the final milling is completed and there is exact replica of the tooth preparation dimensions. The technician then chooses the expected cement line [19]. An intraoral scanner collects the intraoral images of the preparation and recombines the images as a 3D object consisting of a set of triangles or polygons. A polygon is formed by three points which serve as a criterion for

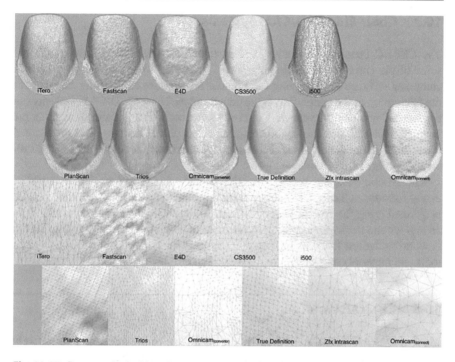

Fig. 10.15 Data acquired with various intraoral scanners for the same abutment tooth [15]

assessing the resolution of the scanned data, the resolution depends on the number of polygons—the higher the number is, the higher the resolution is (Fig. 10.15). Different CAD/CAM systems showed variances in the number of polygons in the same tooth shape (6000–400,000 polygons) [21].

Intraoral scanners have limited optical window size and perform best when the object fills more than half of the optical window; also the algorithm automatically deletes the image when nearby tissues like tongue and lip are included in the scan (this feature often prevents the intraoral scanners from producing normal images of repetitive shapes that can be easily aligned).

The trueness and precision also should be considered and calculated when assessing the accuracy of intraoral scanners. Most of the systems use active triangulation among their principles of scanning or use titanium oxide powder for higher accuracy, where some studies showed no significant difference between image stitching and video sequencing methods used. The limited optical window size is responsible for errors in image recombination in the software scan during certain conditions.

Depending on the different intraoral scanning systems, the scan distance (5–15 mm) or depth varies, i.e., if the abutment tooth is too long or the interdental gap is too narrow, the intraoral scanner must be rotated to the sides of the tooth to scan those areas because of limited focal depth.

10.7 Chair-Side CAD/CAM Systems

The CEREC Omnicam (Sirona dental systems) and the E4D dentist system are some of the currently available chair-side CAD/CAM systems [22]; they include computer software for designing full-contour restorations and milling chamber for the fabrication of the restoration in the dental office. These CAD/CAM systems can produce inlays, onlays, veneers and crowns for both natural teeth as well as the implants and can also fabricate short-span fixed partial dentures and provisional restorations in the dental office. Table 10.5 summarizes their advantages and disadvantages (Fig. 10.16).

The Ivoclar Vivadent has an established chair-side workflow that consists of newly introduced Trios 3 wireless intraoral scanner. The milling/grinding can be performed using the Ivoclar PrograMill cam v4 software which is also available as an app for end devices. According to the manufacturer, the PrograMill (Fig. 10.17) is world's smallest five-axis milling machine and has a tool changer of up to eight tools and material changer for up to five materials.

10.8 Clinical Workflow

Most of the chair-side CAD/CAM systems available in the market have relatively similar functions, cameras, software and milling chambers barring a few changes and patenting of their design features. Table 10.6 gives an overview of the currently available chair-side systems.

Once the tooth preparation has been completed, the scan of the facial surfaces of the dentition in maximum intercuspation is used to align the opposing arches or quadrants of the virtual casts and the margins of the preparation is drawn on the virtual cast to identify the limits or boundary of the restoration within the software program.

Table 10.5 Advantages and disadvantages of chair-side CAD/CAM

Advantages [23]	Disadvantages
• Real-time scanning and visualization of impressions • Easy repeatability • Selective repeatability • Pre-scan option • No impression tray to clean and disinfect • Preparation and restoration analysis options • No cast wear and tear • Rapid communication and availability • Material savings • Patient satisfaction • No temporization • True colour display	• Learning curve • Dry working field • Recording static and dynamic occlusion • Closed systems • Cost factor

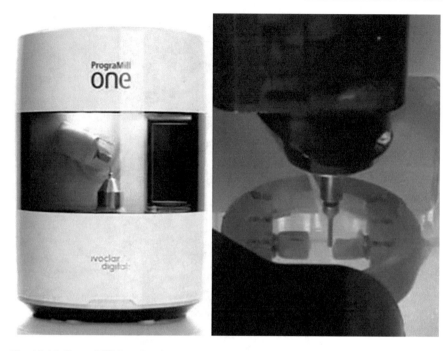

Fig. 10.16   PrograMill One *(Ivoclar Vivadent, Schaan, Liechtenstein)*

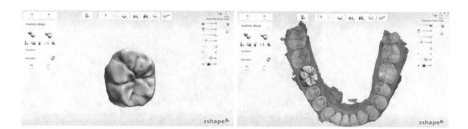

Fig. 10.17   Final design of the prosthesis

The initial design of the restoration on the cast is calculated and proposed by the software using the data of the prepared teeth, adjacent teeth and the opposing teeth. There are various tools for editing and evaluation available in the software which help in refining the specific needs of the case and expectations of the clinician, such as size and the intensity of the proximal contacts and location and intensity of the occlusal contacts and contours (Fig. 10.17).

After finalizing the restoration design, data is transmitted to the milling machine where the previously manufactured block of the desired restorative material is milled to match the full contours of the restoration from the software program.

Table 10.6 Overview of chair-side systems

Milling/CAM unit	Size (L × W × H)	Axes	Spindles/rpm	Wet/dry processing	Milling/ grinding	Water/ compressed air	Materials	Materials used
							Block dimension	
ProgaMill one	380 × 380 × 479 mm	5-axis turn-milling technology (5XT)	1 spindle 80,000 rpm	Wet	Milling and grinding	Both integrated	≤45 mm length	Ivoclar materials: Zirconia, glass ceramic, PMMA, composite
Lyra mill	450 × 470 × 590 mm	4 axes	1 spindle 60,000 rpm	Wet	Grinding	Both integrated	≤40 mm length	Glass ceramic, PMMA, composite, hybrid ceramic
Straumann cares C series	480 × 640 × 540 mm	4 axes	1 spindle 100,000 Rpm	Wet	Milling & grinding	Water: Integrated	≤40 mm length	Glass ceramic, hybrid ceramic

Size depicts the size of machine and rpm depicts the speed

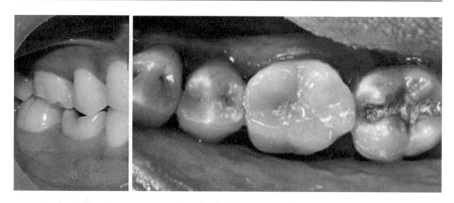

Fig. 10.18 Preoperative and postoperative images of crown cementation

The final cementation is carried out once the fit of the restoration is verified on the tooth preparation; final finishing and polishing are completed using microfine diamonds and polishing instruments (Fig. 10.18).

10.9 Chair-Side Restorative Materials

The chair-side restorative materials are monolithic, that is, the entire restoration is made up of single material than a bilayer restoration which comprises a coping and veneer layer. The advantages of the restoration being monolithic is that it is a dense, homogenous material without porosities and voids which improves the mechanical properties of the restoration. The restorative materials are dispensed in solid block form specific to the individual CAD/CAM milling machine. The chair-side milling machines utilize the subtractive wet grinding process to shape the desired restoration. There are numerous categories of restorative materials available for chair-side CAD/CAM restorations as given in Table 10.7 [24, 25].

CEREC blocs (Sirona dental systems) and VITABLOCS Mark II are made of feldspathic glass porcelain, fine grain and homogenous porcelain. Made up of average particle size of 4 μm; the small particle size gives rise to the high glossy surface and minimum abrasive wear of the opposing teeth. IPS Empress CAD (Ivoclar) has a 35–45% of leucite-reinforced glass ceramic with a particle size of 1–5 μ. Etching can be accomplished with hydrofluoric acid because of the presence of the glass component and treated with a silane coupling agent and adhesively bonded to the tooth with resin cement.

IPS e.max CAD (Ivoclar) consists of 0.2–1.0 μm lithium metasilicate crystals with 40% crystals by volume; after the lithium disilicate restoration is milled, the restoration undergoes a two-stage firing process in a porcelain oven under vacuum for complete crystallization of the lithium disilicate (Fig. 10.19).

This leads to the formation of glass ceramics with 70% crystal volume and fine grain size of 1.5 μm incorporated in a glass matrix. Two types of composite resin blocks are also available, used for long-term provisional and final restorations.

Table 10.7 Chair-side CAD/CAM materials

Materials	Brand
Adhesive ceramic leucite reinforced	IPS empress CAD (Ivoclar)
Adhesive ceramic feldspathic	Viva mark II (Vident)
	Sirona blocks (Sirona)
High-strength ceramic lithium disilicate	IPS Emax CAD (Ivoclar)
Hybrid ceramic	Enamic (Vident)
Nano ceramic	Lava ultimate (3 M ESPE)
Composite	Paradigm MZ100 (3 M ESPE)
Temporary acrylic	Tello CAD (Ivoclar)
	Vita CAD-temp (Vident)

Fig. 10.19 Crystallization of the lithium di-silicate

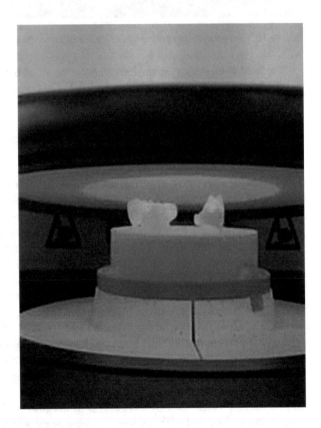

Paradigm MZ100 (3 M/ESPE) is a composite block based on Z100 chemistry and is recommended for permanent resin restorations [26].

Telio CAD (Ivoclar) is a polymethyl methacrylate (PMMA) resin block used for provisional crowns and FPDs. This is a part of Telio system consisting of self-curing composite, desensitizer and cement. It is available in 40 and 55 mm size blocks and in varieties of shades.

10.10 Computer-Assisted Manufacturing

10.10.1 Open and Closed Systems

The data obtained from the CAD application can be utilized in open or closed systems.

In closed systems, e.g. CEREC system, PrograMill PM5 (Fig. 10.20) all the workflow takes place within the in-house equipment like the scanner, software and the milling machine. The drawback of these systems is that the laboratory had to acquire this type of systems which would restrict using only these materials made available by the manufacturer [20]. With the advancement in the technology, there are tools available for each stage in sn independent manner like scanners, software and milling machines from different companies which could be compatible with each other.

An *open* system is where the data acquired from the intraoral scanner can be transferred to any data processing centre for designing and machining of the indirect restoration. The data is digitalized in a standard template file system (STL), so that any computer-aided machine which accepts the STL files can manufacture the indirect restoration. The advantage of open systems is that a large number of professionals have access to this technology [20].

Fig. 10.20 PrograMill milling machine

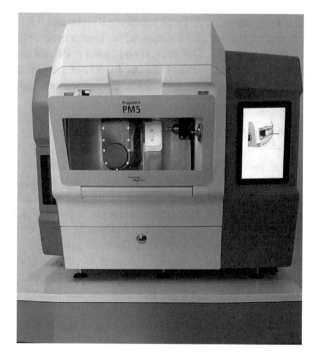

10.11 Subtractive and Additive Processes

10.11.1 Subtractive Process

Nowadays, subtractive technology is the most commonly used manufacturing technology in digital manufacturing. After the final designing of the indirect restoration, the data is processed by the software, and it selects the appropriate size and portion of the block of the restorative material; the milling machine selects the size of the carbide bur or the diamond burs, either in a dry environment or under a water coolant. The milling process begins with the use of coarse grain burs (3 mm) and completing the process with finishing burs (1.6 mm) in diameter [27], e.g. DECSY (Digital Process Ltd., Japan).

There is scope for automatic changing of the burs as well as the position of the block being machined. The COMET SYSTEM (Germany) comes with interchangeable cutters which is driven by computerized speed and multiple axes capable of building an accurate copy of 10 microns marginal fit [28]. Another important parameter is the number of axes. The restoration geometry depends on the number of axes; the more the number is, the finer and more detailed the morphology of the restoration is produced.

The block is stabilized or attached with only one side in the milling machine; this area is devoid of access to the milling unit, so the milling or cutting is achieved manually in some available systems. The milling path is another important parameter to be considered. There are two milling paths, i.e., radial from the centre of the crown and straight in the direction; the former is more suitable for milling the details of the crown [29]. The straight and radial paths are more useful when it comes to zirconia material, because the production of craze lines in addition to the micro-crack can influence the integrity of the restorations [30].

10.11.2 Additive Process

There have been a lot of descriptions of the literature towards the use of additive technology in recent times and has been widely used in some laboratories and practices worldwide [31]. One of the striking features of additive technology is the creation of fine details of complex internal anatomies [31]. There is a complete absence of production of waste in this technique, as the restoration is built layer by layer. The additive process does allow for mass production such as crowns and bridges, using laser-sintering, where high productivity meets quality standards at reduced costs similar to those found in industrial production. The subtractive CAD/CAM technology, in turn, utilizes less time and less human labour, as they are machined one part at a time [31].

There are numerous additive techniques employed:

- Stereolithography (SLA).
- Fused deposition modelling (FDM).
- Selective electron beam melting (SEBM).
- Laser powder forming (SLM or SLS).
- Inkjet printing.

The principle of SLM or SLS technology is based on slicing the restoration digital design and patterns of each layer of the restorations, which are scanned and produced from a computer-generated data from the melted metal powder. The laser beam then melts the non-precious powder alloys like titanium and cobalt-chromium and is called selective laser melting (SLM). If the same is used with porcelain powder, it is called selective laser sintering (SLS).

BEGO MEDIFACTURING® CAD/CAM system uses this technology which produces crowns and bridges using precious metals, CoCr, titanium and porcelain [32].

The SIRONA company has developed EOSINT M 270, which is a direct metal laser sintering machine that fuses metal powder into a solid part by melting it locally using a focused laser beam. Layers of 20 microns are created which in turn is controlled by sophisticated hardware and software leading to frames with high accuracy and detailed resolution, good surface quality and excellent mechanical properties.

The various limitations with this technology include deficient shaping [32]especially in the occlusal areas giving rise to concerns about aesthetic and mechanical properties. The long extension bridges are milled in one piece which might lead to strain development. The veneering technique also might lead to strain development in-spite of the precision of the framework. Monolithic zirconia also has limitation like the wear of antagonistic teeth [19].

10.12 Conclusion

The advancements over the past decades in the therapeutic tools and resources in the field of medicine have seen an exponential rise, particularly in the designing, manufacturing process and prosthetic reconstruction in the field of dentistry. Applying novel methods such as digital impressions, CAD/CAM technology and newer materials, the dentist must provide high-quality dental care. The CAD/CAM technology has shown better mechanical properties, aesthetically pleasing and durable materials, increased efficiency in the laboratory processing and quick fabrication of the restoration as well as accurate fit and predictability [33, 34]of the restorations. The future of dentistry is 'digital'. Dental professionals should be aware of the newer developments and provide high standards of dental care based on extensive research and scientific evidence.

References

1. Kaye. Restorative digital dentistry, part 1: the journey to new paradigms. Dent Today. 2016;35(10):22–7.
2. Logozzo S, Franceschini G, Kilpela A, Caponi M, Governi L, Blois L. A comparative analysis of intraoral 3D digital scanners for restorative dentistry. Internet J Med Technol. 2008;5:1.
3. Holt RD. Advances in dental public health. Prim Dent Care. 2001;8(3):99–102.
4. Al-khateeb S, Oliveby A, et al. Laser fluorescence quantification of remineralization in situ of incipient enamel lesions; influence of fluoride supplements. Caries Res. 1997;31(2):132–40.
5. Kidd EA. The operative management of caries. Dent Update. 1998;25(3):104–8.110.
6. Pretty IA. Caries detection and diagnosis: novel technologies. J Dent. 2006;34:727–39.
7. Longbottom C, Huysmans MC. Electrical measurements for use in caries clinical trials. J Dent Res. 2004;83:spec no.C76-9.
8. Verdonschot EH, Angmar-Mansson B, Ten Bosch JJ, et al. Developments in caries diagnosis and their relationship to treatment decisions and quality of care. ORCA Saturday Afternoon Symposium 1997. Caries Res. 1999;33(1):32–40.
9. Schneiderman A, Elbaum M, Shultz T, et al. Assessment of dental caries with digital imaging Fiber optic transillumination (DIFOTI): in vitro study. Caries Res. 1997;31:103–10.
10. Khalife MA, Boynton JR, Dennison JB, et al. In vivo evaluation of DIAGNOdent for the quantification of occlusal dental caries. Oper Dent. 2009;34(2):136–41.
11. Fasbinder DJ, Neiva GF. Clinical applications of digital dental technology. 1st ed: John Wiley & Sons, Inc; 2015.
12. Freedman GA Contemporary esthetic dentistry. London, England: Mosby 2012, chapter 17, 469–70.
13. Rosenstiel SF, Land MF, Fujimoto J. Contemporary fixed prosthodontics. 3rd ed;2001.p.266–7.
14. Nayar S, Mahadevan R. A Paradigm shift in the concept for making dental impressions. J Pharm Bioallied Sci. 2015;7(5):215.
15. Bhuvaneswaran M, Vekaash CJV. Digital imaging in dental impressions. J Oper Dent Endod. 2018;3(2):63–70.
16. Poticny D, Fasbinder DJ. Accuracy of digital model articulation. J Dent Res. 2011;90:131.
17. Fasbinder DJ. Digital workflow for the LAVA COS system. Insite Dent. 2009:114–7.
18. Park JM, Shim JS. Optical impression in restorative dentistry, computer vision in dentistry. https://doi.org/10.5772/Intechopen.84605.
19. Koutayas SO, Vagkopoulou T, Pelekanos S, et al. Zirconia in dentistry: part 2. Evidence based clinical breakthrough. Eur J Esthet Dent (Review). 2009. Winter;4(4):348–80.
20. Helvey GA. Press-to-zirconia: a case study utilizing CAD/CAM technology and the wax injection method. Pract Proced Aesthet Dent. 2006;18(9):547–53.
21. Kim RJ-Y, Park J-M, Shim J-S. Accuracy of 9 intraoral scanners for complete-arch image acquisition: A qualitative and quantitative evaluation. J Prosthet Dent. 2018;120(6):895–903.e1.
22. Levine N. To the sky and beyond. Dent Prod Rep. 2009;116
23. Zarub M, Mehl A. Chairside systems: a current review. Int J Comput Dent. 2017;20(2):123–49.
24. Fasbinder DJ. Materials for chair side CAD/CAM restorations. Compend Contin Educ Dent. 2010;31:702. 4.706,708
25. Fasbinder DJ, Dennison JB, Heys D, et al. Clinical evaluation of lithium disilicate chair-side CAD/CAM crowns at 4 years. J Dent Res. 2012a;91:645.
26. Rusin RP. Properties and applications of a new composite block for CAD/CAM. Compend Contin Educ Dent. 2001;22:35–41.
27. Miyazaki T, Hotta Y, Kunii J, et al. A review of dental CAD/CAM: current status and future perspectives from 20 years of experience. Dent Mater J (Review). 2009;28(1):44–56.
28. Willer J, Rossbach A. Computer assisted milling of dental restorations using a new CAD/CAM data acquisition system. J Prosthet Dent. 1998;80(3):346–53.
29. Hotta Y, Miyazaki T, Fujiwara T, et al. Durability of tungsten carbide burs for the fabrication of titanium crowns using CAD/CAM. Dent Mater J. 2004;23(2):190–6.

30. Rekow ED, Silva NR, Coelho PG, et al. Performance of dental ceramics: challenges for improvements. J Dent Res. 2011;90(8):937–52.
31. Van Noort R. The future of dental devices is digital. Dent Mater (Review). 2012;28(1):3–12.
32. Sirona the Dental Company (homepage) CAD/CAM materials: global site, 2013 (cited on 2013 Sep 15).
33. Giordano R, Mclaren EA. Ceramics overview: classification by microstructure and processing methods. Compend Contin Educ Dent. 2010;31(9):682–4.
34. Yuksel E, Zaimoglu A. Influence of marginal fit and cement types on microleakage of all ceramic crowns. Braz Oral Res. 2011;25(3):261–6.

Digitization in Periodontics

11

Mihir R. Kulkarni

11.1 Introduction

Periodontology has evolved from the discipline of controlling the diseases of the tooth-supporting structures to the robust science of understanding the physiology of these tissues and exploring the pathogenesis of periodontal and peri-implant diseases. The science of periodontology originated in the early practices of resecting the 'diseased' tissues, progressed through the era of repair and regeneration and is presently pushing the boundaries of technology with experiments of tissue engineering, infecto-genomics, bioinformatics, stem cell research and many other frontier areas. The rapid progress in periodontal research and clinical techniques has been possible largely due to the technology made available to us in the so-called 'digital' age. An anecdotal example to emphasize the sheer magnitude of this rapid progress can be obtained from a review by Teles et al. [1]. In their comprehensive assessment of the concepts of periodontal microbiology, the authors provided interesting data from the Forsyth Institute (Cambridge, MA, USA). They stated that the centre assessed 300 subgingival plaque samples by the culture method in the period between 1982 and 1988. This number increased to 9600 between 1988 and 1993 on the application of the colony lift technique and later increased to a staggering 34,400 between 1993 and 1999 after the advent of the checkerboard DNA-DNA hybridization. A centre that processed 300 samples between 1982 and 1988 was able to process about 5734 samples per year by 1999 [1]. This progress has been the result of scientific ingenuity and method, but the role of digitization and automation cannot be discounted.

The world is moving from the information age to the experience age. This transition has been ushered in with the 'discovery' of the modern currency—the data.

M. R. Kulkarni (✉)
Department of Periodontics, SDM College of Dental Sciences and Hospital, Dharwad, India

© Springer Nature Switzerland AG 2021
P. Jain, M. Gupta (eds.), *Digitization in Dentistry*,
https://doi.org/10.1007/978-3-030-65169-5_11

Data or information is the new currency. This currency can be recorded, generated, analysed, stored and transmitted in digital form, thus making it a very powerful tool for progress. Data about a disease that required meticulous recording on paper, careful filing, cataloguing and analysis can today be recorded on smart devices connected to networks and can be analysed by powerful computers at geographically distant locations in a matter of seconds. This has raised the capabilities of scientific research to gigantic proportions. The measure of the quality of a hospital, clinic, university or laboratory is the amount of data it generates. Data is the backbone of epidemiology and can help to identify the trends and patterns in a disease process that may go unnoticed while treating patients at an individual level. Data can be crucial in medico-legal problems to identify the source of the error if any. It can also be a tool for hypothesis generation, testing and development of new clinical methods, all directed towards the ultimate goal of improving the standard of care for our patients.

Digitization of this data is a key step that allows for greater convenience in handling it. Clinicians can utilize digital data for recording and storing relevant findings in a systematic manner. A network of such clinics can generate valuable information about a disease that a single clinic would not be able to. Such a system of practice-based research networks (PBRNs) is already in use in the United States. It is a network of hundreds of private practitioners and has received funding from the National Institute of Dental and Craniofacial Research (NIDCR). Use of digital patient data in the PBRNs will make it an increasingly efficient instrument for dental research. It has been noted that electronic dental records are increasingly being used in the PBRNs and stated that such electronic data may offer an important resource to support not only clinical care but also quality assurance and research [2].

With all the improvements that digitization has to offer, it does come with its share of problems. Ease in the transmission of clinical data gives rise to concerns of privacy and confidentiality. Sensitive data can be accessed by the pharmaceutical industry or other commercial organizations in order to sell a product or treatment that may not always be in line with evidence-based dentistry (EBD). Use of digital media and techniques for diagnosis, treatment planning and even treatment may lead to an over-reliance on technology before it can be allowed to evolve adequately. Availability of too much data can also be tricky as it would finally be at the disposal of an individual who can be easily perplexed with the sheer volume of it. Finally, the very core trait of digitization and automation, which is its rapid evolution, is also its bane. Rapid change in technology leads inevitably to the need to change the hardware and the network bandwidths. This is presently expensive, especially in the developing world, and may be the only limiting factor for the universal acceptance of digital dentistry.

This chapter will focus on digital advances that have significantly contributed to the advancement of periodontology. Digital and technological aspects of various stages of periodontal management will be examined and the influence of digitization on periodontal research will also be discussed.

11.2   Digital Aids in Clinical Periodontics

Diagnosis is the initial and essential step in the management of a disease. A proper diagnosis helps the clinician to formalize the thought process required to frame the treatment plan. Clinical case record or a case history is an algorithm designed to help a clinician to reach the diagnosis. Periodontal examination is an important part of the clinical case record and has seen remarkable digitization. Periodontal diagnosis requires a detailed recording of several clinical parameters which provide an insight into the status of the periodontal health. These key findings include the following:

1. Gingival inflammation and bleeding on probing.
2. Periodontal pocket charting.
3. Clinical attachment level.
4. Indices for plaque, calculus and gingivitis or periodontitis.
5. Measurement of gingival recession.
6. Detection of furcation involvement.
7. Identification of mucogingival problems.

11.3   Periodontal Probes

The most important tool for all the above-mentioned assessments is the periodontal probe. These are tools designed to measure the periodontal pocket depth. The periodontal pocket is a pathologically deepened gingival sulcus due to the apical migration of the junctional epithelium and has been called a 'cardinal symptom of periodontitis' [3]. The *first-generation periodontal probes* are simple hand instruments with a blunt tip, a calibrated blade and a contra-angled shank (Fig. 11.1). Michigan 'O' Probe with William's markings, the UNC-15 and the WHO probe are a few popular first-generation probes. The first-generation probes are the most widely used instruments for periodontal charting even today. The most commonly stated disadvantages of using these instruments is the lack of standardization of the technique, angulation and the pressure used for probing—all of which can result in significant intra- and inter-examiner variations. This may cast a doubt on the reliability of first-generation probes in periodontal practice, but it has been observed that when used carefully, the first-generation probes can produce meaningful and reasonably reproducible data [4].

Nevertheless, there have been constant efforts to improve the accuracy and reliability of the periodontal probe. The *second-generation probes* were designed to achieve 'gentle probing' and were designed to be pressure sensitive. Gabathuler and Hassell designed the first true pressure-sensitive probe [5]. Another example of this generation is the *Yeaple probe* designed by Polson et al. [6]. This probe has a pen-like handpiece and an electronic control unit that can be used to set the probing force between 0.05 N and 0.5 N. The handpiece is designed to allow a variety of probe tips to be attached to it.

Fig. 11.1 First-generation periodontal probes

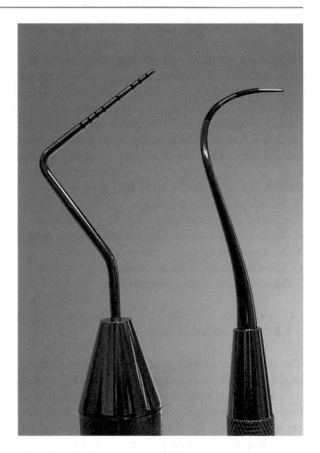

Third-generation probes were designed to have a constant probing force. The Florida Probe system designed by Gibbs et al. is a prototype of third-generation probes and has seen constant changes as per the changing concepts and technology [7]. The original design of the Florida Probe® system included a handpiece, a displacement transducer with a digital readout, a footswitch and a computer. The system incorporated a 0.4-mm probe tip (resembling a Michigan 'O' probe tip) and a standardized force of 25 g. The most important feature of this probe was that it provided a digital output that is directly recorded in a computer [7]. A version of the Florida Probe for use along with an acrylic stent is also available. A common practical issue with periodontal charting is the need for an assistant. A chair-side assistant can help make the charting process faster by noting the findings on a chart or feeding them in a computer system. But this has the disadvantages of requiring more manpower and also the introduction of a source of error. Having the operator record the findings personally has the problem of increasing the appointment time and the need for complex infection control protocols (Fig. 11.2) [8, 9].

To overcome these problems, the Florida probe has been upgraded with a voice recognition tool and is available as *VoiceWorks™*. This enables a single operator

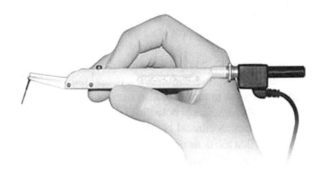

Fig. 11.2 Florida probe
(*Courtesy:* www.
dentalcompare.com) [9]

to carry out the periodontal charting. The software allows the operator to record not only the probing depth but also other clinical variables like recession, bleeding on probing, furcation involvement, exudation and mobility. The Florida probe system has been tested for reproducibility and has been validated by several studies and can be considered as a 'golden standard' for automated probing [7, 8–11]. Combined with a voice assistant, digital charting, controlled pressure and the option of using a stent, the Florida probe system seems to be a good choice for routine clinical use.

The *Toronto automated periodontal probe* [12] is another example of third-generation probes. The Toronto probe uses the occlusal or incisal surface of the tooth as a reference point and has the facility of adjusting the probing pressure with the help of air pressure. The probe also incorporates a mercury column for indicating and guiding the angulation of probing. The Toronto probe was modified by Tessier et al. for the estimation of probing velocity [13]. The probing velocity is intended to be a measure of the integrity of the dento-gingival unit (junctional epithelium and a gingival group of fibres) and may be used to quantify the effect of inflammation on the probing depth. This concept is quite ingenious, especially on account of its simplicity and needs to be explored further in clinical studies for improving probe designs.

The *Interprobe™* electronic probe system comprises an optical encoder and an optical filament that is inserted into the periodontal pocket. The flexible nature of this probe (optical filament) may result in improved patient comfort, but it may also get displaced due to the presence of sub-gingival deposits. The Interprobe too has a connected digital interface for recording the findings on a computer with graphically illustrated charts [14].

Disadvantages of the third-generation probes [14] are as follows:

1. The probe may penetrate the periodontal tissues deeper than the junctional epithelium, especially in inflamed tissues. This may cause more discomfort to the patient.
2. Reduced tactile sense.
3. The issue of obstruction to the probe by anatomic/pathologic factors is not resolved.

4. All of the above affect the accuracy and reproducibility of the measurements.
5. The probes do not provide a three-dimensional (3D) data about the pocket.

In order to overcome these disadvantages, a need was felt for a device that can generate a 3D representation of the periodontal pocket. The probing depth varies not only from tooth to tooth but also from one point to another point on the same tooth. It is often the practice to note the highest probing depth (~ deepest pocket) for every tooth for routine clinical charting. A better technique is to measure six points per tooth, but that too does not provide complete information about the pocket morphology. Accurate *3D imaging* of the pocket offers the following *advantages:*

1. The variability of manual probing, in terms of angulation, force and choice of the probe, is eliminated.
2. The lack of intuitiveness of the constant-force probes is avoided.
3. Patients could be more comfortable as the actual physical act of 'probing' inflamed tissues is avoided.
4. The 3D images can be a better tool for patient education than just numbers.

Several attempts have been made to device a periodontal probe that can generate a 3D representation of a periodontal pocket. *Fourth-generation* probes are a step in this direction and employ ultrasound technology. The principle of these probes is the simple concept of reflection of ultrasonic waves. A device is used to generate ultrasonic waves that are directed towards the base of the pocket and are expected to be reflected by the gingival and periodontal groups of supra-crestal fibres. The reflected waves are picked up by a receiver, and the signal is transferred to a processor. The processor then uses pre-coded algorithms (software programmes) to decode the signal and generate an estimation of the pocket dimensions. This technology has not become mainstream due to some *disadvantages* such as the following: [14].

• Ultrasound imaging has poor contrast.
• The mechanism of interpreting the generated waveforms is complex.
• The technology is expensive.
• The clinical feasibility of the technology has not been established.

With advances in technology, several new methods have been employed to determine the depth and 3D configuration of periodontal pockets (Table 11.1).

Imaging of the periodontal pocket can also be combined with therapeutic strategies. Elashiry et al. conducted an in vitro study to explore this concept [15]. The authors combined calcium tungstate micro-particles with an antibacterial compound (K 21) and observed that this enhanced the antibacterial action of this mixture against *Porphyromonas gingivalis* and *Streptococcus gordonii*. This combined strategy can prove beneficial by facilitating periodontal charting and therapy in a single procedure.

Table 11.1 Different periodontal pocket imaging technologies currently in use. *(Table modified from Elashiry* et al. *2018)* [15]

Technology	Advantages	Disadvantages
Periodontal pocket CBCT-based imaging (using radiopaque contrast agents)	• High resolution • Lower radiation exposure • Fast scanning • Broad application • CBCT is widely available	• Ionizing radiation • Metallic image artefacts
Optical coherent tomography (OCT)	• Non-ionizing radiation • High tissue contrast • High resolution	• Deep tissue imaging limited by light waves scattering
Photoacoustic imaging tomography	• Non-ionizing radiation • High-resolution deep tissue imaging vs OCT • Higher contrast vs ultrasound imaging • Faster scanning vs MRI	• ~5-cm tissue penetration • Poor penetration of gas cavities • Thick bones attenuate and distort signals
Endoscopic capillaroscopy	• Non-ionizing radiation • Image pocket through microcirculation	• Not clear if pocket depths, area or volumes possible
MRI	• Non-ionizing radiation • Soft and hard tissue imaging with short-echo-time MRI generations	• Only soft tissue imaging and low resolution with conventional MRI • Long scanning time • Short-echo-time MRI systems not broadly available for clinical MRI or routine dental imaging • Not clear if new MRI can image periodontal pockets

Probing a pocket is a fundamental clinical procedure and is a part of basic oral examination. From the available evidence, it may be prudent to say that a manual probe (first-generation) in the hands of a trained clinician is still a reliable and efficient tool for pocket charting. With this in mind, it is necessary to include adequate training sessions for periodontal probing in the dental graduate curriculum. It has been suggested that dental students should be exposed to actual periodontal probing in patients during preclinical training [16]. Furthermore, this training should be checked by a faculty member and any discrepancy in measurement in excess of 1 mm has to be demonstrated to the student [17].

11.4 Detection of Sub-Gingival Calculus

Dental calculus is the mineralized form of dental plaque. Based on its location on the tooth and with reference to the location of the gingival margin in health, dental calculus is classified as supra-gingival calculus and sub-gingival calculus. While calculus may by itself not be the cause of periodontal disease, it is the most important plaque retentive factor and hence is a key player in the pathogenesis of plaque-induced periodontal diseases. Sub-gingival calculus is a bigger threat to periodontal health than supra-gingival calculus due to crucial differences in the nature of its formation and organization. Sub-gingival calculus derives its mineral content from the gingival crevicular fluid (GCF). It is tenaciously attached to the tooth surface and is sometimes seen to merge with cementum to form the 'calculo-cementum'. It is often greenish or brown in colour and harbours on its surface an un-mineralized layer of sub-gingival plaque that can be rich in putative periodontal pathogens. Indeed, it has been known for a long time that teeth with sub-gingival calculus lose attachment faster than teeth without sub-gingival calculus [18].

Detection of sub-gingival calculus can be very difficult especially during closed debridement (non-surgical periodontal therapy) due to its location below the gingival margin. An effective closed debridement of a diseased root surface can help to avoid the need for periodontal surgery. This can be vital in avoiding complications of periodontal surgery such as gingival recession and dentinal hypersensitivity. Management of periodontal disease by non-surgical therapy can also have the positive effect of minimizing patient morbidity and simplifying the convalescence period. The most commonly used tool to detect sub-gingival calculus is the explorer—a sharp instrument that provides tactile feedback. But it may not be useful when the root surface has already been instrumented and harbours 'burnished' calculus. Advanced techniques and digital devices have been introduced to enable the detection of such elusive sub-gingival calculus (Table 11.2) [18].

11.4.1 Fibre-Optic Endoscopy

The Perioscopy device (Perioscopy Inc., Oakland, CA, USA) is the only fibre-optic endoscopy-based device available for calculus detection (Fig. 11.3) [19, 20]. The device is a miniaturized version of the medical endoscope and permits a direct visual examination of the tooth wall of a periodontal pocket. The system consists of a 1-mm fibre-optic bundle with illumination, irrigation and a digital display. A randomized controlled trial using this endoscope for sub-gingival scaling showed that use of the Perioscopy device resulted in a statistically significant calculus removal, but this effect was limited to interproximal sites deeper than 6 mm [21].

Table 11.2 Types of calculus detection technologies

Technology	Clinical applications
Fibre-optic endoscopy (Perioscopy)	Calculus detection only
Spectro-optical technology (DetecTar)	
Autofluorescence (DIAGNOdent)	
Ultrasound (PerioScan)	Combined calculus detection and removal
Laser and auto-fluorescence (Keylaser3)	

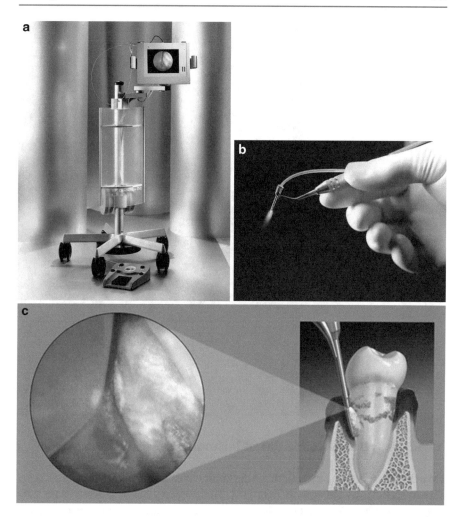

Fig. 11.3 (**a**, **b**) Perioscopy system *(Courtesy of Dentalview, Inc.)*. (**c**) Visualization of subgingival calculus using perioscopy system [19, 20]

11.4.2 Spectro-Optical Technology (Differential Reflectometry)

This technology is based on a sensor used to detect the variations in the absorption, reflectance or emission of light by dental calculus. A red-light-emitting diode (LED) is used in combination with a fibre-optic 'spectroscope' to detect the 'spectral signature' of sub-gingival dental calculus. The device (DetecTar; Dentsply Professional, York, PA, USA) consists of a portable, cordless handpiece that picks up the signal and conveys it to a computer which then decodes it using certain algorithms. The instrument also has a curved periodontal probe with millimetre markings and provides audible and visible signals to the operator on detecting calculus (Fig. 11.4) [18, 22].

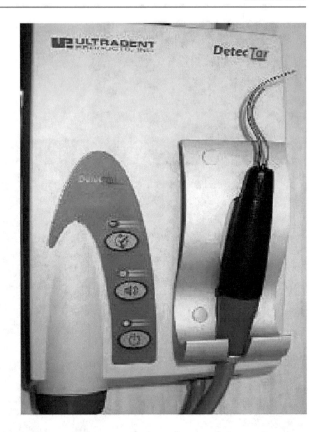

11.4.3 Autofluorescence-Based Technology

Dental root surface and calculus have the ability to emit fluorescent light after exposure to specific wavelengths of light [18]. This property can be used to detect sub-
gingival calculus. The DIAGNOdent caries detection instrument (*refer to Chap. 2
for more details on the device*) (KaVo, Biberach, Germany) has been adapted for
sub-gingival calculus detection (Fig. 11.5). Light is delivered on to the root surface
with an optical fibre, and the resulting fluorescence is captured [18]. The intensity
of fluorescence is measured and scored on a relative value scale of 0–99 (Table 11.3).

In vitro studies have shown promising results for using laser fluorescence
(DIAGNOdent) for the detection of sub-gingival calculus [23, 24].

11.4.4 Keylaser3

The same diode (InGaAsP) laser unit used in the DIAGNOdent device has been
combined with an Er:YAG laser in the Keylaser3™ (KaVo, Biberach, Germany)
(Fig. 11.6). The 2940-nm Er:YAG laser can be used for removal of the sub-gingival
calculus. The Keylaser3 has shown better results as compared to a differential

Fig. 11.5 The DIAGNOdent TM Pen (KaVo, Biberach, Germany) (*Reproduced with permission from John Wiley & Sons*) [17]

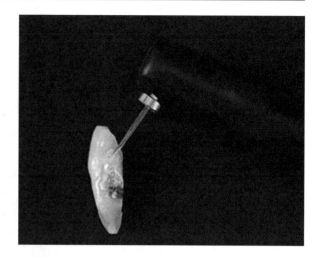

Table 11.3 DIAGNOdent values (as per the manufacturer)

Value	Interpretation
≤5	Clean root surface
5–40	Very small calcified plaque sites
≥40	Mineralized deposits

reflectometry-based device (DetecTar) for the detection of sub-gingival calculus in an in vitro study [25]. The Er:YAG laser has been shown to be comparable to ultra-sonic devices for sub-gingival scaling [18] and in combination with a calculus-detection system can be a useful albeit expensive clinical tool.

11.4.5 Ultrasonic Technology

Ultrasonic technology, used widely for scaling has been adapted for the detection of sub-gingival calculus. The PerioScan (Sirona Dental Systems, Bensheim, Germany) device incorporates this technology along with a conventional ultrasonic scaler device. The device has a detection mode and a treatment mode and indicates the detection of calculus by light and sound signals (Fig. 11.7) [26]. A clinical study has demonstrated that the PerioScan device is a reasonably reliable tool for the detection of sub-gingival calculus [27]. This study also observed that the repro-ducibility of the device was higher in areas of deeper probing depths and furcation involvement.

More recently, *optical coherence tomography* (OCT) has also been used for the detection of calculus and root cementum. Proposed to be a non-contact, non-invasive, high-resolution and real-time method, this is a promising technology that needs to be investigated further for the detection of sub-gingival calculus [28]. For a clinician, it is important to have a device that is convenient to use, delivers predict-able, clinically relevant results and does not levy an unreasonable demand on the cost and duration of treatment. Though the above-mentioned devices have

Fig. 11.6 Keylaser3
(KaVo, Biberach,
Germany) (*Reproduced
with permission from John
Wiley & Sons*) [17]

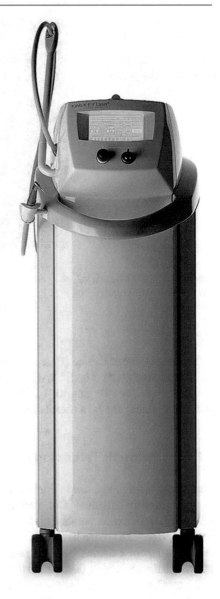

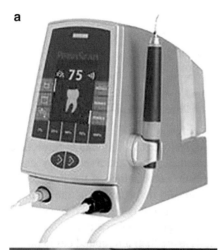

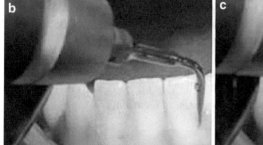

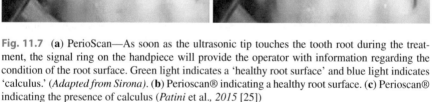

Fig. 11.7 (**a**) PerioScan—As soon as the ultrasonic tip touches the tooth root during the treatment, the signal ring on the handpiece will provide the operator with information regarding the condition of the root surface. Green light indicates a 'healthy root surface' and blue light indicates 'calculus.' (*Adapted from Sirona*). (**b**) Perioscan® indicating a healthy root surface. (**c**) Perioscan® indicating the presence of calculus (*Patini* et al., *2015* [25])

demonstrated good results in a few studies, a clear clinical benefit has not been demonstrated for any technology [18].

11.5 Measurement of Tooth Mobility

Measurement and recording of the mobility of teeth is an important part of the periodontal case history record. Assessment of tooth mobility provides important clues regarding periodontal health and can also be useful for assessment of response to

Table 11.4 Miller's tooth mobility index

Grade	Interpretation [29]
1	The first distinguishable sign of movement greater than normal
2	A movement of the tooth which allows the crown to move 1 mm from its normal position in any direction
3	Allows the tooth to move more than 1 mm in any direction. Teeth which may be rotated or depressed in their alveoli are classified as mobility #3

treatment. All teeth have a certain degree of physiologic mobility that is considered to be normal. This mobility has an initial intra-socket stage and a secondary stage. The intra-socket mobility is due to a viscoelastic deformation of the periodontal ligament, and the secondary stage is due to elastic deformation of the alveolar socket. Traditionally, tooth mobility is assessed by using two metallic instruments or one instrument and one finger to hold a tooth followed by an attempt to move it in all directions [28]. The findings of this exercise are then interpreted based on the Miller tooth mobility Index [29], (Table 11.4) based on the following scoring system:

Although this has been a very popular method and continues to be the most widely used one, few disadvantages of this method are:

- Subjective variations in the magnitude and direction of the applied force.
- Subjective variations in interpretation.
- No specialized instrument is available to assist in recording.
- Limited sensitivity.

In order to overcome these disadvantages, several devices have been invented to accurately record tooth mobility. These consisted of the Muhlemann's micro and macro Periodontometer and O'Leary and Rudd's Periodontometer. They came with their own set of limitations such as the Muhlemann's Periodontometer was a large and uncomfortable device for routine use, the technique for its use is tedious and time-consuming, and the macro-periodontometer can only be used for the anterior teeth. Also, measurements of micro-periodontometer are less reproducible than other devices. On the other hand, full mouth recording with the O'Leary and Rudd's Periodontometer is time-consuming and may require as long as 40 min. They also require diagnostic casts to be fabricated in advance to locate the occlusal points to be engaged by the pin.

These attempts were followed by several others including the Korber's transducer, Pameijer's device, Ryden's laser reflection method, Dental holographic interferometry and Persson and Svensson loading/sensing devices among others. But none of these methods has achieved mainstream clinical acceptance due to practical limitations like having a complicated technique, being uncomfortable to the patient and requiring expensive equipment [30]. Between 1972 and 1984, a group of researchers devised the *Periotest* method to examine periodontal function [31]. The Periotest device measures the periodontal damping and was found to indirectly enable the recording of tooth mobility. Studies have demonstrated that the Periotest device is a reliable tool for measurement of tooth mobility, especially in teeth affected with periodontal disease [32]. It is not a very sensitive method in cases of minimal or physiologic mobility [33] and has also been noted to cause physical damage to a tooth [34]. *Resonance Frequency Analysis (RFA)* is the currently favoured technique to examine the stability of osseointegrated dental implants. Though the technique is unsuitable for measuring tooth mobility, it may provide clinically relevant information in the diagnosis of ankylosed teeth [35].

With advances in technology, a few promising devices have been recently invented for assessment of the mobility of teeth. A no-contact *electromagnetic vibration device* has been developed [34]. This device has three parts, the vibrator, the detector and the analyser. The vibrator generates electromagnetic waves and the resulting tooth vibrations are picked up by the acceleration sensors in the detector which is then interpreted by the analyser and a tooth mobility value is generated. This instrument has the advantage of a non-contact mechanism. This makes it an atraumatic method to detect tooth mobility and may also be a boon for infection control. Further adaptation and testing of this device are necessary before it can be introduced for routine clinical use.

Another novel device to measure tooth mobility was introduced by Konerman et al. [36] This *intraoral measurement device* consists of a piezoelectric actuator to generate tooth movement, a force sensor and a microcontroller board for receiving the signal. An individualized acrylic splint fabricated using diagnostic casts is required to position the device intraorally. The device has been demonstrated to generate precise measurements and has been used to measure tooth mobility after orthodontic treatment [36]. Complexity of fabrication and use may limit the applications of this device to research areas and it may not be suitable for daily clinical diagnostic use in its present form. More recently, the successful and reliable application of an intra-oral scanner to record tooth mobility has also been demonstrated [37].

Clinical tooth mobility is often a cause of concern for the clinician as well as the patients. A reduction in tooth mobility after treatment is an important sign of the effectiveness of the therapy. Sometimes the tooth mobility shows a transient increase after periodontal flap surgery, followed by a reduction. Furthermore, higher mobility for teeth that have been treated for periodontitis and have a reduced periodontium is also physiologic; and such teeth can be maintained in acceptable function [38]. Tooth mobility is considered to be a predictor for tooth loss [39] but is not recommended to be used as a sign of periodontal health or disease [40]. A clinicians understanding of the concepts of tooth mobility and its utility in patient management should be complemented with a device that can accurately measure and record tooth mobility. Such a device backed by clinical evidence is not available at present and remains an important goal of clinical periodontal research.

11.6 Digital Occlusal Analysis in Periodontal Therapy

Occlusion is the dynamic relationship of the maxillary and mandibular teeth which is controlled by neuro-muscular co-ordination and is guided by the anatomy of the temporomandibular joint and teeth; for the primary function of mastication. The concept of occlusion is interpreted differently by different specialists. While one professional may concentrate on intercuspation, another may deal with principles of articulation and concepts like centric occlusion and balanced occlusion. A third professional may be more interested in proximal contacts and cuspal guidance as to the guiding principles for occlusion, whereas another may focus on the ability of the periodontium to sustain the eccentricities of occlusal contacts. In health, there exists an equilibrium between the generated occlusal forces and the adaptive capacity of the periodontium. Any disturbance to this equilibrium—either due to abnormal forces or due to a reduced periodontium can lead to injury of the periodontal tissues. This injury is known as *trauma from occlusion (TFO)* and is an important clinical consideration in periodontal therapy.

To understand the role of digital methods of occlusal analysis in periodontics, it is important to first know the relationship between TFO and periodontal disease. The role of occlusal trauma in the initiation and progression of inflammatory periodontal disease has been a topic of controversy for over 6 several decades. There have been a few studies that have found a positive association between the two while others that have failed to find any. The current evidence-based concepts regarding the role of TFO in periodontal disease can be summarized as follows: [41, 42].

- Trauma from occlusion does not cause periodontitis.
- Traumatic forces may facilitate the extension of inflammation into the periodontium and may lead to an advance in the plaque front, deepening of a periodontal pocket and attachment loss.
- Interferences in the movement from centric occlusion to maximum intercuspation are responsible for trauma from occlusion.
- Proximal contact relationships are as important as occlusal contacts for the integrity of the periodontium.
- Occlusal corrections have an important role to play in periodontal therapy and can help minimize the progression of periodontal breakdown.

It is essential to accurately record the occlusal relationships to identify areas of excessive occlusal load or to detect areas or points of eccentric contacts. Presently, the most popular tool used for digital occlusal evaluation is the *T-scan* (Tekscan, Inc., S. Boston, MA, USA). The main advantage of this device is the ability to get real-time readings of occlusal contacts that can then be used to guide the patient to occlude as per requirement. The current version available is the *T-scan 10* which incorporates several improvements in software and sensor design. Although there are studies documenting the use of the T-scan for diagnosis of trauma from occlusion [43], there is a lack of good quality evidence to suggest the routine use of T-scan for the same. Another instrument for digitally recording the occlusal relationships is the *OccluSense®* (Bausch, Germany). This device has a thinner sensor than the T-scan (60 microns). However, there are no studies to substantiate the sensitivity, specificity and reproducibility of the device for the diagnosis of traumatic occlusal contacts and hence it cannot be suggested for clinical use.

From the current state of evidence for the use of digital diagnostic aids, it is clear that these tools are adjuncts to the more traditional clinical techniques like the use of bite registration pastes, articulating papers or silk strips. While these devices can provide valuable real-time information in an intuitive way, they do not always agree with the traditional tests [44]. This places the onus of decision-making on the clinician—again rendering the diagnostic process subjective or based on anecdotal evidence.

11.7   Digital Periodontal Treatment Planning and Database Maintenance

To continue the argument presented in the introduction to this chapter, 'data' is now assuming importance as a clinical tool. Traditionally considered to be the device of researchers, data is now considered to be an important part of clinical decision-making—the backbone of evidence-based decision-making (EBDM). EBDM is the basis of modern medicine and dentistry. It is the duty of a clinician to document relevant data of the encountered clinical situations in a systematic manner. It is also her/his duty to base clinical decisions on sound peer-reviewed literature whenever possible. In this context, a periodontist can be said to have four (4) important objectives for the maintenance of a database.

- To assess maintenance and prognosis at an individual level for every patient.
- To contribute to clinical research and EBDM.
- For the requirements of medico-legal and insurance proceedings.
- To generate data for the association of periodontal diseases with systemic diseases and conditions—the 'perio-systemic interlink'.

A digital database of periodontal examination can be easily maintained by using computer software. The computer software for periodontal charting can either be a stand-alone software programme or can come bundled with an automated periodontal probing system. An example of a stand-alone software is the *Consult-PRO* (North York, Canada) dental education software [45]. This enables the clinician to record the patients' dental findings as well as to educate the patients about the disease and treatment. The software has a Consult-PRO Perio option for detailed periodontal charting and to monitor the patients' response to treatment and adherence to the maintenance schedule and home care procedures. The patient education tools in the Consult-PRO software are quite intuitive and allow the clinician to demonstrate common procedures to patients via animations and diagrams.

An example of software bundled along with an automated probing system is the FP32 software that is available for use with the *Florida probe*® system [46]. The FP32 software incorporates a 'talking assistant' capable of providing audio instruction in 15 languages. The software can also generate post-treatment personalized hand-outs and incorporates a personalized risk-assessment module. The GoProbe software is a stand-alone version of the FP32 software, designed for use with other probe systems.

The acceptance of digital dental records has been on the rise among dental practitioners. A study about electronic dental records in 2013 [2] found that 74% of the practitioners in the USA and 90% of the practitioners in the Scandinavian countries of Denmark, Norway and Sweden used electronic database maintenance. Another encouraging finding of this study was that half of the interviewed practitioners (51%) were willing to re-use the data for the purpose of research [2]. For a dentist, a visual interface to communicate with the patient has several advantages. A patient is much more likely to be attracted to a graphic or animation depicting the treatment plan as compared to just a description or a rough hand-drawn sketch. A printed chart or an application with reminders can be a powerful tool to reinforce the maintenance instructions and thereby maximize the treatment outcomes.

With the rapid pace of digitization and the wide range of available options, there is a need to ensure a certain amount of basic standardization in periodontal screening and recording software. This standardization may be achieved by:

- Use of the same indices to record periodontal status (e.g. community periodontal index or periodontal screening and recording system).
- Mandatory recording of systemic disease along with relevant laboratory findings (e.g. HbA1c in diabetes mellitus, lipid profile in patients with coronary artery disease etc.).
- An in-built mechanism to allow only fully completed charts to be saved.
- A common file format for easy data exchange and retrieval.
- Facility to back-up the data on a network (e.g.: Cloud).
- A common licence and distribution format for permissions regarding the use of clinical data for research.

Ensuring such uniformity in practice-based dental networks is of utmost importance for improvements in patient care protocols and research. A recent review failed to find any substantial role of supportive periodontal therapy (SPT) on the maintenance of adult dentition [47]. This was attributed the lack of conclusiveness of the study to heterogeneity in the reported literature, among other reasons [47].

11.8   Digital Advances in Periodontal Therapy

The evidence-based principles and practice of periodontal therapy have remained largely the same since the 1980s. Non-surgical periodontal therapy continues to be the most widely employed approach in the management of periodontitis in most practices. Short-term improvement of the periodontal status that occurs after a non-surgical therapy prevents the treating dentist and the patient to realize the need for more invasive instrumentation. Many of the short-comings of traditional periodontal surgery have been addressed by minimally invasive approaches and should help allay the fears about surgical periodontal therapy, but the technology remains underutilized. This may be due to the steep learning curve associated with minimally invasive therapy, the inherent resistance of practitioners to adapt to the advances and the expensive nature of the required equipment [48].

11.9   Minimally Invasive Periodontal Surgery

Advances in optical instruments and endoscopes have made it possible to visualize the diseased root surfaces through very small incisions. The endoscope-assisted periodontal therapy and later the videoscope-assisted minimally invasive periodontal surgery have evolved from the original minimally invasive periodontal surgery technique described by Harrel and Rees in 1995 [49].

The minimally invasive periodontal surgery (MIS) was originally performed using surgical loupes. The loupes were later replaced with a glass fibre endoscope and, more recently, a videoscope. The video-scope assisted minimally invasive periodontal surgery (VMIS) permits the use of higher magnification and smaller incisions than the MIS and enables the removal of 'micro islands' of calculus. Excellent clinical results have been reported in a longitudinal clinical study employing the MIS with adjunctive use of enamel matrix derivative (EMD). The study also reported minimal post-operative recession with the use of MIS [50]. The main principles of the MIS and the VMIS are: [51].

- Preservation of periosteal blood supply to the tissues and the interdental papilla.
- Causing minimal trauma to the periodontal tissues.
- A tension-free closure of the flap at or above the original gingival level with minimal suturing (Fig. 11.8).

The simplified papilla preservation flap (SPPF) was introduced by Cortellini et al. in 1999 [52]. Taking this concept a bit further, Cortellini and Tonneti introduced the minimally invasive surgical technique (MIST) in 2007 [53] and the modified-minimally invasive surgical technique (M-MIST) in 2009 [54]. More recently the 'entire papilla preservation flap' technique has also been introduced [55]. The main difference between the MIST and the M-MIST is that in the MIST, the interdental papilla associated with the osseous defect is reflected using principles similar to the SPPF, whereas in the M-MIST, the interdental papilla is left intact and a horizontal sub-papillary incision is used to access the bone defect.

All the above-mentioned surgical techniques have been possible only due to the modernization of surgical tools and the advent of magnification in clinical dental practice. Though these techniques have shown favourable results in expert hands in the management of infra-bony defects [56, 57], a real benefit over the traditional techniques has yet not been quantified due to the lack of adequate comparative studies [58]. Considering the advantages of minimally invasive approach especially with respect to patient comfort, it may be recommended to employ these techniques whenever possible but only after adequate training. An important concept that has been revisited due to the minimally invasive surgical approach is that of the role clot stabilization in periodontal regeneration. Evidence may soon emerge prompting a shift from the use of traditional bone grafts and GTR membranes to the use of growth factors, lasers and enamel matrix derivatives in combination with minimally invasive surgery.

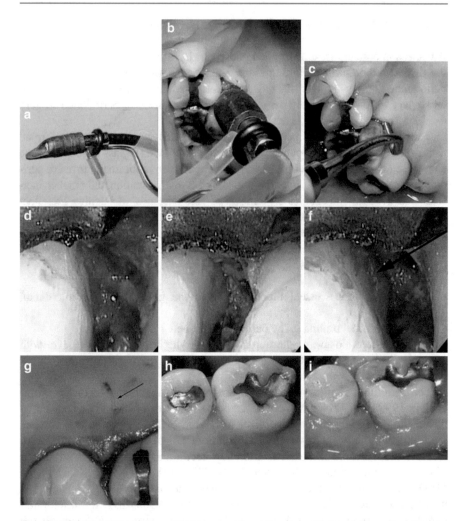

Fig. 11.8 (**a**) Dental Videoscope. (**b**) Videoscope in use for minimally invasive surgery. (**c**) Palatal incision placed with a modified knife. (**d**) Granulation tissue in the periodontal defect. (**e**) Periodontal defect after debridement and root preparation. (**f**) Remnants of calculus visible using the videoscope. (**g**) Flap closed with a single vertical mattress suture. (**h**, **i**) Before and after photos of the surgical site *(Reproduced with permission from John Wiley & Sons)* [50]

11.10 Three-Dimensional Imaging and Scaffolds

A scaffold needs to have several mechanical and biological characteristics to be useful clinically. It should physically conform to the defect, maintain the clot in the defect for the desired duration, allow biological re-modelling and have a favourable internal structure to suit the complexities of the growing tissue. Three-dimentional (3D) imaging and 3D printing has probably been the most significant improvement in clinical dentistry in recent times. 3D imaging allows a comprehensive visualization of a periodontal defect prior to surgical intervention. This permits more accurate planning and execution of the surgery thereby improving operator efficiency and patient-related outcomes. A 3D scan of a periodontal defect can be used to fabricate a 3D scaffold. This scaffold can then be inserted to accurately fit the defect and provide the desired architecture for the planned tissue regeneration.

Computer-assisted designing and computer-assisted manufacturing (CAD-CAM) can utilize state of the art technologies like selective laser sintering, inkjet printing, stereolithography and extrusion printing to generate 3D scaffolds [59]. Various materials have been investigated for the fabrication of the scaffold. Examples include collagen, alginate, chitosan, polymers like polycaprolactone, polyglycolic acid and polylactic acid, bioceramics like hydroxyapatite, β-Tricalcium phosphate and bioactive glass, and metals like titanium and magnesium alloys [59].

For optimum clinical outcomes, a scaffold alone is not sufficient. It needs to be complemented by growth factors, anti-microbial agents, stem cells or autologous platelet concentrates wherever indicated. Technological advances in centrifugation have ushered in the rapid evolution of platelet-rich fibrin (PRF) as an adjunct to wound healing and tissue engineering [60]. This exciting autologous biomaterial can be an excellent adjuvant to 3D printed scaffolds with its ability to stabilize a clot and release growth factors.

11.11 Exploring Digital Solutions to Periodontal Research Problems

The importance of digital database maintenance for research cannot be understated. Meticulous recording and interpretation of available data can go a long way in addressing important research issues and this has been emphatically demonstrated by John Snow in his analysis of the Cholera epidemic of London in 1854. In his extraordinary analysis of the data of the affected cases, John Snow not only provided deep insights into the (then unknown) germ theory of disease but also helped to end to the epidemic itself [61]. This remarkable feat was achieved by the means of only a pen, a paper and a logical approach. With this in mind, the power of the current tools of observation and data management and machine learning in the right hands can be imagined to be limitless.

There are several challenges facing periodontal research at present. Key areas of periodontal research that can have immediate clinical implications are:

- Characterization of the complete human periodontal microflora.
- Quantifying the impact of periodontal infection on systemic health.
- Predictable regeneration of the lost periodontal tissues.

The aetiology of periodontitis has been a constantly changing narrative since the elaboration of the specific and non-specific plaque hypotheses. It was soon observed that bacterial aetiology alone cannot explain the initiation of periodontitis. Increasing understanding about the host response to the microbial challenge and elaboration of the concepts of plaque as a biofilm led to the introduction of the ecological plaque hypothesis by Marsh [62]. Subsequent advances in the understanding of the microbial composition of the periodontitis associated dental biofilm (sub-gingival plaque) have led to the advent of the hypothesis of dysbiosis—for the causation of periodontitis [63].

Ever since the advent of the germ theory of disease and the observation of bacteria in the dental plaque samples, periodontal microbiology has been an important area of research. The concept of bacterial causation of periodontitis received more credence with the identification of putative periodontal pathogens like *Porphyromonas gingivalis*, *Aggregatibacter actinomycetemcomitans*, *Fusobacterim nucleatum*, *Prevotella intermedia* and *Treponema denticola*. Characterization of these bacteria led to the identification of several virulence factors that play a critical role in the establishment of periodontitis. With the invention of modern research tools like the polymerase chain reaction (PCR), our knowledge about periodontitis associated bacteria bloomed and several putative pathogens were identified. PCR made it possible to identify pathogens that were previously ignored—as they could not be easily cultured.

At present, several molecular techniques are available for microbiological research. These include the checkerboard DNA-DNA hybridization, 16 s rRNA sequencing, ribotyping, heteroduplex analysis and whole-genome sequencing. More open-ended techniques like RNA oligonucleotide qualification, Human oral microbiome identification microarray (HOMIM) and the Human oral microbiome database are now pushing the research boundaries at an unprecedented rate [1] and enable the identification of all the bacterial species in a given sample in a single test, something that is impossible with the traditional culture techniques.

Such research will drastically improve our understanding of the composition of the oral microflora. Biochemical analyses too have advanced rapidly due to tools like multilocus enzyme electrophoresis and MALDI-tof (proteomics). Genetic studies are important to identify the genetic risk factors for the initiation and progression of periodontitis. Current research designs like the genome-wide association studies (GWAS) are providing important insights into this very important aspect of 'host susceptibility [64].

Rapid advances in research techniques have made it possible to not only broaden the spectrum of periodontal research but also broaden our perspective of the disease process. This will soon lead to a confluence of various 'branches' of periodontal research into a single and productive stream leading to rapid clinical advances in the treatment of periodontal diseases.

11.12 Advances in Periodontal Care at Home

Advances in the *toothbrush* have probably been one of the most important improvements in periodontology from the patients' perspective. A toothbrush is the most important tool for the maintenance of oral health and the prevention of dental caries, gingivitis and periodontitis.

Broxodent® was the first *powered toothbrush* to be made and was invented by Dr. Philippe-Guy Woog in 1954. Over the years, many variants of the powered toothbrush have been introduced and can be classified as follows: [65].

A. Based on the type of movement.
  (a) Vibration.
  (b) Rotation-oscillation.
B. Speed of movement.
  (a) Sonic.
  (b) Ultrasonic.

Powered toothbrushes have transitioned from bulky devices to more ergonomic designs almost identical to manual toothbrushes. The vibrations or oscillations-rotations of the bristles generated by the automated toothbrush can help patients to maintain oral hygiene more effectively as such fine movements may not be possible with manual toothbrushes. Studies have often demonstrated that the results of the powered toothbrushes are comparable to manual toothbrushing [65]. It is usually accepted that the powered toothbrushes with rotation-oscillation motion are more effective than the vibratory ones which in-turn are more effective than manual toothbrushing. A recent study analysed the effects of powered toothbrushing after a follow-up of 11 years. Over 1500 participants completed the 11 years' follow-up and were analysed for probing depth, clinical attachment loss, dental caries and tooth retention. The study concluded that powered toothbrushing was effective in reducing the progression of probing depth and clinical attachment loss and also for preventing tooth-loss [66]. The powered toothbrush is also an effective oral hygiene aid for plaque control among individuals who depend on care-givers for oral hygiene maintenance or have limited dexterity. Hence, they are particularly indicated for oral hygiene maintenance of differently-abled individuals or in the geriatric age group. Additional intervention using adaptive devices, videoconferencing and in collaboration with occupational therapists has shown to improve the gingival health in such dependent population groups [67].

The *ionic toothbrush* is another innovation based on the principle of ion exchange. It changes the ionic charge of the tooth surface to make it repel dental plaque and may even be effective in inaccessible areas. While based on a solid concept, the ionic toothbrush has not been found to be as effective as a powered toothbrush in the limited available literature [68].

Interdental cleaning is an important adjunct to toothbrushing. Dental floss is the most commonly used interproximal aids but their popularity is reducing after the advent of interdental brushes (Fig. 11.9). The European Federation of Periodontology has also recommended that the use of dental floss be limited to periodontally healthy areas that do not allow the passage of an interdental brush [69]. The limited efficiency of dental flossing in maintaining interdental plaque control has been noted by another recent network meta-analysis [70]. This observed inferiority of dental floss to other interdental cleaning aids may be due to the fact that it is extremely technique-sensitive and may provide the desired results only in controlled or supervised situations.

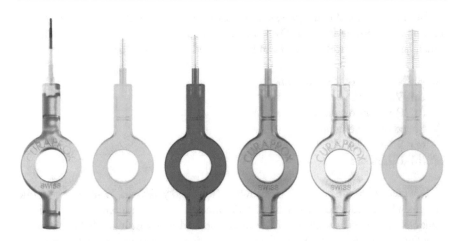

Fig. 11.9 Interdental brushes with different sizes and colour codes

Interdental brush design has seen rapid development. Many brands have been marketing interdental brushes made of fine filaments that can negotiate Type 1 embrasures—areas that traditionally were recommended to be flossed. Several brands are now available in the market and have been shown to be very effective in the maintenance of inter-proximal plaque control and in the reduction of gingival inflammation [70, 71]. A Cochrane Database Systematic review published in 2020 evaluated the efficacy of various interdental cleaning aids as adjuncts to toothbrushing [72]. The review noted that there was some evidence (low level) that interdental brushes and oral irrigators were better than dental floss or toothpicks for the reduction of interdental plaque and gingivitis. The authors further observed that the better results seen with the use of interdental brushes and oral irrigators were observed to be short-term and may not be clinically important [72]. *Oral irrigators*, popularly known as water-flossers (e.g. WaterPik, Philips Sonicare) (Fig. 11.10) are also effective in the maintenance of oral hygiene around prostheses and dental implants.

Though there is a lack of substantial evidence for the routine prescription of interdental aids, studies continue to show a modest but consistent benefit. A lot of the literature demonstrating positive results also needs to be evaluated critically for being influenced by conflicting interests or industrial sponsorships. With the increasing variety of available devices, it is the responsibility of a clinician to choose the most appropriate device based on the clinical situation and also to train the patients to effectively use the device.

11.13 Future Prospects and Conclusion

The periodontium is the support system for the teeth. The health of the periodontal tissues is an important factor affecting the stability and longevity of the human dentition. Challenges like the regeneration of lost alveolar bone and interdental gingival

Fig. 11.10 WaterPik oral
irrigator

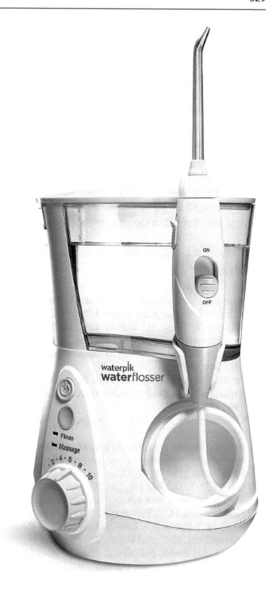

papillae are fitting examples to demonstrate the importance of a healthy periodontium. Digital advances in dentistry have revolutionized the field of Periodontology in the past decade. The improvements in probing systems have allowed the tedious process of periodontal charting to become more comfortable and fast. Digital tools for assessment of tooth mobility and occlusal discrepancy have made this part of the periodontal diagnosis more objective. Digital tools for patient education and home care have improved patient compliance and may lead to an overall improvement in the community oral health standard.

Digital advances in research, especially in the field of bioinformatics has revolutionized medical research. A large amount of data is being generated every day in the areas of periodontal regeneration, biomarker analysis, microbiology, genetics and epidemiology. All this data can be integrated into meaningful information for the development of new treatment methods and drugs by using advanced tools like the systems biology approach [73].

All the advances, from those in basic laboratory research to those in clinical trials and techniques, are ultimately aimed at improving the oral and periodontal health of the individual and of the community. Digitization and automation if used to improve the standard of care and convenience can only be a positive thing. With the rapid acceptance of technology, it is not long before the periodontal maintenance schedule is managed by virtual voice assistants, periodontal treatment is aided by digital clinical assistants and the efficacy of home care is monitored by 'smart' devices.

References

1. Teles R, Teles F, Frias-Lopez J, Paster B, Haffajee A. Lessons learned and unlearned in periodontal microbiology. Periodontol. 2013;62:95–162.
2. Schleyer T, Song M, Gilbert GH, Rindal DB, Fellows JL, Gordan VV, Funkhouser E. Electronic dental record use and clinical information management patterns among practitioner-investigators in The Dental Practice-Based Research Network. J Am Dent Assoc. 2013;144:49–58.
3. Hefti AF. Periodontal probing. Crit Rev Oral Biol Med. 1997;8:336–56.
4. Armitage GC. Manual periodontal probing in supportive periodontal treatment. Periodontol. 1996;12:33–9.
5. Gabathuler H, Hassell T. A pressure-sensitive periodontal probe. Helv Odontol Acta. 1971;15:114–7.
6. Polson AM, Caton IB, Yeaple RN, Zander HA. Histological determination of probe tip penetration into gingival sulcus of humans using an electronic pressure sensitive probe. I. Clin Periodontol. 1980;7:479–88.
7. Gibbs CH, Hirschfeld JW, Lee JG, Low SB, Magnusson I, Thousand RR, Yemeni P, Clark WB. Description and clinical evaluation of a new computerized periodontal probe—the Florida Probe. J Clin Periodontol. 1988;15:137–44.
8. Manz MC, Morris HF, Ochi S. Evaluation of the inter probe electronic periodontal probe. Implant Dent. 1992;1:284–7.
9. The Florida Probe. Periodontal disease—teaching and motivating patients with the Florida Probe [Internet]. 2008 [cited 09/08/2020]. https://www.dentalcompare.com/Featured-Articles/2203-Periodontal-Disease-Teaching-and-Motivating-Patients-with-the-Florida-Probe
10. Osborn J, Stoltenberg J, Huso B, Aeppli D, Pihlstrom B. Comparison of measurement variability using a standard and constant force periodontal probe. J Periodontol. 1990;61:497–503.
11. Reddy MS, Palcanis KG, Geurs NC. A comparison of manual and controlled-force attachment-level measurements. J Clin Periodontol. 1997;24:920–6.
12. Birek P, McCulloch CA, Hardy V. Gingival attachment level measurements with an automated periodontal probe. J Clin Periodontol. 1987;14:472–7.
13. Tessier JF, Kulkarni GV, Ellen RP, McCulloch CA. Probing velocity: novel approach for assessment of inflamed periodontal attachment. J Periodontol. 1994;65:103–8.
14. Elashiry M, Meghil MM, Arce RM, Cutler CW. From manual periodontal probing to digital 3-D imaging to endoscopic capillaroscopy: Recent advances in periodontal disease diagnosis. J Periodontal Res. 2019;54:1–9.

15. Elashiry M, Meghil MM, Kalathingal S, et al. Development of radiopaque, biocompatible, antimicrobial, micro-particle fillers for micro-CT imaging of simulated periodontal pockets. Dent Mater. 2018;34:569–78.
16. Drucker SD, Prieto LE, Kao DW. Periodontal probing calibration in an academic setting. J Dent Educ. 2012;76:1466–73.
17. Anerud A, Loe H, Boysen H. The natural history and clinical course of calculus formation in man. J Clin Periodontol. 1991;18:160–70.
18. Meissner G, Kocher T. Calculus-detection technologies and their clinical application. Periodontol. 2010;55:189–204.
19. Kamath DG, Umesh NS. Detection, removal and prevention of calculus: literature review. Saudi Dent J. 2014;26(1):7–13.
20. Osborn J. Role of the dental endoscope in calculus detection. Dimens Dent Hyg. 2016;14(02):40,42–4.
21. Geisinger ML, Mealey BL, Schoolfield J, Mellonig JT. The effectiveness of subgingival scaling and root planing: an evaluation of therapy with and without the use of the periodontal endoscope. J Periodontol. 2007;78:22–8.
22. Walsh LJ. Optical diagnostic methods: current status and future potential. Australas Dent Pract Mag. 2008;19(5):64–70.
23. Krause F, Braun A, Frentzen M. The possibility of detecting sub-gingival calculus by laser-fluorescence in vitro. Lasers Med Sci. 2003;18:32–5.
24. Shakibaie F, Walsh LJ. Laser fluorescence detection of subgingival calculus using the DIAGNOdent classic versus periodontal probing. Lasers Med Sci. 2016;31:1621–6.
25. Shakibaie F, Law K, Walsh LJ. Improved detection of subgingival calculus by laser fluorescence over differential reflectometry. Lasers Med Sci. 2019;34:1807–11.
26. Patini R, Zunino B, Foti R, Proetti L, Gallenzi P. Clinical evaluation of the efficacy of Perioscan® on plaque-induced gingivitis in paediatric age. Senses Sci. 2015;2(3):98–103.
27. Tsubokawa M, Aoki A, Kakizaki S, et al. In vitro and clinical evaluation of optical coherence tomography for the detection of sub-gingival calculus and root cementum. J Oral Sci. 2018;60(3):418–27.
28. Carranza FA, Newman MG, Takei HH, Klokkevold PR. Carranza's clinical periodontology. 11th ed. St. Louis, MO: Elsevier Saunders; 2012.
29. Miller S. C: textbook of periodontia. 1st ed. Philadelphia, PA: Blakiston; 1938.
30. Varadhan KB, Parween S, Bhavsar AK, et al. Tooth mobility measurements- realities and limitations. J Evol Med Dent Sci. 2019;8:1342–50.
31. Schulte W, Lukas D. The perio-test method. Int Dent J. 1992;42:433–40.
32. Chakrapani S, Goutham M, Krishnamohan T, Anuparthy S, Tadiboina N, Rambha S. Periotest values: its reproducibility, accuracy, and variability with hormonal influence. Contemp Clin Dent. 2015;6:12–5.
33. Goellner M, Schmitt J, Holst S, Petschelt A, Wichmann M, Berthold C. Correlations between tooth mobility and the Periotest method in periodontally involved teeth. Quintessence Int. 2013;44:307–16.
34. Yamane M, Yamaoka M, Hayashi M, Furutoyo I, Komori N, Ogiso B. Measuring tooth mobility with a no-contact vibration device. J Periodontal Res. 2008;43:84–9.
35. Bertl MH, Weinberger T, Schwarz K, Gruber R, Crismani AG. Resonance frequency analysis: a new diagnostic tool for dental ankylosis. Eur J Oral Sci. 2012;120:255–8.
36. Konermann A, Al-Malat R, Skupin J, et al. In vivo determination of tooth mobility after fixed orthodontic appliance therapy with a novel intraoral measurement device. Clin Oral Investig. 2017;21:1283–9.
37. Meirelles L, Siqueira R, Garaicoa-Pazmino C, Yu SH, Chan HL, Wang HL. Quantitative tooth mobility evaluation based on intraoral scanner measurements. J Periodontol. 2019; https://doi.org/10.1002/JPER.19-0282.
38. Nyman SR, Lang NP. Tooth mobility and the biological rationale for splinting teeth. Periodontol. 1994;4:15–22.

39. Martinez-Canut P. Predictors of tooth loss due to periodontal disease in patients following long-term periodontal maintenance. J Clin Periodontol. 2015;42:1115–25.
40. Lang NP, Bartold PM. Periodontal health. J Clin Periodontol. 2018;45(Suppl20):S9–S16.
41. Hallmon WW, Harrel SK. Occlusal analysis, diagnosis and management in the practice of periodontics. Periodontol. 2004;34:151–64.
42. Passanezi E, Sant'Ana ACP. Role of occlusion in periodontal disease. Periodontol. 2019;79:129–50.
43. Zhou S, Mahmood H, Cao C, Jin L. Teeth under high occlusal force may reflect occlusal trauma-associated periodontal conditions in subjects with untreated chronic periodontitis. Chin J Dent Res. 2017;20:19–26.
44. Baba K, Tsukiyama Y, Clark GT. Reliability, validity, and utility of various occlusal measurement methods and techniques. J Prosthet Dent. 2000;83:83–9.
45. Consult-PRO. https://www.consult-pro.com/about.html. Accessed on 20/04/2020.
46. Florida Probe. http://www.floridaprobe.com/fp32software.htm. Accessed on 20/04/2020.
47. Manresa C, Sanz-Miralles EC, Twigg J, Bravo M. Supportive periodontal therapy (SPT) for maintaining the dentition in adults treated for periodontitis. Cochrane Database Syst Rev. 2018;(1):CD009376. https://doi.org/10.1002/14651858.CD009376.pub2.
48. Rethman MP, Harrel SK. Minimally invasive periodontal therapy: will periodontal therapy remain a technologic laggard? J Periodontol. 2010;81:1390–5.
49. Harrel SK, Rees TD. Granulation tissue removal in routine and minimally invasive surgical procedures. Compend Contin Educ Dent. 1995;16:960–7.
50. Harrel SK, Wilson TG Jr, Nunn ME. Prospective assessment of the use of enamel matrix proteins with minimally invasive surgery: six year results. J Periodontol. 2010;81:435–44.
51. Harrel SK, Wilson TG Jr, Rivera-Hidalgo F. A video scope for use in minimally invasive periodontal surgery. J Clin Periodontol. 2013;40:868–74.
52. Cortellini P, Pini-Prato GP, Tonetti MS. The simplified papilla preservation flap. A novel surgical approach for the management of soft tissues in regenerative procedures. Int J Periodontics Restorative Dent. 1999;19:589–99.
53. Cortellini P, Tonetti MS. A minimally invasive surgical technique (MIST) with enamel matrix derivate in the regenerative treatment of defects: a novel approach to limit morbidity. J Clin Periodontol. 2007;34:87–93.
54. Cortellini P, Tonetti MS. Improved wound stability with a modified minimally invasive surgical technique in the regenerative treatment of isolated interdental intrabony defects. J Clin Periodontol. 2009;36:157–63.
55. Aslan S, Buduneli N, Cortellini P. Entire papilla preservation technique: a novel surgical approach for regenerative treatment of deep and wide Intrabony defects. Int J Periodontics Restorative Dent. 2017;37:227–33.
56. Cortellini P, Tonetti MS. Clinical and radiographic outcomes of the modified minimally invasive surgical technique with and without regenerative materials: a randomized-controlled trial in intra-bony defects. J Clin Periodontol. 2011;38:365–73.
57. Harrel SK, Nunn ME, Abraham CM, Rivera-Hidalgo F, Shulman JD, Tunnell JC. Videoscope assisted minimally invasive surgery (VMIS): 36-month results. J Periodontol. 2017;88:528–35.
58. Clementini M, Ambrosi A, Cicciarelli V, De Risi V, de Sanctis M. Clinical performance of minimally invasive periodontal surgery in the treatment of infrabony defects: systematic review and meta-analysis. J Clin Periodontol. 2019;46:1236–53.
59. Asa'ad F, Pagni G, Pilipchuk SP, Giannì AB, Giannobile WV, Rasperini G. 3D-printed scaffolds and biomaterials: review of alveolar bone augmentation and periodontal regeneration applications. Int J Dent. 2016;2016:1239842.
60. Miron RJ, Chai J, Zheng S, Feng M, Sculean A, Zhang Y. A novel method for evaluating and quantifying cell types in platelet rich fibrin and an introduction to horizontal centrifugation. J Biomed Mater Res A. 2019;107:2257–71.
61. Cameron D, Jones IG. John snow, the broad street pump and modern epidemiology. Int J Epidemiol. 1983;12:393–6.

62. Marsh PD, Moter A, Devine DA. Dental plaque biofilms: communities, conflict and control. Periodontol. 2011;55:16–35.
63. Yost S, Duran-Pinedo AE, Teles R, Krishnan K, Frias-Lopez J. Functional signatures of oral dysbiosis during periodontitis progression revealed by microbial metatranscriptome analysis. Genome Med. 2015;7:27. https://doi.org/10.1186/s13073-015-0153-3.
64. Masumoto R, Kitagaki J, Fujihara C, Matsumoto M, Miyauchi S, Asano Y, Imai A, Kobayashi K, Nakaya A, Yamashita M, Yamada S, Kitamura M, Murakami S. Identification of genetic risk factors of aggressive periodontitis using genomewide association studies in association with those of chronic periodontitis. J Periodontal Res. 2019;54:199–206.
65. Ng C, Tsoi JKH, Lo ECM, Matinlinna JP. Safety and design aspects of powered toothbrush—a narrative review. Dent J. 2020;8:15.
66. Pitchika V, Pink C, Völzke H, Welk A, Kocher T, Holtfreter B. Long-term impact of powered toothbrush on oral health: 11-year cohort study. J Clin Periodontol. 2019;46:713–22.
67. Yuen HK. Effect of a home telecare program on oral health among adults with tetraplegia: a pilot study. Spinal Cord. 2013;51:477–81.
68. Singh G, Mehta DS, Chopra S, Khatri M. Comparison of sonic and ionic toothbrush in reduction in plaque and gingivitis. J Indian Soc Periodontol. 2011;15(3):210–4.
69. Chapple IL, Van der Weijden F, Doerfer C, et al. Primary prevention of periodontitis: managing gingivitis. J Clin Periodontol. 2015;42(Suppl 16):S71–6.
70. Kotsakis GA, Lian Q, Ioannou AL, Michalowicz BS, John MT, Chu H. A network meta-analysis of interproximal oral hygiene methods in the reduction of clinical indices of inflammation. J Periodontol. 2018;89(5):558–70.
71. How to use interdental brushes to clean between teeth. https://www.dentaly.org/en/oral-hygiene/interdental-brushes/
72. Worthington HV, MacDonald L, Poklepovic Pericic T, et al. Home use of interdental cleaning devices, in addition to toothbrushing, for preventing and controlling periodontal diseases and dental caries. Cochrane Database Syst Rev. 2019;4(4):CD012018.
73. Abhyankar V, Bland P, Fernandes G. The role of systems biologic approach in cell Signaling and drug development responses-a mini review. Med Sci (Basel). 2018;6(2):43. https://doi.org/10.3390/medsci6020043.

Dental Implants and Digitization

12

Nitish Surathu, Ali Tunkiwala, and Udatta Kher

12.1 Introduction

The last couple of decades have seen a tremendous increase in the use of computer-driven technology to automate several processes in the dental industry. The use of computer-aided design (CAD) and computer-aided manufacturing (CAM) have transformed the process of design, manufacture, and delivery of many dental services [1]. Restorative dentistry has probably been the largest gainer of this transformation. Dental implantology however comes a close second and digital technology has brought dental radiology, implant surgery, and implant prosthodontics together in a manner that few could have envisioned possible.

12.2 History and Development

In the late 1980s, the osseointegrated root-form implant began to see extensive clinical use as a modality to replace teeth. Professor Branemark had completed several years of clinical research that saw the modality become popular clinically [2]. The root-form implant held several geometric advantages over other forms of previously practiced endosseous implants such as blade implants and ramus frames. A cylindrical shape with a screw thread of definitive diameter and length quickly became the most popular. The geometry of this type of implant lent itself very easily to large-scale commercial manufacturing.

Several companies began to manufacture implants using computer numeric controlled (CNC) lathes which are still the mainstay of the industry. These CNC lathes themselves became extremely accurate and in time were able to

N. Surathu
Private practice, Gisborne, New Zealand

A. Tunkiwala · U. Kher (✉)
Private Practice, Mumbai, India

© Springer Nature Switzerland AG 2021
P. Jain, M. Gupta (eds.), *Digitization in Dentistry*,
https://doi.org/10.1007/978-3-030-65169-5_12

manufacture extremely high accuracy tolerances. This allowed for excellent componentry fit and restorative predictability (R). Once endosseous root-form implants had established themselves as an accepted modality of treatment, the industry began to face challenges with clinical demands for restorative customization. A growing esthetic demand for implant restorations to be as natural as possible drove this increased demand for customization as well. The industry stepped up to the challenge and invested in CNC manufacturing of customized restorative componentry. The early 2000s saw the creation of large facilities dedicated to CAD/CAM design of custom abutments, restorations, and other restorative componentry such as bars [3]. These facilities provided multilocation high-end computer-aided manufacturing and served to eliminate expensive investment in the equipment required.

As implant restorative dentistry itself became more customized, it became obvious to the industry that control of the surgical process would be the next challenge. Specialists with surgical skills and general dentists with sufficient surgical aptitude had already taken to offering dental implant services to their patients. There still remained a large cohort of clinicians who could consider implant services, if surgical predictability became a reality. A demand for greater surgical predictability also came to be a result of implants being used for more complex rehabilitation. Full arch implant rehabilitations were particularly surgically challenging and demanded better anatomical understanding. Implants also began to be used in bone deficient situations with increased grafting [4, 5]. The development of techniques that incorporated angled implants also saw a greater demand for surgical skill in terms of accommodation of the patient's anatomy [6, 7] (Fig. 12.1).

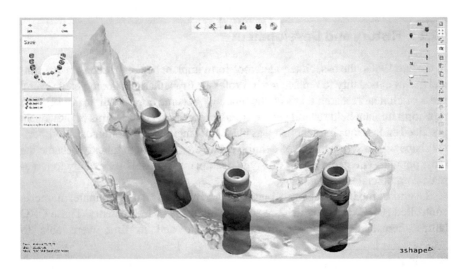

Fig. 12.1 Customized angled overdenture design

The development of cone beam computerized tomography at around the same time also made three-dimensional radiographic visualization of anatomy a reality [8, 9]. It remained up to the industry to marry these digital technologies together and develop a protocol for more accurate surgery.

Much research in the late 90s and early 2000s eventually saw the development of guided implant surgery. The development of surgical guides and instrumentation that allowed accurate preparation of bone for a dental implant became very popular over time [10, 11]. Several dentists with a moderate surgical skill set as well as clinicians demanding greater planning accuracy for complex cases, became supporters of guided implant surgery. The surgical guides themselves were made at the time in centralized CAM facilities that employed rapid prototyping technology [12, 13]. The gradual erosion of the cost of computer-aided manufacturing, both in milling and rapid prototyping, eventually made the consideration of chair-side use of these technologies a reality.

The industry as it stands today has completely decentralized these technologies and moved them into the dentist's office [14, 15]. The evolution of better milling technology has also seen chair-side milling of custom titanium and zirconia componentry become a possibility. The development of low-cost 3D printing has also meant that the manufacture of surgical guides with complex geometries can also become chair-side [16–18] (Fig. 12.2).

Software business models that had once focused on centralized manufacturing for a fee, have now largely become low cost or even free, sometimes allowing a cost to be incurred only when needed. We are therefore at a very exciting juncture with regard to the digitization of implant dentistry and the future is bright.

This chapter seeks to chronologically elaborate on several aspects of this digitization process that have come to be a reality today. The idea is to educate the reader about multiple digital technologies that are currently available with regard to multiple aspects of the delivery of clinical implant dentistry.

Fig. 12.2 A safe guide with lateral access from *Simplant*

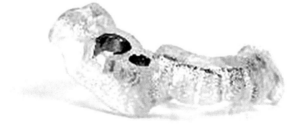

12.3   Implant Manufacturing

The earliest root-form implants were hand manufactured from titanium rods. Over the years, the process became mechanized, and large industrial precision lathes began to be used for the manufacture of root-form implants. The advent of computer-aided design and manufacturing saw this process become more and more digitized [19–21]. Computer numeric controlled lathes today are capable of manufacturing dental implants and componentry with as little as a 2-micron tolerance. Advances in computer numeric control lathe technology have also allowed the manufacture of more and more specialized restorative componentry that has needed multiaxis machining. The industry is today capable of producing high precision componentry that allows the restorability of implants in multiple difficult situations. Examples include the manufacture of zygomatic [22, 23] and nasal floor implant as well as angulated screw channel [24, 25] restorative components and the use of materials such as zirconia titanium alloys in the manufacture of dental implants. Advances have also meant an advancement of production efficiencies and quantities and implant companies are today able to service a multibillion-dollar worldwide industry that sees hundreds of thousands of implants placed annually. The future is likely to see the evolution of newer implant material types and the customization of dental implants for unique situations (Fig. 12.3).

12.4   Restorative Componentry

The late eighties saw the development of restorative CAD and CAM technologies in Europe. Companies began to be able to manufacture custom restorations in ceramics and custom componentry in titanium. Large industry players moved to acquire this technology and the nineties saw the introduction of either centralized manufacturing facilities for restorations or their componentry or the advent of early

Fig. 12.3 Azento concept all-inclusive implant solution

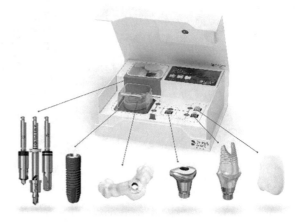

chair-side milling solutions [14, 26–28]. Computer-aided designing came to start to replace what was traditionally handcrafted by dental technicians. The quality of custom implant componentry actually began to enhance restorative outcomes. Dental technicians themselves moved to automate their own design manufacturing processes and sought to outsource much of what they produced to large centralized manufacturing facilities that invested in multimillion-dollar multiaxis milling machines. Manufacturing capabilities of these machines began to include full arch restorations in zirconia and titanium as well, including full-arch bridges, titanium substructures, and titanium bars.

The quality and passivity of fit even in cross-arch situations were often exemplary and computer-aided manufacturing helped address many of the weaknesses of conventional restorative manufacturing. Many cross-arch cast restorative solutions were heavy, expensive, and sometimes inaccurate [29, 30]. Milled single- and multiple-unit restorative componentry slowly began to become the mainstay of the implant industry [31, 32]. The real advances in the manufacture of restorative componentry however began to come when manufacturing began to become decentralized. Computer-aided manufacturing technologies gradually became more portable and the industry began to develop desktop milling solutions that returned control to the dental technician. Dental technicians themselves needed to adapt to technological change and move to learn and use digital software to replace conventional manufacturing. Multiaxis manufacturing lathes are now easily available as desktop solutions and mill ceramics, zirconia, titanium, cobalt chrome, wax, techno polymers, acrylics, and composite [33, 34]. The wide range of capability of these machines has also meant that dental laboratories have become extensively digitized.

Chair-side milling technology has also seen significant change over the last decade. Dentists are able to provide chair-side milling solutions in ceramics, composite, and zirconia that often see them able to deliver restorations in one appointment. Newer milling machines are also capable of milling titanium abutments and non-precious metal restorations, giving today's digital dentist many more additions to his clinical repertoire [35–37]. Chair-side design technologies have also put the clinician more in power of single-unit restorations, in particular, giving a dentist the ability to design crowns, veneers, implant abutments, implant restorations, and inlays and onlays. The sheer range of materials that have become available for chair-side milling is also impressive with materials such as composites, feldspar ceramics, leucite reinforced ceramics, ceramic-composite hybrids, zirconia, acrylics, non-precious alloy and lithium silicates/disilicates/zirconia reinforced silicates, all being available in the form of blocks that are accepted by chair-side mills. Advances have also included the ability of these machines to dry mill and wet mill, thus reducing processing times for post milling sintering or crystallization [38, 39].

Technologies in furnace development have also kept pace and provided dentists with chair-side solutions that are capable of an extremely rapid rise in sintering/crystallization temperatures as well as rapid cooling. The fastest mills are capable of milling some materials in less than 5 min with sintering/crystallization taking only another 10 min [40, 41]. These technologies have therefore resulted in the creation of chair-side restorations while the patient waits. The expansion of the envelope of single appointment dentistry is a reality of dental practice today and dentists have no alternative but to embrace computer-aided design and manufacturing to be able to offer it.

12.5 Digital Impression in Implant Dentistry

Chair-side intraoral scanning has also seen significant evolution in the last decade. The use of contrast sprays and 2D photography that stitched images together is something of the past and the scanners of today are capable of full color realistic 3d imagery. Exceptional speeds of data acquisition have also resulted in greater acceptance for intraoral scanners [41–43]. The trueness of intraoral scans has also been scientifically assessed with a variety of scanners. It is interesting to see that intraoral scanners are today capable of cross arch accuracy that is comparable to or better than dental impressions with the best impression materials (Fig. 12.4).

It is realistically possible today to consider the elimination of conventional impressions, at least in most dentate cases if not all cases. Intraoral scanners of today are also able to accurately image to a depth of 20 millimeters, allowing a large envelope for the size of restorations possible and their sub-gingival extent. Some advanced intraoral scanners are also capable of accounting for fluids such as blood and saliva and compensating for refractive error that may otherwise result.

More information on the types of scanners and their descriptions/uses is given in Chap. 11.

Dynamic intraoral scanning has also become a reality today and it is actually possible to generate genuine articulation between intraoral scans of opposing arches as long as static and excursive bite records are obtained. Software advances have also resulted in an increased ability to integrate various digital data sets. Intraoral scans are therefore integratable not just with cone beam computed tomography volumes but also facial scans and impression generated models or wax-ups [44, 45] (Fig. 12.5).

Fig. 12.4 STL wireframes that form the basis of most 3D images

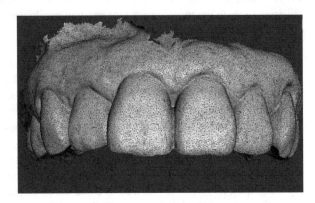

Fig. 12.5 Integrated facial and intraoral scans

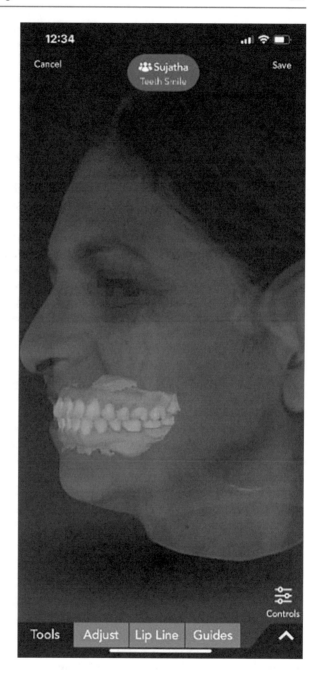

Integration of this nature allows substantial cross over between the digital and analog worlds. Clinicians and technicians are therefore able to choose workflows that they prefer and still manage continuity of flow from a digital workspace to an analog workspace and vice versa. Data sizes of intraoral scans have also become far more efficient with the evolution of newer file formats that allow greater mesh compression. This directly translates into ease of digital transfer and allows clinicians and technicians and other providers in various parts of the world to come together in one workspace.

The laboratory equivalent of intraoral scans is the model scanner that uses largely similar scanning principles. Model scanners typically scan impressions or poured-up dental models. In general, the direct scanning of impressions has always presented difficult challenges, with undercuts in an impression allowing limited access to a scanner. This is still best addressed by pouring up an analog model that can be scanned. It however continues to compel an analog step in a workflow that can otherwise be completely digital. The best digital solution offered for this problem continues to be the CBCT scanning of impressions and their inversion using 3D rendering software [46–48]. To some degree, the access of intraoral scanner heads does limit the amount of data that can be acquired by an intraoral scanner. It is expected that the size of intraoral scanners and their field of view will continue to see the improvement that will overcome these obstacles. The power consumption of intraoral scanners has also meant the development of models that can be battery supported, thus allowing greater portability.

This is a tremendous advantage in multioperatory dental offices and can serve to reduce a practice's investment. The weight of intraoral scanners has also come down with time, despite the incorporation of heating of fans to reduce fogging. If anything, the pace of development continues to pose a challenge for rapid technological redundancy, and this can be an issue if the investment is not a well-thought-out decision. New generation intraoral scanners are also attempting to integrate other emerging technologies such as subtractive superimpositional techniques that allow for assessment of changes in a dentition such as wear, migration, or recession. Some scanners have also incorporated caries detection and transillumination modalities that allow for illuminative structural assessment of teeth.

12.5.1 Scan Bodies

In effect, the dramatic advances in intraoral scanning have meant that all impression procedures in implant dentistry can be truly and completely digitized. This has led to the development of multiple scan bodies that are really replacements for conventional impression copings in implant dentistry [49]. Scan bodies have tended to be unique to commercially developed digital workflows in order to ensure sanctity in the workflow with minimal room for error [50, 51]. Some have however become more popular than others, driven largely by their acceptance by commercial CAD design software packages. Many scan bodies offer a titanium base, a polymer replaceable post, and digital libraries that can be imported into popular CAD software. These digital libraries allow the creation of digital or physically printed 3D models that become working models for dental laboratories. The accuracy of scan bodies has meant that their use in cross arch situations is also possible. Indeed, scan bodies have also been employed in full arch situations for the development of milled multi-unit prosthesis in titanium, zirconia, and techno polymers. Some companies have also offered integration between scan bodies and custom abutment manufacturing (Figs. 12.6 and 12.7).

These custom abutments are often fabricated with a high degree of accuracy on either 5 axis lathes or computer numeric controlled lathes that are capable of

Fig. 12.6 Acuris conometric concept

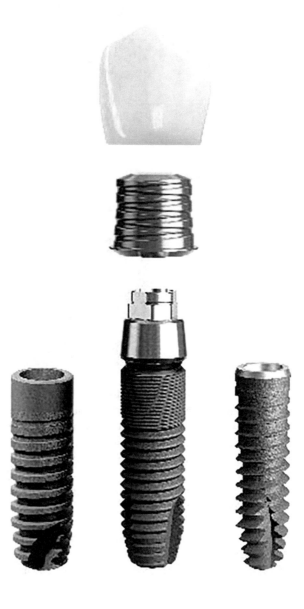

Fig. 12.7 Custom
abutments from Atlantis

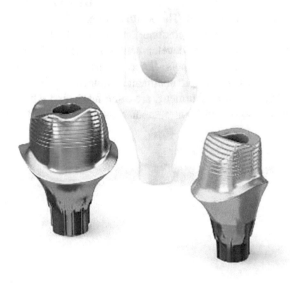

Fig. 12.8 Photogramme-
try scan markers in an All
on 4 (*Courtesy of Dr Han
Choi, Auckland*)

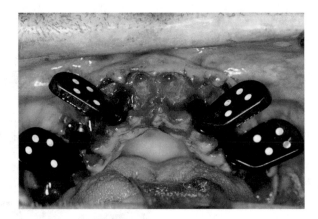

generating custom abutments with a quality that is similar to prefabricated stock
implant componentry. Some of these manufacturers even allow dentists to mill their
restorations from core restoration files supplied by them(R). This ensures that costs
are further curbed, and dentists are able to have well designed implant restorations
that offer a quality fit on custom implant abutments.

12.5.2 Photogrammetry

The other dramatic improvement in implant impressions has come about with
the use of photogrammetry (Fig. 12.8). This technique allows the registration
of the exact three-dimensional location of the implants using 3D coordinate

measurements to record geometric properties. Photogrammetry [52, 53] has been shown to be highly accurate in implant dentistry and ensures the minimization of inaccuracies in cross arch digital impressions. At least two systems are now commercially available and offer a package that includes specially designed implant mounts with geometric imagery and a photogrammetry camera that accurately records three-dimensional orientation. It is anticipated that photogrammetry may well become the technique of choice for accurate impressions in restorative full-arch dentistry.

12.6   Guided Implant Surgery

The longest-standing digitization protocol in implant dentistry has for long been the field of computer-guided implant surgery [54] (Fig. 12.9). The technique fundamentally integrates digital restorative data with radiographic data in order to provide a clinician with a restorative guideline. This allows the use of this guideline over a radiographic representation of bone at a proposed site, to accurately plan an implant's position. The earliest versions of this technology either utilized diagnostic wax-ups that were scanned using model scanners or acrylic partial/complete dentures with radiographic gutta-percha markers. In its earliest days, the technique also used conventional medical-grade axial tomography that resulted in significant radiation exposure. The development of cone beam computed tomography brought about a significant change with regard to reduced radiation exposure levels. It gradually becomes cost realistic for dental practices as well to incorporate cone beam computed tomography into their practices. This one development alone has resulted in an explosion of the use of guided implant surgical techniques.

The earliest software packages were developed in Belgium and were tested extensively in multi-center clinical trials. At the time, most guided surgical stents were developed using stereolithographic techniques for rapid prototyping in centralized facilities. The cost of these stents was prohibitive, but they added significantly to the accuracy of implant placement. Companies also moved to develop surgical instrumentation that was specific to guided surgery and surgical protocols that incorporated these stents quickly became popular with strong marketing.

Fig. 12.9 Planning image with color intraoral scan import

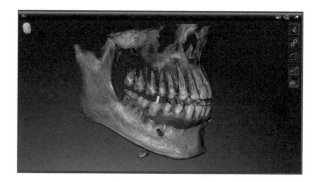

The development of intraoral scanning and new software for cone beam computed tomography saw integration taken to a whole new level. Dentists were able to plan implant restorations chair-side on digital models, although they were limited to single restorations and short edentulous spans. These planned implant restorations were easily incorporated into guided surgery software resulting in very accurate implant planning. Recent Software packages include libraries for multiple implant systems, thus broadening the scope for use of guided surgery. Software packages have now become increasingly intuitive as well, allowing users to slice data in a variety of custom planes that went beyond conventional multi-planar radiology [55–57]. This allowed users to place implants at any angle of their choice while still being able to assess distances, angles, and parallelism between multiple implants. Clinicians were also offered the ability to clearly delineate anatomical landmarks such as nerves in order to allow for accurate planning of implants in proximity to them. The ability to detect some of these landmarks has become increasingly more accurate with time as well, given high-resolution voxel sizes in current cone beam computed tomography machines. Some software today also allow volumetric planning of grafts in deficient sites [58–60]. It has also become possible to generate accurate three-dimensional models from radiographic data and integrate this with data from intraoral scans, facial scans, and soft tissue scans. The generation of new file formats is also opening up possibilities for incorporation of full color in these data sets, adding a whole new dimension to aesthetically driven digital treatment planning that involves implants.

Significant improvement in guided surgery tooling has also meant that some of the initial difficulties with guide implant surgery are better addressed. One of the early limitations often used to be the size of drills and consequent limitations with regard to mouth opening in certain patients. Lateral access sleeves have allowed for easier access to guided surgery drills into a surgical guide, especially in posterior sites (Fig. 12.10). Many manufacturers have also moved to eliminate "Spoons" or "Keys" and attempted to incorporate a metal sleeve in the guide (Fig. 12.11). This

Fig. 12.10 Spoon or key-based guided surgery

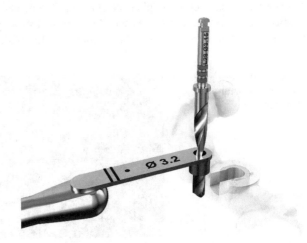

Fig. 12.11 Incremental keys or spoons in guided surgery

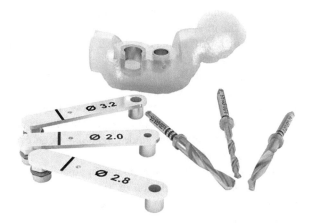

Fig. 12.12 Sleeve-on-drill Astratech guided drills

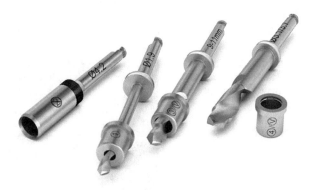

approach has sometimes resulted in some loss of axial control but newer instrumentation incorporating sleeves directly on drills has addressed this (Fig. 12.12). Most instrumentation will likely become keyless in the future resulting in greater ease of use of surgical guides.

The largest limitation of guided implant surgery continues to be the generation of restorative data for treatment planning in edentulous patients. In the absence of a significant number of teeth to allow integration of various data sets involved, it becomes necessary to scan acrylic partial or complete prostheses and use these as restorative guides as well as templates for surgical guide design. Most conventional guided surgery stents are designed to fit on teeth, thus allowing for excellent stability during surgery [61–63]. In edentulous situations, these surgical guides either have to be mucosa or bone supported. Regardless, the use of removable prostheses as scanning templates introduces a potential for error as the fit of these prostheses is sometimes less than optimal or the prosthesis is simply not fully seated during a CBCT scan. Given the limited radiopacity of acrylic, it also becomes important to ensure that soft wares adequately recognize and position these prostheses in their correct 3D orientation. The use of gutta-percha markers to facilitate this has often been cumbersome and while the evolution of adhesive radiopaque glass beads has helped this situation somewhat, it still remains cumbersome.

The accuracy of scanned polymer data is also highly variable, and varying degrees of radio-opacity of different brands affect this parameter as well. In any case, edentulous guides have evolved significantly to go beyond early generation mucosa supported guides that were based on the morphology of an existing prosthesis. It is today possible to generate bone level guides that can be used for extremely accurate bone reduction. It is also possible to accurately stack implant surgery guides over bone reduction guides, resulting in an even greater degree of surgical accuracy [64, 65] (Figs. 12.13–12.15).

The single most significant change in guided implant surgery has however been brought about by the evolution of 3D printing. 3D printers used to be extremely expensive even until 5 years ago. Recently however there has been extensive development in 3D printing and many dentists can now realistically consider the incorporation of inexpensive 3D printers into their practices. New generation chair-side dental 3D printers are capable of fabricating surgical guides with a 50-micron accuracy level [66]. This means that dentists are able to inexpensively print highly

Fig. 12.13 Digitally simulated bone reduction for All on X treatment planning

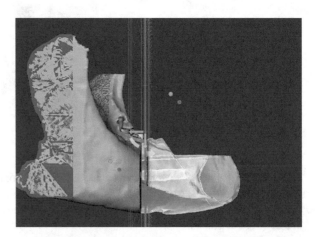

Fig. 12.14 Mesh software designed custom bone reduction guide

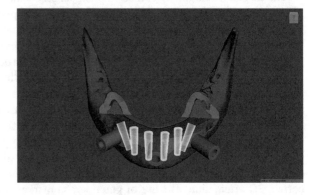

Fig. 12.15 Superimposable bone reduction and implant placement guides

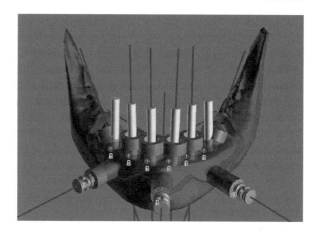

Fig. 12.16 3D Printed implant OVD base

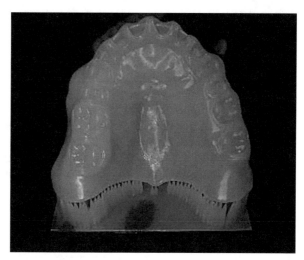

accurate tooth, mucosa and bone supported surgical guides. 3D printing also allows for the fabrication of extremely accurate temporary implant prostheses that can be linked to a surgical guide (Fig. 12.16). New generation software also allows significant customization of these surgical guides, offering unlimited control over the dimensions of surgical componentry and offset distances. Surgical guides have therefore never been more customizable, and they continue to push the accuracy of surgical implantology to significantly higher levels.

12.7   Navigational Surgery

Another significant advance in guided surgery is navigational surgery. This technology does not even employ surgical guides as we know them but instead uses computed tomography in conjunction with a computer-guided navigation system that guides the operator in real time. The principal advantage of navigational surgery is that the technology is dynamic as opposed to conventional guided surgery which is static. This means that any changes to a treatment plan in conventional guided surgery demand freehand use of instrumentation and rejection of the planned surgical guide. Navigational surgery on the other hand is able to allow the operator to make dynamic changes to a treatment plan and yet continue to have the advantages of computer navigated guidance. Several companies have become involved with the development of computer-guided navigational surgery and the technology is finding application in multiple fields in addition to surgical implantology.

12.8   Clinical Cases

This section will present cases where digital planning has been used for implant surgery and in implant prosthodontics.

Case 1   Figures 12.17–12.36 describe a case managed with implant guided surgery *(Courtesy Dr. Ali Tunkiwala).*

A 60-year-old, medically fit patient reported with a failed upper bridge. On examination, the upper right cuspid was broken. The first premolar was already missing and the second premolar was healthy. It was decided to do a partial extraction therapy (Socket Shield) with guided implant placement and immediate provisional restoration. The preparation of the shield is a technique sensitive procedure and once that is accomplished it is important to get the implant in the perfect 3D position such that it does not contact the shield.

Initially, an intraoral scan was done of the preoperative status followed by a CBCT. The data from the CBCT and the patient's STL file was merged to plan the

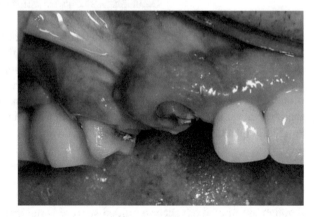

Fig. 12.17 Preoperative status of fractured #13. The treatment plan was to do a partial extraction of 13 followed by an implant placement. And a delayed placement in 15

Fig. 12.18   Intraoral scans of preoperative status that will be converted to an STL format and sent along with the CBCT to the planning software

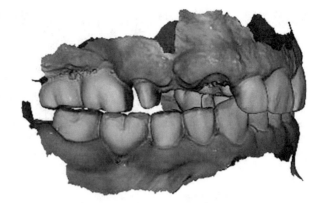

Fig. 12.19   Preoperative radiograph

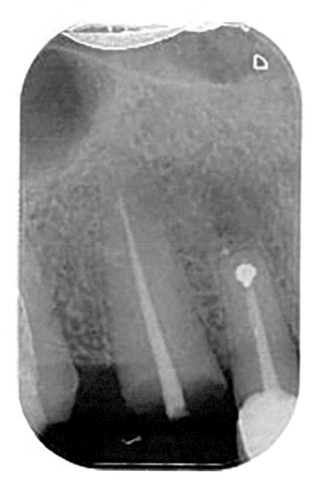

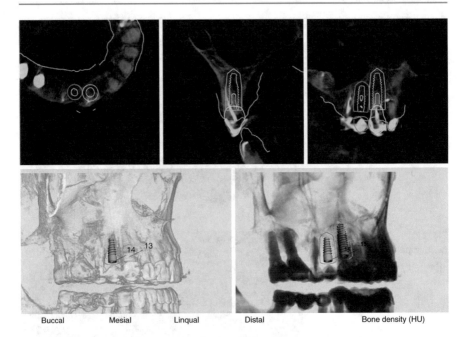

| Buccal | Mesial | Linqual | Distal | Bone density (HU) |

Fig. 12.20 The CBCT and STL files are merged in the software to allow virtual implant placement in #13 and #14 region based on the available bone

Fig. 12.21 A 3D printed stent is generated from the virtual plan and sleeves inserted to aid in implant placement in the planned positions

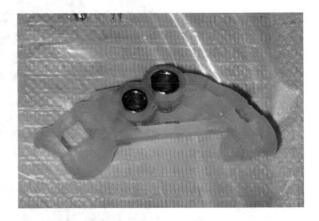

optimal, prosthetically driven implant placement on the software. Once approved, a tooth-supported surgical guide was 3D printed and provided for the implant placement.

During the surgical process, partial extraction was done for the cuspid followed by the placement of a surgical stent. Guided surgery was performed for both, the cuspid as well as the first premolar. A putty index was made from the preoperative

Fig. 12.22 #13 Partial
extraction therapy done
before utilization of the
stent to place the implant

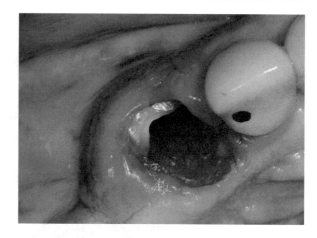

Fig. 12.23 #13 Stent
utilized for pilot drill

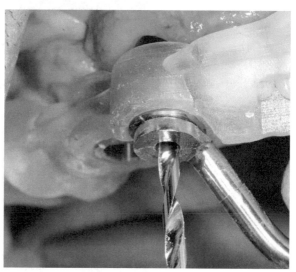

wax-up model, which was used to carry the material to the temporary cylinders on the implants to make an immediate screw-retained provisional restoration.

After 4 months, the provisional restoration was removed and an implant level impression was done. To get a perfect subgingival geometry on the final custom-made zirconia abutment, the provisional restoration was extra-orally attached to the implant replica and the assembly was scanned with an intraoral scanner. The laboratory was then able to merge the subgingival contour around the implant replica in the software and replicate the contour of provisional restoration perfectly on the final custom abutment with well-placed margins for the final cement-retained restorations. On these abutments, individual zirconia crowns were fabricated (Figs. 12.17–12.36).

Fig. 12.24 #13 Implant insertion

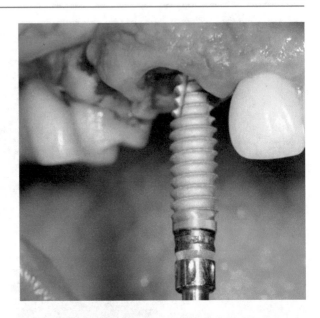

Fig. 12.25 #13, #14 implant placed in final position

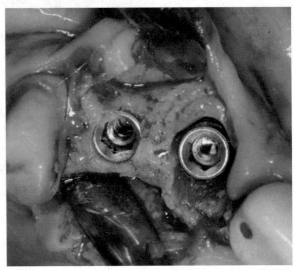

Fig. 12.26 Immediate screw-retained provisional restoration placed on the implants

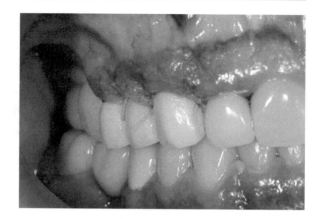

Fig. 12.27 Post-surgical radiograph

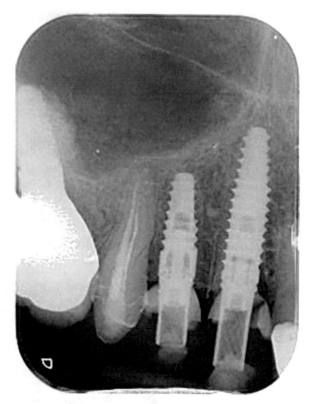

Fig. 12.28 Healed sites at
4 months after implant
placement

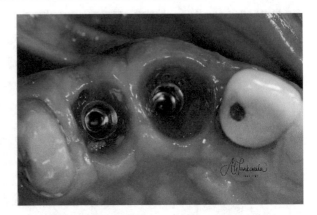

Fig. 12.29 Scan body
utilized to make digital
impressions of the implants
and of #15

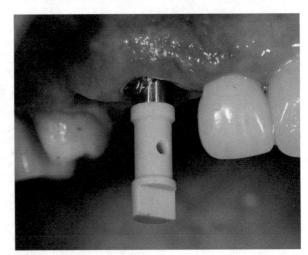

Fig. 12.30 Provisional
Restorations fixed to
implant replica

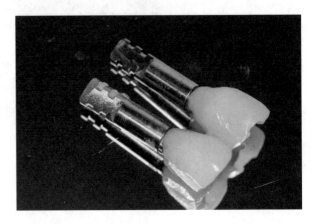

Fig. 12.31 Final digital
impressions

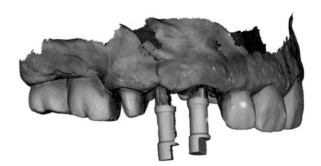

Fig. 12.32 Scanned
provisional restorations
that will be used to
customize the subgingival
abutment contours

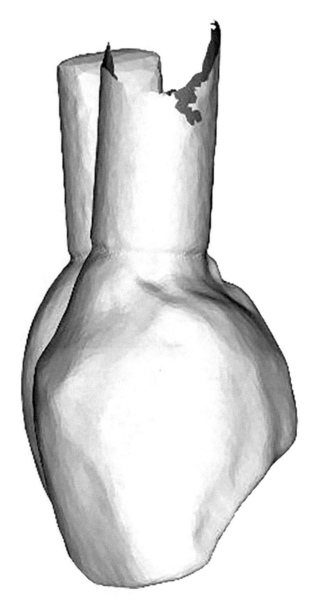

Fig. 12.33 Customized
Zirconia abutment

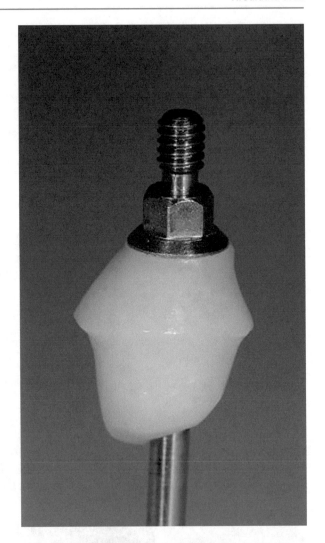

Fig. 12.34 Zirconia
Abutment in position

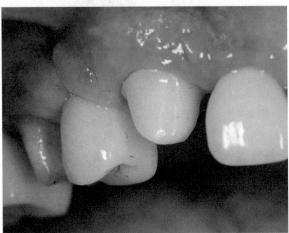

Fig. 12.35 Final Individual zirconia crowns for #13 and #14 Implants and #15 natural tooth *(Courtesy for laboratory work—Mr. Danesh Vazifdar, Adaro Dental Lab)*

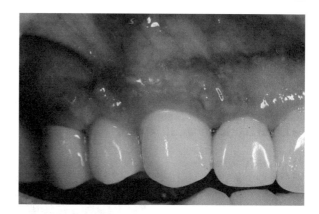

Fig. 12.36 Postoperative radiograph

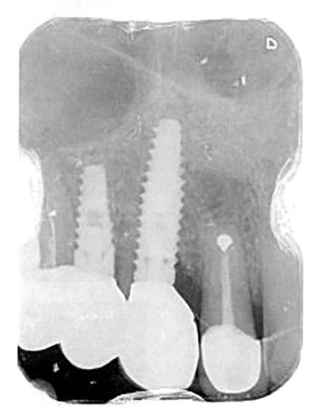

Case 2 Case 2 describes implant placement for congenitally missing lateral incisors *(Courtesy Dr. Udatta Kher).*

A 24-year-old healthy male reported with congenitally missing maxillary lateral incisors. The treatment plan agreed upon was to replace the missing incisors with implant-supported fixed restoration. The narrow mesiodistal space posed a challenge for ideal three-dimensional implant placement. Hence, a guided surgery strategy was planned. A guided surgery stent was fabricated by merging the intraoral scan data and cone beam CT scan data. Prefabricated PMMA screw-retained restorations on a PEEK abutment were prepared.

Two narrow-diameter implants (Biohorizons Tapered Internal 3.0 X12) were placed flapless, using the surgical guide. The prefabricated provisional restorations were screwed onto the implants soon after placement. Digital protocols enabled accurate prosthetically driven implant placements along with perfectly contoured immediate provisional restorations. The restorations were kept out of any protrusive or lateral contacts (Figs. 12.37–12.47).

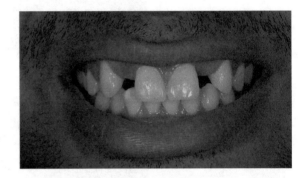

Fig. 12.37 Congenitally missing maxillary lateral incisors

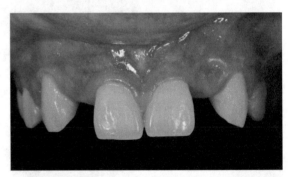

Fig. 12.38 Preoperative situation

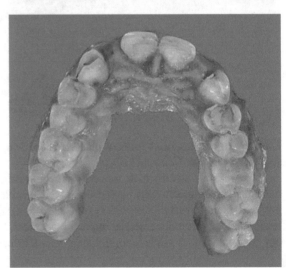

Fig. 12.39 Intraoral scan

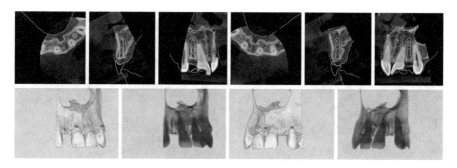

Fig. 12.40 CBCT data used for stent fabrication

Fig. 12.41 Digital planning for provisional restoration

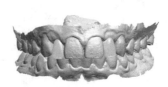

Fig. 12.42 Surgical stent

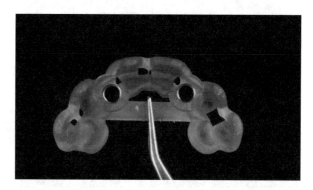

Fig. 12.43 Intraoral view of the surgical stent

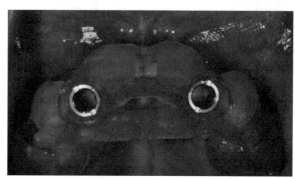

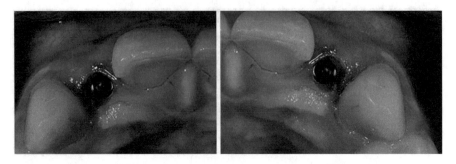

Fig. 12.44 Immediate postoperative view after flapless implant placement

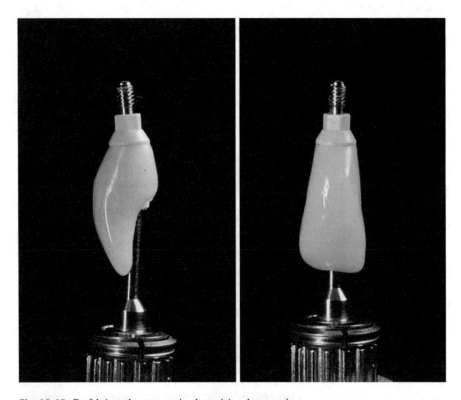

Fig. 12.45 Prefabricated screw-retained provisional restoration

Case 3 Case 3 describes a maxillary full-arch implant-supported restoration *(Courtesy Dr. Udatta Kher).*

A 47-year-old *edentulous* male with controlled diabetes mellitus reported to have dental implants and immediate fixed restorations after the surgical procedure. He already had a mandibular implant-supported fixed restoration.

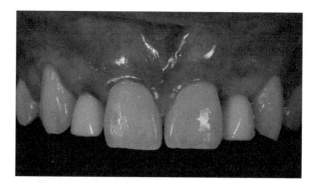

Fig. 12.46 Immediate postoperative view of the PMMA screw-retained provisional restorations for the missing lateral incisors. *(Courtesy for laboratory work- Katara Dental, Pune, India)*

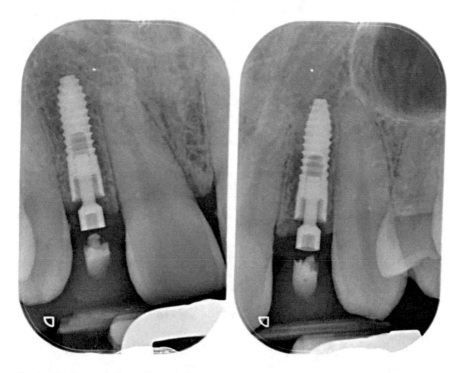

Fig. 12.47 Postoperative radiograph displaying accurate implant positioning

CBCT revealed good bone volume in all areas except the right posterior maxilla. The treatment plan consisted of placing eight implants (*Bio Horizons Inc, USA*) across the arch in a prosthetically driven position. A guided surgery stent was fabricated using *dual-scan* technique. A prefabricated prosthetic shell was kept ready for the immediate loading protocol after implant placement.

An indirect sinus lift with putty bone grafting material (*Novabone putty, USA*) was performed in the right maxilla after raising a mucoperiosteal flap.

Using the surgical stent, eight implants were placed across the arch in strategic locations using a flapless approach. The prefabricated prosthetic shell was connected to the implants using temporary titanium abutments. The intaglio surface was kept convex and highly polished. The finished temporary prosthesis was screwed onto the implants on the same day. Occlusal adjustments were done to achieve uniform contacts across the arch. The temporary prosthesis was replaced with a definitive screw-retained restoration after a period of 6 months (Figs. 12.48–12.58).

Fig. 12.48 Edentulous maxilla

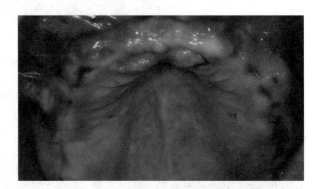

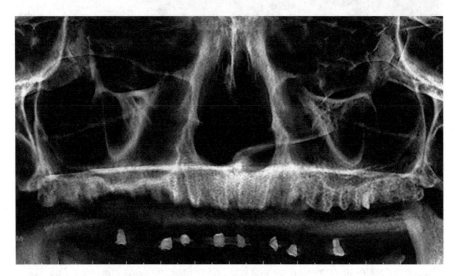

Fig. 12.49 Edentulous maxilla with radiographic markers incorporated in denture which represent implant site locations

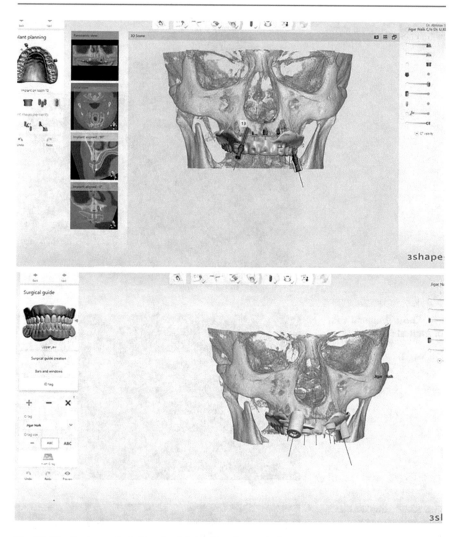

Fig. 12.50   Dual-scan technique for fabrication of a surgical stent

Fig. 12.51 Surgical stent

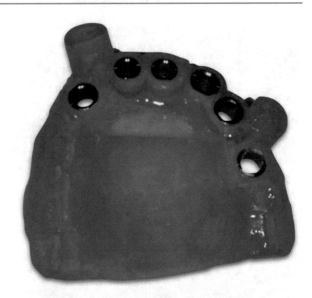

Fig. 12.52 Intraoral view
of surgical stent

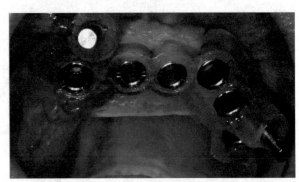

Fig. 12.53 Implant site
preparation using a
surgical stent

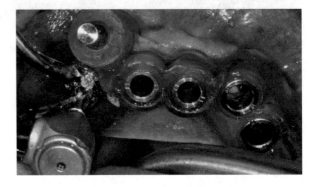

Fig. 12.54 Prefabricated prosthetic shell with titanium temporary abutments

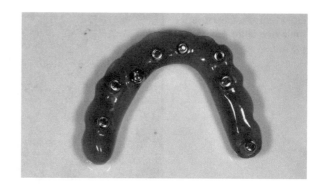

Fig. 12.55 Immediate postoperative view of the screw-retained maxillary restoration against a Metal ceramic mandibular implant-supported restoration

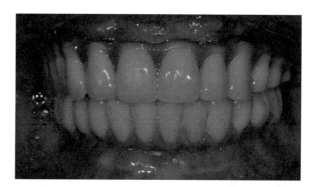

Fig. 12.56 Definitive screw-retained metal-ceramic restoration. *(Courtesy for laboratory work- Katara Dental, Pune, India)*

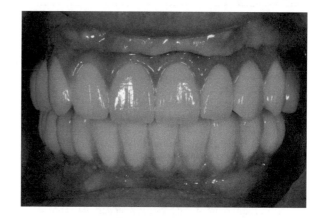

Fig. 12.57 Postoperative view of the definitive restoration

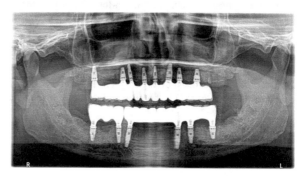

Fig. 12.58 Postoperative
smile view of the patient

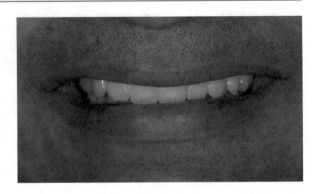

12.9   Conclusion

The digitization of implant dentistry has seen exponential growth over the last
decade. The most significant advantages have been the increased level of surgical
and restorative accuracy, the degree of predictability of pretreatment planning, and
a new level of technologically inspired confidence for the implant dentist. There is
no doubt that the level of digitization is only set to grow further. The future may
possibly see the development of customized implants and the development of
extremely accurate prefabricated restorations.

References

1. Davidowitz G, Kotick PG. The use of CAD/CAM in dentistry. Dent Clin N Am.
   2011;55(3):559–70. ix
2. Brånemark PI. Osseointegration and its experimental background. J Prosthet Dent.
   1983;50(3):399–410.
3. Ortorp A, Jemt T. Clinical experience of € cnc-milled titanium frameworks supported
   by implants in the edentulous jaw: a 3-year interim report. Clin Implant Dent Relat Res.
   2002;4:104–9.
4. Bahat O, Fontanesi RV, Preston. Reconstruction of the hard and soft tissues for optimal placement of osseointegrated implants. Int J Periodontics Restorative Dent. 1993;13:255–75.
5. Seibert JS, Salama H. Alveolar ridge preservation and reconstruction. Periodontology.
   1996;2000(11):69–84.
6. Krekmanov L, Kahn M, Rangert B, Lindstrom H. Tilting of posterior mandibular and maxillary implants of improved prosthesis support. Int J Oral Maxillofac Implants. 2000;15:405–14.
7. Maló P, Rangert B, Nobre M. "All-on-four" immediate-function concept with Brånemark system implants for completely edentulous mandibles: a retrospective clinical study. Clin Implant
   Dent Relat Res. 2003;5(Suppl 1):2–9.
8. Hounsfield GN. Computerized transverse axial scanning (tomography). 1. Description of system. Br J Radiol. 1973;46(552):1016–22.
9. Todd AD, Gher ME, Quintero G, Richardson AC. Interpretation of linear and computed tomo-
   grams in the assessment of implant recipient sites. J Periodontol. 1993;64:1243–9.
10. Becker CM, Kaiser DA. Surgical guide for dental implant placement. J Prosthet Dent.
    2000;83(2):248–51.

11. Akça K, Iplikçioğlu H, Cehreli MC. A surgical guide for accurate mesiodistal paralleling of implants in the posterior edentulous mandible. J Prosthet Dent. 2002;87(2):233–5.
12. Bibb RJ, Bocca A, Sugar A, Evans P. Planning Osseointegrated implant sites using computer aided design and rapid prototyping. J Maxillofac Prosthet Technol. 2003;6:1–4. ISSN: 1366-4697
13. Ganz SD. Presurgical planning with CT-derived fabrication of surgical guides. J Oral Maxillofac Surg. 2005;63(9 Suppl 2):59–71.
14. Mörmann WH, Brandestini M, Lutz F, Barbakow F. Chairside computer-aided direct ceramic inlays. Quintessence Int. 1989;20(5):329–39.
15. Poticny DJ, Klim J. CAD/CAM in-office technology: innovations after 25 years for predictable, esthetic outcomes. J Am Dent Assoc. 2010;141(Suppl 2):5S–9S.
16. Whitley D 3rd, Eidson RS, Rudek I, Bencharit S. In-office fabrication of dental implant surgical guides using desktop stereolithographic printing and implant treatment planning software: a clinical report. J Prosthet Dent. 2017;118:256–63.
17. Deeb GR, Allen RK, Hall VP, Whitley D 3rd, Laskin DM, Bencharit S. How accurate are implant surgical guides produced with desktop stereolithographic 3-dimensional printers? J Oral Maxillofac Surg. 2017;75:2559.e1-8.
18. Yeung M, Abdulmajeed A, Carrico CK, Deeb GR, Bencharit S. Accuracy and precision of 3D-printed implant surgical guides with different implant systems: an in vitro study. J Prosthet Dent. 2020;123(6):821–8.
19. Mangano F, Chambrone L, van Noort R, Miller C, Hatton P, Mangano C. Direct metal laser sintering titanium dental implants: a review of the current literature. Int J Biomater. 2014;2014:461534.
20. Schulze C, Weinmann M, Schweigel C, Keßler O, Bader R. Mechanical properties of a newly additive manufactured implant material based on Ti-42Nb. Materials. 2018;11:124.
21. Oliveira TT, Reis AC. Fabrication of dental implants by the additive manufacturing method: a systematic review. J Prosthet Dent. 2019;122(3):270–4.
22. Branemark PI, Gröndahl K, OhrnellL O, Nilsson P, Petruson B, Svensson B, Engstrand P, Nannmark U. Zygoma fixture in the management of advanced atrophy of the maxilla: technique and long-term results. Scand J Plast Reconstr Surg Hand Surg. 2004;38:70–85.
23. Aparicio C, Manresa C, Francisco K, et al. Zygomatic implants: indications, techniques and outcomes, and the zygomatic success code. Periodontol. 2014;66(1):41–58.
24. Garcia-Gazaui S, Razzoog M, Sierraalta M, Saglik B. Fabrication of a screw-retained restoration avoiding the facial access hole: a clinical report. J Prosthet Dent. 2015;114(5):621–4.
25. Sakamoto S, Ro M, Al-Ardah A, Goodacre C. Esthetic abutment design for angulated screw channels: a technical report. J Prosthet Dent. 2018;119(6):912–5.
26. Duret F, Preston JD. CAD/CAM imaging in dentistry. Curr Opin Dent. 1991;1:150–4.
27. Van der Zel JM. Ceramic-fused-to-metal restorations with a new CAD/CAM system. Quintessence Int. 1993;24:769–78.
28. Andersson M, Oden A. A new all-ceramic crown: a dense-sintered, high purity alumina coping with porcelain. Acta Odontol Scand. 1993;51:59–64.
29. Carr AB, Stewart RB. Full-arch implant framework casting accuracy: preliminary in vitro observation for in vivo testing. J Prosthodont. 1993;2(1):2–8.
30. Tan KB, Rubenstein JE, Nicholls JI, Yuodelis RA. Three-dimensional analysis of the casting accuracy of one-piece, osseointegrated implant-retained prostheses. Int J Prosthodont. 1993;6(4):346–63.
31. Paniz G, Stellini E, Meneghello R, Cerardi A, Gobbato EA, Bressan E. The precision of fit of cast and milled full-arch implant-supported restorations. Int J Oral Maxillofac Implants. 2013;28(3):687–93.
32. Örtorp A, Jemt T. CNC-milled titanium frameworks supported by implants in the edentulous jaw: a 10-year comparative clinical study. Clin Implant Dent Relat Res. 2012;14:88–99.

33. Beuer F, Schweiger J, Edelhoff D. Digital dentistry: an overview of recent developments for CAD/CAM generated restorations. Br Dent J. 2008;204(9):505–11.
34. Abduo J, et al. Trends in computer-aided manufacturing in prosthodontics: a review of the available streams. Int J Dent. 2014;2014:783948.
35. Kapos T, Ashy LM, Gallucci GO, Weber HP, Wismeijer D. Computer-aided design and computer-assisted manufacturing in prosthetic implant dentistry. Int J Oral Maxillofac Implants. 2009;24(Suppl):110–7.
36. Parpaiola A, Norton MR, Cecchinato D, Bressan E, Toia M. Virtual abutment design: a concept for delivery of CAD/CAM customized abutments—report of a retrospective cohort. Int J Periodontics Restorative Dent. 2013;33(1):51–8.
37. Parpaiola A, et al. CAD/CAM implant abutments: peri-implant hard and soft tissue response with up to 4 years of follow-up- a retrospective cohort study evaluation. Int J Periodontics Restorative Dent. 2020;40(2):193–201.
38. Denry I, Kelly JR. State of the art of zirconia for dental applications. Dent Mater. 2008;24(3):299–307. https://doi.org/10.1016/j.dental.2007.05.007.
39. Alao A-R, Stoll R, Song X-F, Miyazaki T, Hotta Y, Shibata Y, Yin L. Surface quality of Yttria-stabilized tetragonal zirconia polycrystal in CAD/CAM milling, sintering, polishing and sandblasting processes. J Mech Behav Biomed Mater. 2016;65 https://doi.org/10.1016/j.jmbbm.2016.08.021.
40. Zaruba M, Mehl A. Chairside systems: a current review. Int J Comput Dent. 2017;20(2):123–49.
41. Blatz MB, Conejo J. The current state of chairside digital dentistry and materials. Dent Clin N Am. 2019;63(2):175–97.
42. Zimmermann M, Mehl A, Mörmann WH, Reich S. Intraoral scanning systems—a current overview. Int J Comput Dent. 2015;18(2):101–29.
43. Vandeweghe S, Vervack V, Dierens M, De Bruyn H. Accuracy of digital impressions of multiple dental implants: an in vitro study. Clin Oral Implants Res. 2016;28:648.
44. Mangano F, Mangano C, Margiani B, Admakin O. Combining intraoral and face scans for the design and fabrication of computer-assisted design/computer-assisted manufacturing (CAD/CAM) polyether-ether-ketone (PEEK) implant-supported bars for maxillary overdentures. Scanning. 2019;2019:4274715.
45. Harris BT, Montero D, Grant GT, Morton D, Llop DR, Lin WS. Creation of a 3-dimensional virtual dental patient for computer-guided surgery and CAD-CAM interim complete removable and fixed dental prostheses: a clinical report. J Prosthet Dent. 2017;117:197.
46. Ender A, Mehl A. Accuracy of complete-arch dental impressions: a new method of measuring trueness and precision. J Prosthet Dent. 2013;109:121–8.
47. Kihara H, Hatakeyama W, Komine F, et al. Accuracy and practicality of intraoral scanner in dentistry: a literature review. J Prosthodont Res. 2020;64(2):109–13.
48. Cicciù M, Fiorillo L, D'Amico C, Gambino D, Amantia EM, Laino L, Crimi S, Campagna P, Bianchi A, Herford AS, Cervino G. 3D digital impression systems compared with traditional techniques in dentistry: a recent data systematic review. Materials (Basel, Switzerland). 2020;13(8):1982.
49. Grossmann Y, Pasciuta M, Finger IM. A novel technique using a coded healing abutment for the fabrication of a CAD/ CAM titanium abutment for an implant-supported restoration. J Prosthet Dent. 2006;95:258–61.
50. Lin WS, Harris BT, Morton D. The use of a scannable impression coping and digital impression technique to fabricate a customized anatomic abutment and zirconia restoration in the esthetic zone. J Prosthet Dent. 2013;109(3):187–91.
51. Motel C, Kirchner E, Adler W, Wichmann M, Matta RE. Impact of different scan bodies and scan strategies on the accuracy of digital implant impressions assessed with an intraoral scanner: an in vitro study. J Prosthodont. 2020;29(4):309–14.
52. Jemt T, Bäck T, Petersson A. Photogrammetry—an alternative to conventional impressions in implant dentistry? A clinical pilot study. Int J Prosthodont. 1999;12(4):363–8.

53. Peñarrocha-Oltra D, Agustín-Panadero R, Bagán L, Giménez B, Peñarrocha M. Impression of multiple implants using photogrammetry: description of technique and case presentation. Med Oral Patol Oral Cir Bucal. 2014;19(4):e366–71.
54. Cunha RM, Souza FÁ, Hadad H, Poli PP, Maiorana C, Carvalho P. Accuracy evaluation of computer-guided implant surgery associated with prototyped surgical guides. J Prosthet Dent. 2020; S0022-3913(19)30486-X. Advance online publication
55. Parel SM, Triplett RG. Interactive imaging for implant planning, placement, and prosthesis construction. J Oral Maxillofac Surg. 2004;62(9 Suppl 2):41–7.
56. Spector L. Computer-aided dental implant planning. Dent Clin N Am. 2008;52(4):761–vi.
57. Block MS, Emery RW. Static or dynamic navigation for implant placement-choosing the method of guidance. J Oral Maxillofac Surg. 2016;74(2):269–77.
58. Venet L, Perriat M, Mangano FG, Fortin T. Horizontal ridge reconstruction of the anterior maxilla using customized allogeneic bone blocks with a minimally invasive technique—a case series. BMC Oral Health. 2017;17(1):146.
59. Schlee M, Rothamel D. Ridge augmentation using customized allogenic bone blocks: proof of concept and histological findings. Implant Dent. 2013;22(3):212–8.
60. Kloss FR, Offermanns V, Donkiewicz P, Kloss-Brandstätter A. Customized allogeneic bone grafts for maxillary horizontal augmentation: a 5-year follow-up radiographic and histologic evaluation. Clin Case Rep. 2020;8:886–93.
61. Ozan O, Turkyilmaz I, Ersoy AE, McGlumphy EA, Rosenstiel SF. Clinical accuracy of 3 different types of computed tomography-derived stereolithographic surgical guides in implant placement. J Oral Maxillofac Surg. 2009;67(2):394–401.
62. Geng WF, et al. Accuracy of different types of computer-aided design/computer-aided manufacturing surgical guides for dental implant placement. Int J Clin Exp Med. 2015;8(6):8442–9.
63. Ramasamy M, Giri RR, Subramonian K, Narendrakumar R. Implant surgical guides: from the past to the present. J Pharm Bioallied Sci. 2013;5(Suppl 1):S98–S102. https://doi.org/10.4103/0975-7406.113306. PMID: 23946587; PMCID: PMC3722716
64. Costa AJDM, Teixeira Neto AD, Burgoa S, Gutierrez V, Cortes ARG. Fully digital workflow with magnetically connected guides for full-arch implant rehabilitation following guided alveolar ridge reduction. J Prosthodont. 2020;29:272–6.
65. Nickenig HJ, Safi AF, Matta RE, Zöller JE, Kreppel M. 3D-based full-guided ridge expansion osteotomy—a case report about a new method with successive use of different surgical guides, transfer of splitting vector and simultaneous implant insertion. J Craniomaxillofac Surg. 2019;47(11):1787–92.
66. Yuan F, Sun Y, Zhang L, Sun Y. Accuracy of chair-side fused-deposition modelling for dental applications. Rapid Prototyp J. ahead-of-print. 2019; https://doi.org/10.1108/RPJ-04-2018-0082.

Digital Smile Design

13

Suprabha Hooda and Geeta Paul

13.1 Introduction

An attractive smile is always a desire of an individual for his or her social well-being and confidence. Aesthetics, being one of the most important pillars of dentistry, has always been a part of the research for better outcomes. Smile analysis and designing have been under focus in dentistry since last decade and necessitates a comprehensive approach to patient care.

Knowledge of interrelationships between dental anatomy and physiology and patient's soft-tissue treatment limitations [1]. From the first generation when hand drawing on printed photos of the patient was used to communicate and explain the final outcome, it has now progressed into complete digital drawing on DSD software on a computer.

The chapter is divided into three parts for ease of understanding. The first part starts with explaining the analysis of dental and facial components required in a smile design followed by the digital shade matching instruments and its advantages over conventional technique and the various systems available commercially. It then goes on to discuss the requirements for a digital smile design technique (and the different software) which is a tool to design and modify the smile of patients and helps them to visualize it beforehand the final outcome. This section also includes information on photographic views required for smile designing. Various devices are now being used to visualize diagnosis and improve communication and enhance predictability throughout treatment. The chapter concludes with the future advancements in this field.

S. Hooda (✉) · G. Paul
Department of Prosthodontics, Inderprastha Dental College, Ghaziabad, India

© Springer Nature Switzerland AG 2021
P. Jain, M. Gupta (eds.), *Digitization in Dentistry*,
https://doi.org/10.1007/978-3-030-65169-5_13

13.2   Historical Perspective

Smiles have been evidenced as early as 300 BC. In 1938, Dr. Charles Pincus described a technique in which porcelain veneers were retained by a denture adhesive during cinematic filming [2].

Introduction of veneers to the dentistry has resulted in the most aesthetic, least invasive treatment modality as these showed most demanding clinical performance in respect of strength, longevity, conservative nature and biocompatibility. Dr. Christian Coachman has been given credit for presenting smile designing in a digital means and proposed generations for the evolution of smile designing [3]. The *first generation* consisted of analogue drawings (with a pen) on a printed copy of photographs to visualize the treatment outcome. Digital dentistry was still not introduced, and there was no use of a study model. The *second generation* benefitted from 2D drawings and visual connection to the analogue model. This made it more accurate and less time-consuming. Although digitization had been introduced, it was still not specific to dentistry. The *third generation* was the era of the digital analogue connection when the first drawing software specific to digital dentistry was introduced. This linked the 2D smile design to a 3D wax mock-up. However, connection to 3D digital world was still not possible. The *fourth generation* progressed from 2D to 3D analysis involving facial integration and predetermined dental aesthetic parameters. The *fifth generation* was the complete 3D workflow followed by the latest *sixth generation* of the 4D concept by adding motion to the smile design process.

13.3   Principles of Smile Design

To obtain desired aesthetic outcomes, diagnostic data from questionnaires and checklists which are obtained from patients should be transferred adequately to the design of the restorations. The diagnostic data must guide the subsequent treatment phases, integrating all of the patient's needs, desires and functional and biologic issues into an aesthetic treatment design. Recent advances in technology allow the clinician to measure dynamic lip-tooth relationships and incorporate that information into the orthodontic problem list and biomechanical plan.

The principles of smile design require integration of dento-facial composition and dental composition. The dental facial composition includes the hard and soft tissues of the face (lips and the smile as they relate to the face). The dental composition relates more specifically to the teeth (size, shape and positions) and their relationship to the alveolar bone and gingival tissues. Both the analyses are required for a smile design.

13.4   Facial Composition

There are two basic types of smiles (Fig. 13.1): social smile and enjoyment smile.

Proper alignment, symmetry and proportion of face are believed to be the basic principles in facial aesthetics. When viewed from the frontal aspect, the basic shape

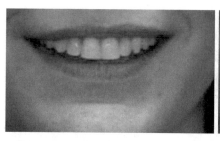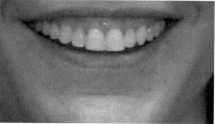

Fig. 13.1 Anterior tooth display in social and enjoyment smiles; note difference in gingival show *(Reproduced with permission from Journal of Clinical Orthodontics: Ackerman MB, Ackerman JL. Smile analysis and design in the digital era. J Clin Orthod. 2002;36(4):221–236)*

Fig. 13.2 Smile components *(Reproduced with permission from Journal of Clinical Orthodontics: Ackerman MB, Ackerman JL. Smile analysis and design in the digital era. J Clin Orthod. 2002;36(4):221–236)*

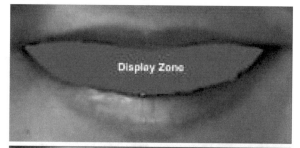

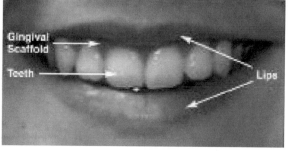

of the face can either be square, square tapering, tapering or ovoid. When viewed from the lateral aspect, facial profile can either be convex, concave or straight. These facial features contribute to deciding the morphology of tooth.

The two facial features significant in a smile design are the inter-pupillary line and the lips [4]. The inter-pupillary line should be perpendicular to the midline of the face and parallel to the occlusal plane while the lips create the boundaries of the smile design.

The upper and lower lips form the border of the display zone of the smile. Within this zone lies the components of the smile i.e. teeth and the gingival scaffold (Fig. 13.2). The soft-tissue components of the display zone include lip thickness, inter-commissure width, inter-labial gap, smile index (width/height), and gingival architecture. Although the commissures of the lips form the lateral borders of the smile, the eye can perceive inner and outer commissures, (Fig. 13.3).

Fig. 13.3 Anatomy of commissures *(Reproduced with permission from Journal of Clinical Orthodontics: Ackerman MB, Ackerman JL. Smile analysis and design in the digital era. J Clin Orthod. 2002;36(4):221–236)*

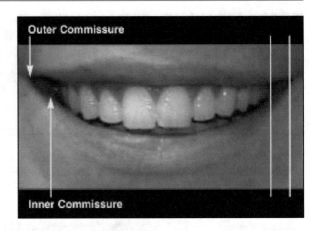

Fig. 13.4 Horizontal dimension of the face *(Courtesy Dr. Mohan)*

Hair

Brows
Eyes

Nose
Lips

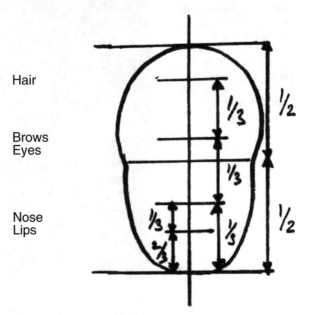

The face can be divided into horizontal and vertical dimensions. The horizontal dimensional aspect (width of the face) should be the width of five 'eyes' and the distance between the eyebrow and chin should be equal to the width of the face (Fig. 13.4).

The vertical aspect (facial height) is divided into three equal parts from the forehead to the eyebrow line, namely from the eyebrow line to the base of the nose and from the base of the nose to the base of the chin. The full face is divided into two parts with the eyes being the midline while the lower part of the face (from the base of the nose to the chin) is divided into the upper lip and the lower lip with the chin (Fig. 13.5).

Fig. 13.5 Vertical
dimensions of the face
(Courtesy Dr. Mohan)

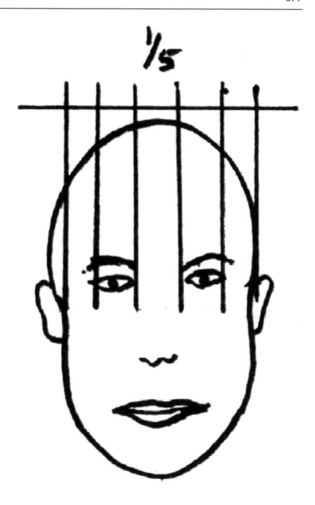

13.5   Dental Composition

I. Tooth Components
(a) Dental midline.
(b) Incisal length.
(c) Tooth dimensions.
(d) Axial inclination.
(e) Zenith Points.
(f) Incisal embrasures.
(g) Interproximal contact area and interproximal contact points.
(h) Sex, personality and age.

II. Soft Tissue Components
(a) Gingival health.
(b) Gingival level.
(c) Smile line.
(d) Interdental embrasure.

13.6   Tooth Components

13.6.1 Dental Midline

The midline, the vertical contact interface between maxillary central incisors, is evaluated by its location and alignment. Ideally, it should be perpendicular to the incisal plane and parallel to the long axis of the face. It should drop straight down from the papilla.

However, some minor discrepancies between facial and dental midlines (up to 4 mm) may either be sometimes not noticed or considered acceptable [5, 6]. Studies have suggested that 75% of maxillary midline do not coincide with the mandibular midline. Maxillary midline is considered as a reference point than mandibular midline as mandibular incisors either do not show or show minimal in smile position.

Midline should be:

(a) Parallel to the long axis of the face.
(b) Perpendicular to the incisal plane.
(c) Over the papilla.

13.6.2 Incisal Length

Maxillary incisal edge position is the most important determinant in smile creation because once set, it serves as a reference point to decide the proper tooth proportion and gingival levels. This is related to labial and lingual contours of the tooth, anterior guidance and lip support which are vital in achieving both aesthetics and function. Patient's input, phonetics and the amount of tooth display help us to locate this position. Phonetics is evaluated by asking the patient to pronounce alphabets like M, E, F, V and S in an erect sitting or standing position. In young individuals, incisal tooth display is more, approximately 3.5 mm, with decreases with age.

13.6.3 Tooth Dimensions

Correct dental proportion is related to facial morphology and is essential in creating an aesthetically pleasing smile. Central dominance dictates that the centrals must be the dominant teeth in the smile, and they must display pleasing proportions. They are the key to the smile. The proportions of the centrals must be aesthetically and mathematically correct.

Tooth proportion is related to facial morphology with central incisors playing the dominant role in a smile. Hence, the proportions of central incisors must be both mathematically correct and aesthetically pleasing. The width to length ratio of the centrals should be approximately 4:5 (0.8–1.0); a range for their width of 75–80% of their length is most acceptable.

The lateral incisors and canines have their form and placement depending on the shape, size and location of the central incisors. The shape and location of the centrals influence the appearance and placement of the laterals and canines. Various guidelines for establishing correct proportions are [4].

1. *Golden proportion (Lombardi)*—This principle states that the width of each anterior tooth is 60% of the width of the adjacent tooth (the mathematical ratio being 1.6:1:0.6) (Fig. 13.6). Its applicability in clinical practice is limited due to differing arch forms, lip and facial proportions [7].
2. *Recurring aesthetic dental proportions (RED) (Ward)*—According to this, as we move posteriorly from the midline, the width proportion should remain constant from the facial aspect (Fig. 13.7).
3. *M proportions (Methot)*—is a comparison of the tooth width with the facial width.
4. *Chu's aesthetic gauges*—is in support of the RED concept and refutes the golden proportion.

Fig. 13.6 Golden proportion based on apparent width from the frontal view *(Courtesy Dr. Mohan)*

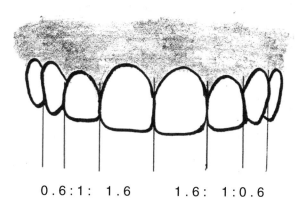

0.6 : 1 : 1.6   1.6 : 1 : 0.6

Fig. 13.7 Recurring aesthetic dental proportion *(Courtesy Dr. Mohan)*

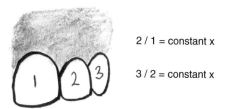

2 / 1 = constant x

3 / 2 = constant x

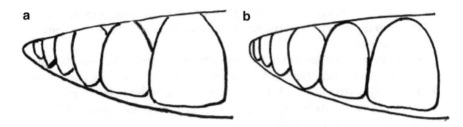

Fig. 13.8 (a) Insufficiently developed buccal corridor; (b) properly developed buccal corridor (*Courtesy Dr. Mohan*)

The author recommends using these as a guide rather than a rigid mathematical formula. Another important aspect to consider is the buccal corridor. This refers to the dark space (negative space) visible during smile formation between the corners of the mouth and the buccal surfaces of the maxillary teeth (Fig. 13.8). This space should be kept to a minimum during the smile design process and is minimized by restoring the premolars. However, it should not be completely eliminated because a hint of negative space imparts to the smile a suggestion of depth.

13.6.4 Axial Inclinations

In this, we compare the central vertical midline to the vertical alignment of maxillary teeth that is visible in the smile line. As we move from central incisor to canine, the progressive increase in the mesial inclination of each subsequent anterior teeth should appear natural i.e. central incisors should be least noticeable, lateral incisors slightly more pronounced and canines the most pronounced. It also refers to the degree of tipping of the tooth.

13.6.5 Zenith Points

This is the most apical position of the cervical tooth margin. It is located distal to the long axis of the maxillary centrals and canines (Fig. 13.9). Location of these points is important in cases of diastema closure and correction of tooth angulation.

13.6.6 Incisal Embrasures

The size and depth of incisal embrasures must progress naturally from central incisors to canines. The apical contact point moves apically as we progress towards canines, mimicking the smile line (Fig. 13.10a). If this depth and variation in the embrasures is not achieved, then the dentition may impart to have a box-shaped appearance with teeth appearing too uniform and contact areas too long.

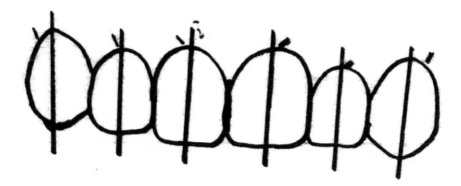

Fig. 13.9 Zenith points and its relation to midline *(Courtesy Dr. Mohan)*

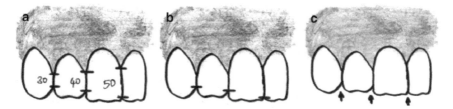

Fig. 13.10 (**a**, **b**, **c**) (**c**) ICAs—50:40:30 rule, (**b**) ICPs—moves apically as we move from central to canine, (**a**) Incisal embrasure—increase in size and depth from central to canine *(Courtesy Dr. Mohan)*

13.6.7 Interproximal Contact (ICA) Area and Interproximal Contact Points (ICP)

ICA is the broad zone where two adjacent teeth touch. The zone coronal to ICA is called the spillway spaces or embrasures. The embrasures are important as they make a spillway for the escape of food during chewing and prevent food from being forced through the contact area. The area apical to ICA forms the interproximal spaces. The most incisal aspect of ICA is the interproximal contact point (ICP) [8]. As a general rule, as we go posteriorly, the ICP moves apically (Fig. 13.10b). The increasing ICA helps to create the illusion of longer teeth by wider and also extend apically to eliminate black triangles.

The design of the above zone varies with the form and alignment of teeth. ICA of maxillary teeth helps in defining the pink aesthetics for patients who have a high smile line. Tarnow et al. introduced the 'mm rule', which states that when the distance from the contact point to the interproximal osseous crest is 5 mm or less, there would be a complete fill of the gingival embrasures with interdental papilla. The chance of complete fill is progressively reduced by 50% for each millimetre increase above the 5 mm distance (the 50:40:30 rule) (Fig. 13.10c) [9].

Table 13.1 Characteristics of SPA

Characteristics	
Sex	Maxillary incisors • Females: Round smooth, soft delicate • Males: Cuboidal, hard vigorous
Personality	Maxillary canine • Aggressive, hostile angry: Pointed long 'fangy' cusp form • Passive, soft: Blunt, rounded, short cusp
Age	Maxillary central incisor • Youthful teeth: Unworn incisal edge, defined incisal embrasure, low chroma and high value • Aged teeth: Shorter; so less smile display, minimal incisal embrasure, high chroma and low value

13.6.8 Sex, Age and Personality

Differences in the length, shape and positioning of the maxillary teeth allow for different characterization (Table 13.1).

13.7 Soft Tissue Components

13.7.1 Gingival Health

The gingiva frame symmetry of the smile. The health, colour and texture of the gingival tissues are paramount for long term success and the aesthetic value of the treatment.

The gingival height of contour of both maxillary central incisors should be at the same level, i.e. symmetrical. Cuspids may also have the same gingival level. If all the anterior teeth have the same height of contour, the smile may appear too uniform, thus appear un-aesthetic [10].

The amount of gingiva displayed is another key factor that is noted. A patient can have a gummy smile with teeth either being too short, at normal height or teeth that are too long [11]. When planning the smile makeover, interproximal papillae must have symmetry across the arch and black triangles avoided.

13.7.2 Gingival Level

Establishing the correct gingival levels for each individual tooth plays a vital role in the smile design process. The cervical gingival height (position or level) of the centrals should be symmetrical. The gingival margin of the lateral incisor is 0.5–2.0 mm below that of the central incisors. The least desirable gingival placement over the laterals is for it to be apical to that of the centrals and or the canines and is instead preferred to be located toward the incisal level (Fig. 13.11a). The darkness of the

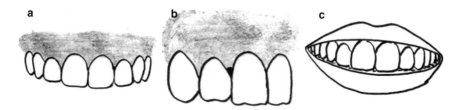

Fig. 13.11 (a, b, c) (a) Ideal gingival level—centrals and canines same level and laterals cervical to them, (b) Interdental embrasure—showing black triangle, (c) Smile line that follows the superior border of the lower lip *(Courtesy Dr. Mohan)*

oral cavity should not be visible in the interproximal triangle (black triangle) between the gingiva and the contact area. A healthy and pointed papilla is preferred instead of a blunted tissue form that accomplishes a black triangle [12] (Fig. 13.11b).

13.7.3 Smile Line

Smile line refers to an imaginary line along the incisal edges of the maxillary anterior teeth which should mimic the curvature of the superior border of the lower lip while smiling. Centrals should appear slightly longer or, at least, not any shorter than the canines along the incisal plane (Fig. 13.11c). Under ideal conditions, the gingival margin and the lip line should be congruent or there can be a 1–2 mm display of the gingival tissue. Showing 3–4 mm or more of the gingiva (gummy smile) often requires cosmetic periodontal re-contouring to achieve an ideal result [13]. Based on the number of maxillary teeth displayed, smile line can be high, medium and low (Fig. 13.12).

13.8   Shade Selection

Current technologies in shade selection have been developed to increase colour matching, communication, reproduction and verification in clinical dentistry. Aesthetic restorative efforts in achieving beautiful smiles are defined and guided by certain universal principles. This necessitates the thorough knowledge and understanding of the concept of shade selection which is an important basis for achieving superior aesthetics [10].

The next section of the chapter will provide a review of the current shade matching technologies with their clinical application.

The later part of the 1990s saw the introduction of colour measurement systems, with the development of the ShadeScan system (Cortex Machina, Montreal, Canada) [14]. This was the first attempt for a shade analysis system. Several studies have evaluated the clinical application of the ShadeScan prototype which employed digital camera technology, in a case report comparing visual vs. instrument-based shade information in the restoration of a single maxillary central incisor [15].

Fig. 13.12 Smile lines

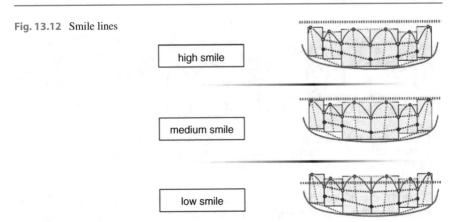

The most commonly used conventional method for shade selection is the visual method making use of various commercially available shade guides such as Vitapan Classical (Vita Zahnfabrik, Bad Sa¨ckingen, Germany). These conventional shade guides have their own drawbacks. The colours of shade guides vary with different guides and manufacturers. Moreover, they are arbitrarily arranged with less consideration given to the volume of the colour space of natural teeth. The porcelain used in the guide may be different from the porcelain being used for the restoration. The shade tabs are thicker and more translucent than natural teeth. This may affect the aesthetic outcome of the final restoration. In addition, assessing shade visually has been characterized by several difficulties such as metamerism, suboptimal colour matching conditions, methods, patient's age fatigue, and drugs/medications [16]. Despite these difficulties, the human eye can discern very small differences in colour. However, the ability to communicate the degree and nature of these differences is lacking.

13.9 Digital Shade Analysis

Dental shade-matching instruments have been brought to market to reduce or overcome imperfections and inconsistencies of traditional shade matching. These devices consist of, a detector, signal conditioner and software that process the signal.

The advantages include mapping the tooth in three parts: gingival, gingival, body and incisal making colour analysis more objective. A virtual try-in can be achieved with the technician verifying the shade and making the necessary changes, including characterising the restoration, as required. In addition, they 'average out' colour data over the complete tooth surface or larger defined areas which can lead to inaccurate shade information [17–21]. The quality control aspect is a real advantage. The reading can be translated into materials that can reproduce those characteristics in the fabricated restorations [22–26].

The types of devices used for shade selection are (Table 13.2).

Table 13.2 Instruments and devices for colour matching

Product	Device	Measurement area
ClearMatch *(Clarity Dental, Salt Lake City, UT)*	Software, digital image analysis	Complete tooth image
CrystalEye *(Olympus America, Center Valley, PA)*	Imaging spectrophotometer	Complete tooth image
Easyshade compact *(Vident, Brea, CA)*	Spectrophotometer	5-mm probe diameter
SpectroShade micro *(MHT, Niederhasli, Switzerland)*	Spectrophotometer/digital colour imaging	Complete tooth image
ShadeVision *(X-Rite, Grandville, MI)*	Digital colour imaging/colorimeter	Complete tooth image

- *Spectrophotometer:* These flexible instruments measure the amount of light energy reflected from an object at 1–25 nm intervals along the visible spectrum and then these measurements are converted to shade tab equivalent. They consist of a detector, dispersing light-medium, optical system and a medium that converts light obtained into a signal that can be analysed, e.g. Crystaleye (Olympus, Tokyo, Japan) and Spectro- Shade (Fig. 13.13) [27]. These mappings are two dimensional and they do not necessarily take into account consider the shape, texture, thickness of the restoration, type of abutment and different core material (metal or ceramic) [28–30].
- *Calorimeter:* These instruments measure tristimulus values and filter light in red, green and blue areas of the visible spectrum. Spectral reflectance is not registered. The tooth image has three components: gingival, middle and incisal third. However, they are considered to be less accurate than spectrophotometers, e.g. ShadeVision (X-Rite, Grandville, MI) [31, 32].
- *Digital cameras and imaging systems:* As described earlier in the chapter. These devices combine the red, green and blue light and translate them into the desired image, e.g. ClearMatch (Smart Technology, Hood River, OR) [33].

However, digital shade analyses have their own limitations. Edge loss may lead to inaccuracy and translucency mapping is inadequate. The position of the probe requires knowledge and expertise and the subsequent laboratory procedures and models are specific to their own systems and costly [2, 34, 35].

13.10 Digital Smile Designing Process (DSD)

As mentioned at the beginning of the chapter, the historical method of smile design was hand drawing on photographs of the patients which were then used for communicating to the patient about the final outcome. In recent times, with the introduction of DSD, it has progressed into a complete digital drawing which can easily be manipulated/ edited, stored, to achieve the final result balancing patients aesthetic concerns and functional needs.

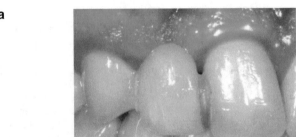

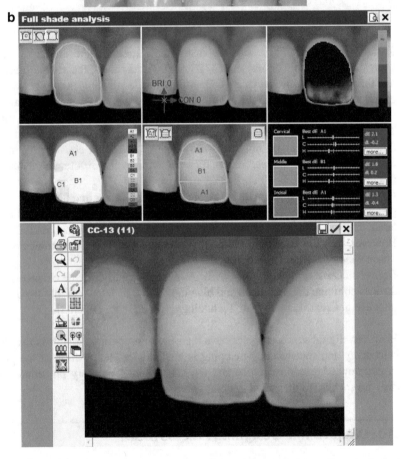

Fig. 13.13 Clinical application of SpectroShade Micro spectrophotometer. (a) Tooth #7 of a congenitally missing lateral incisor to be replaced with an implant [3i, Palm Beach, FL] and metal ceramic full-coverage restoration. (b) The SpectroShade Micro system creates a colour map which can be converted to several shade guide systems, this being the Classic Vita Shade Guide. It provides either an overall shade or the shade can be broken down into three distinct areas, cervical, middle and incisal, and provides detailed shade information in each of these areas and will provide a mathematical analysis resulting in a DE* value. (c) Virtual shade verification can be formed with this system so that shades can be assured prior to time-consuming patient visits. (d) Final restoration of tooth #7 with an implant and crown with an excellent aesthetic and functional outcome (*Reproduced with permission from Elsevier Publishing*)

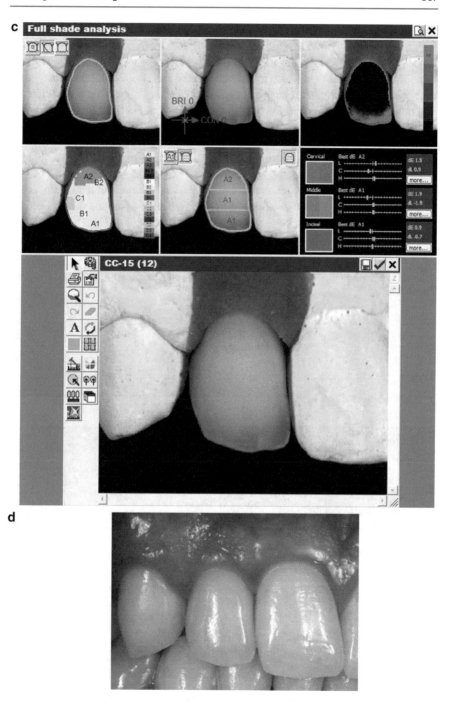

Fig. 13.13 (continued)

The digital smile design (DSD) is a treatment planning for aesthetic dentistry which uses digital software as an effective tool, in which the evaluation of the aesthetic relationship among the teeth, gingiva, smile, and face is obtained through lines and digital drawings which are marked on the facial and intraoral photographs of the patient on computer. The use of digital tools offers a futuristic perspective for diagnosis and treatment planning to both clinician and patient that further facilitates and improves the communication (Figs. 13.14–13.16).

The Digital Smile Design (DSD) is a multi-use conceptual tool that can strengthen diagnostic vision, improve communication, and enhance predictability throughout treatment.

The DSD allows for careful analysis of the patient's facial and dental characteristics along with any critical factors that may have been overlooked during clinical, photographic, or diagnostic cast–based evaluation procedures [34].

Fig. 13.14 Initial digital intraoral scanner with Carestream®

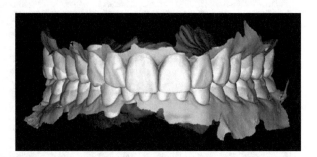

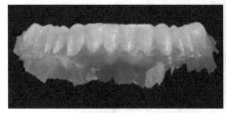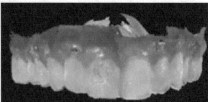

Fig. 13.15 Pretreatment intraoral scan with Carestream

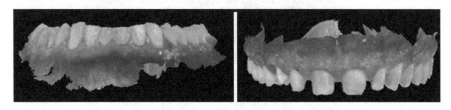

Fig. 13.16 Digital scan of the abutment teeth preparation with Carestream®

13.10.1 Requirements for DSD

Prior to beginning with the treatment procedures, thorough dental screening is a must to rule out any medical, dental, psychological or financial problems. The treatment needs of the patient should be correlated with the patient's past and present dental soft and hard tissues conditions which if been ignored may complicate the smile designing planning. Any surgical, periodontal, orthodontic, restorative procedures should be performed prior to the digital smile designing treatment.

DSD technique is carried out by digital equipment (computer, laptops, tablets or a phone) with any commercially available DSD software installed and a digital SLR. Digital intraoral scanner for digital impression, a 3D printer and CAD/CAM are additional tools for digital 3D workflow. An accurate photographic and video documentation is essential for complete facial and dental analysis and dynamic analysis of teeth, gingiva, lips and face during smiling, laughing and talking in order to integrate facially guided principles into the smile design.

13.10.2 Photography

As mentioned, a proper photography protocol should be followed with photographs taken of good quality, precision, correct posture and good techniques (Fig. 13.17). This is important as the facial reference lines drawn and used for the smile design will be based on the photographic quality. Seven basic photographic views in a fixed head position are required. This includes three frontal views and two profile views (Table 13.3).

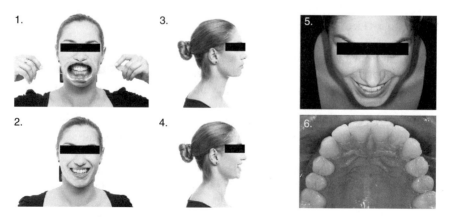

Fig. 13.17 Basic photographic shots *(Reproduced with permission from Dental Photo Master)*

Table 13.3 (a) Basic recommended images. (b) Photographic views needed for DSD

(a)

Extraoral images	Frontal profile
	Frontal smiling
	Oblique/three quarter view
	Oblique smiling
	L-R profile view
Intraoral images	Frontal
	Left buccal
	Right buccal
	Maxillary occlusal
	Mandibular occlusal

(b)

Frontal views	• Full face with a wide smile and the teeth apart
	• Full face at rest
	• Retracted view of the full maxillary and mandibular arch with teeth apart.
Profile views	• Side profile at rest
	• Side profile with a full smile

A 12 o'clock view with a wide smile and incisal edge
of maxillary teeth visible and resting on the lower lip
An intra-occlusal view of maxillary arch from the
second premolar to the second premolar

13.10.3 Videography

Recent advances in technology allow the clinician to measure dynamic lip-tooth relationships and incorporate that information into the orthodontic problem list and biomechanical plan. Digital videography and various software are particularly useful in both smile analysis and in doctor-patient communication.

According to Coachman [13], focus should be adjusted towards the mouth. Ideally, four videos from specific angles should be taken:

1. A facial frontal video with retractor and without retractor smiling.
2. A facial profile video with lips at rest and wide-E smile.
3. A 12 o'clock video above the head at the most coronal angle that still allows the visualization of the incisal edge.
4. An anterior occlusal video to record the maxillary teeth from the second premolar to the second premolar with the palatine raphe as a straight line.

Short complementary videos are also be recommended, capturing possible smile positions, including 45-degree and profile views for facial, phonetic, functional and structural analysis and better treatment outcomes.

Benefits of videos are that they can be paused and a screenshot can be taken of the best recorded moment and converted into a photo. Tarantili et al. studied the smile on video and observed that the average duration of a spontaneous smile was 500 ms, which emphasizes the difficulty of recording this moment in photographs [36].

13.10.4 DSD Software

Factors such as dentofacial aesthetic parameters, ease of use, case documentation ability, cost, time efficiency, systematic digital workflow and organization, and compatibility of the program with CAD/ CAM or other digital systems may influence the user's decision [37].

The clinician may use any of the commercially available DSD software such as Keynote (iWork, Apple, Cupertino, California, USA), Microsoft PowerPoint (Microsoft Office, Microsoft, Redmond, Washington, USA), Photoshop C6, Planmeca Romexis, VisagiSmile, CEREC, Smile Designer Pro, Exocad Smile Creator, Dental Treatment Simulation Pro, Clinicians, etc.

13.11 Steps in Smile Designing Treatment

The basic procedure of smile designing remains the same in spite of the inclusion of different aesthetic parameters in different DSD software. Digital smile designing protocol can be carried out using software for simple manipulation of the digital images, the addition of lines, shapes, and measurements over the clinical and laboratory images.

Reference lines are placed on the centre of the slide, forming a cross, one horizontal and other vertical (Fig. 13.18), followed by facial analysis. The next most important step is to relate the facial photograph to the horizontal reference line. The inter-pupillary line should be the first reference line to establish a horizontal plane along with inter-pupillary and inter-commissural lines. After determining this reference line, the facial midline is outlined according to facial features such as the

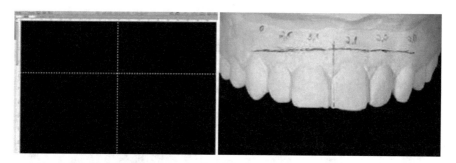

Fig. 13.18 Reference Lines

glabella, nose, and chin. The horizontal and vertical lines are crossed against each other to measure symmetry and cant of the face [38].

Grouping of the lines and the facial photographs is done for better analysis of smile. Midline discrepancy, occlusal plane shifting and canting can be easily detected. Dento gingival analysis is done next to establish the smile curve.

Three transferring lines are drawn over the retracted smile view as:

(a) *Line 1:* From the tip of one canine to the tip of the contralateral canine.
(b) *Line 2:* From the middle of the incisal edge of one central incisor to the middle of the incisal edge of the contralateral central incisor.
(c) *Line 3:* Over the dental midline, from the tip of the midline interdental papillae to the incisal embrasure.

These lines help in calibrating four features on the photograph: size, canting, incisal edge position, and midline position. Line 1 will guide the two first aspects (size and canting), line 2 will guide the incisal edge position, and line 3 will guide the midline position. The width/ length proportion of the central incisors is measured, and a rectangle is then placed over the edges of both central incisors on a digital image. The proportions of the patient's central incisors can be compared to the ideal proportions described in the literature.

As required, more lines may be drawn to evaluate both teeth and gingiva of the patient's maxillary arch, including tooth proportions, interdental relationship, relationship between the teeth and smile line, discrepancy between facial and dental midlines, midline and occlusal plane canting, soft tissue disharmony, relationship between the soft tissues and teeth, papillae heights, gingival margin levels, incisal edge design, and tooth axis. These lines may either be drawn over the photograph or copied and pasted from the software.

Required changes can be accomplished with the help of a digital ruler (Fig. 13.19) which is calibrated against the photograph by measuring the width of the central incisors in the study model. Figure 13.20 shows the procedure of digital smile designing on a DSD 3D software [39].

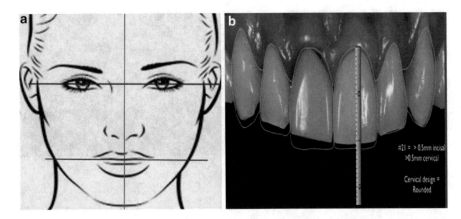

Fig. 13.19 (a) Facial view with horizontal and vertical reference lines, (b) Digital ruler *(Reproduced with permission from Elsevier Publishing)*

This digitally approved smile design at this stage can be used to create physical mock-up which can be tested aesthetically in the patient's mouth. After drawing the lines and markings on the cast, it is possible to transfer any necessary information, such as gingival margins, root coverage, crown lengthening, incisal edge reduction, and tooth width. At this stage, information that includes all the measurements and markings are hand over to the technician, which will be required to develop a precise wax-up on both the slides and cast.

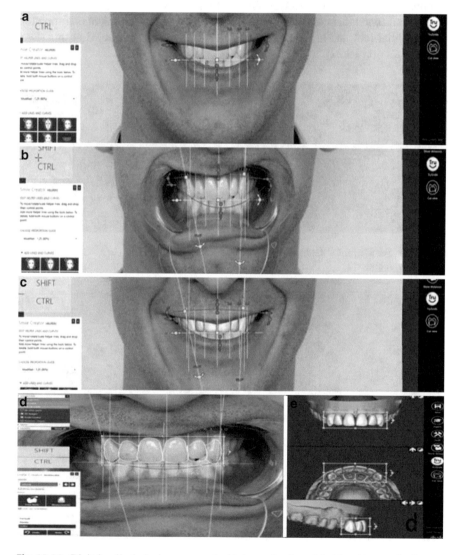

Fig. 13.20 Digital smile designing process. (**a**, **b**) shows drawing of facial and intraoral reference lines. (**c**) shows integration of facial with dental analysis. (**d**) represents incorporation of ideal dental contours in 3D. (**e**) shows digital designed smile compared with original smile (*Reproduced with permission from Elsevier Publishing*)

The guided diagnostic wax-up will be an important reference for any surgical, orthodontic, and restorative procedures. Several guides can be produced over this wax-up to control the procedures, such as surgical stents, orthodontic guides, implant guides, crown lengthening guides, and tooth preparation guides. The next important step is to evaluate the precision of the DSD protocol and the wax-up which is to be used for clinical try-in.

While DSD presents many advantages over more traditional treatment planning methods, the mock-up technique is still regarded as an objective and efficient tool in treatment planning, communication and used to confirm the treatment plan before the final preparations and evaluate final restorations within the limitations of biological and functional considerations. The mock-up can be a clinical confirmation of the digital tool and any occlusion discrepancies can be corrected at this stage (Figs. 13.21 and 13.22).

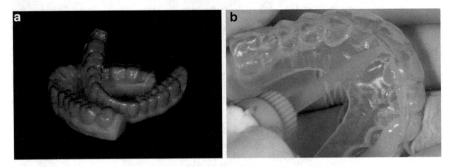

Fig. 13.21 (a) Matrix for the motivational mock-up and digital models. (b) Motivational mock-up made with bisacryl

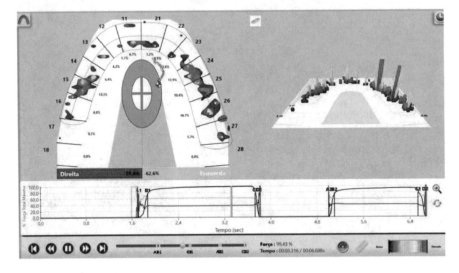

Fig. 13.22 Occlusion confirmed using T-scan technology

13.12 Advantages of DSD [34]

The DSD protocol offers advantages in the following areas:

13.12.1 Aesthetic Diagnosis

A digital photography and digital analysis protocol enables the dentist to visualize and analyze issues that may not be noticeable clinically. Drawing of reference lines and shapes over extra- and intraoral digital photographs can easily be performed using presentation software.

13.12.2 Communication

There are four main issues that must be controlled to improve predictability and meet patient expectations in a smile design process: the horizontal reference plane, facial midline, smile design (tooth shape and arrangement) and colour. The challenge is to transfer this information from the face to the mouth, to the cast, and to the final restoration. The primary goal of the DSD protocol is to facilitate this process of handling the information to the dental technician more efficiently and to fabricate a three-dimensional wax-up, focusing on developing anatomical features within the parameters provided, including the planes of reference, facial and dental midlines, recommended incisal edge position, lip dynamics, basic tooth arrangement, and incisal plane.

It not only improves communication between clinician and patient but also between the interdisciplinary team members, clinician and lab technician. All the professionals involved in the smile design can access the information as required at any time to review, change, or add components during the diagnostic and treatment phases, without being available in the same place or at the same time. This improves transparency, creates better teamwork, and treatment planning. Figure 13.23 shows a clinical case using this software.

A study conducted by *Gabriele Cervino* et al. [40] on DSD published evaluated the effectiveness of the use of Digital Smile Design techniques. They considered the 'communicative' utility of the software, the therapeutic planning, and the aesthetic and functional rehabilitation of the patients and concluded that DSD provides important information to the clinician and patient. Patients can view their rehabilitations even before they start, which is significant from a medico-legal standpoint.

13.12.3 Feedback

The DSD method allows for precise evaluation of the results obtained in every treatment phase as every step in the treatment procedure is systematically and

Fig. 13.23 Clinical case

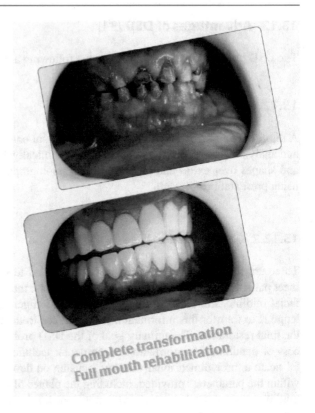

Complete transformation
Full mouth rehabilitation

sequentially organized with photographs, videos, and notes. This helps in comparing pre- and posttreatment photographs.

13.12.4 Patient Management

Its use as a marketing tool to motivate and educate the patient in addition to being used as an evaluative tool for comparisons between before and after is well evidenced in the literature.

In addition, DSD aids in patient acceptance by helping them visualize and understand both past and future treatments.

13.12.5 Education

The clinical cases can also be shared with colleagues, DSD can increase the visual impact of a lecture where the audience can better understand the concepts discussed.

13.13 Limitations of DSD

There are certain drawbacks to the use of DSD as well. The complete diagnosis and treatment planning is dependent on the photography and videography protocol and any discrepancy in their documentation may lead to incorrect or failure of the treatment plan [41]. Moreover, with the requirement of all the equipment for a complete 3D workflow, it makes the use of DSD expensive in clinical settings, in addition to the training and handling needed, thus adding to the cost [42].

13.14 Advances in DSD

In recent years, newer technologies like digital intraoral scanners, CAD-CAM and software programs, has arrived and dominated the dental markets which ultimately has led to the increased pace of digital workflow in dentistry. These newer technologies with their advanced operating features advanced have contributed to improving communication between the clinician and the dental technician and furthermore, reduces the treatment duration. With all these advancements, over the next few years, it will be possible to address facial aesthetics in advanced cases (in certain implant cases) by superimposing the files coming from a CT scan or a Cone Beam, along with 3D files of an oral impression or a facial scan and a photo [37].

There also is a possibility of incorporating 4D concept in which motion can be added to the smile design concept, by the time this book goes into printing [43]. With ever-evolving fast-paced technology a time, not so far, may come, when a digitally designed smile can be projected to virtual reality glasses to foresee the desired smile in actual reality.

13.15 Conclusion

The ever-increasing aesthetic demands of the patients lead to the continuous need to increase the bar of the detailed accuracy. The main objective of aesthetic treatment is always focused on the patient's expectation to improve his or her facial outlook and smile within normal physiological limits. A thorough investigation of patient expectations, biological and functional requirements along with the other restorative needs and a careful evaluation of all factors together are fundamentals to begin any treatment procedures. Dentistry is no way behind in technology as having advantages of today's shade-matching technology, accurate perception of colour, and thus, results can be easily achieved.

References

1. Ward DH. The vision of digital dental photography. Dent Today. 2007;26:100, 102, 104–105
2. Peumans M, Van Meerbeek B, Lambrechts P, Vanherle G. Porcelain veneers: a review of the literature. J Dent. 2000;28(3):163–77.
3. Evolution of Smile Design. (Accessed on 29th June 2020). https://media.digitalsmiledesign.com/christian-coachman-thoughts/smile-designevolution.
4. Coachman C, Calamita MA, Sesma N. Dynamic documentation of the smile and the 2D/3D digital smile design process. Int J Periodontics Restorative Dent. 2017;37:183–93.
5. Terry DA, Snow SR, McLaren EA. Contemporary dental photography: selection and application. Compend Contin Educ Dent. 2008;29:432–49.
6. Manjunath SG, Raju Ragavendra T, Sowmya K, Jayalaksshmi K. Photography in clinical dentistry—a review. Int J Dent Clinics. 2011;3:40–3.
7. Levin EI. Dental esthetics and Golden proportion. J Prosthet Dent. 1978;40:244–52.
8. Mahn E. Clinical digital photography. Part 1 equipment and basic documentation. Int Dent Aust Ed. 2013;3:18–26.
9. Pani S. A review on clinical digital photography. Int J Appl Res. 2017;3:10–7.
10. Sikri VK. Color: implications in dentistry. J Conserv Dent. 2010;13(4):249–55.
11. Duane RD, Jane BD. Acceptability of shade differences in metal ceramic crowns. J Prosthet Dent. 1998;79:254–60.
12. Tarnow DP, Magner AW, Fletcher P. The effect of the distance from the contact point to the crest of the bone on the presence or absence of the interproximal papilla. J Periodontol. 1992;63:995–6. [PubMed: 1474471]
13. Coachman C, Calamita MA, Sesma N. Dynamic documentation of the smile and the 2D/3D digital smile design process. Int J Periodontics Restorative Dent. 2017;37(2):183–93.
14. Evolution of materials. J Dent Technol. 2000;3:9–10.
15. Chu SJ, Tarnow DP. Digital shade analysis and verification: a case report and discussion. Pract Proced Esthet Dent. 2001;13:129–36.
16. Ahmad I. Three-dimensional shade analysis: perspectives of color. Part II. Pract Periodontics Esthet Dent. 2000;12:557–64.
17. Kielbassa AM, Beheim-Schwarzbach NJ, Neumann K, Zantner C. In vitro comparison of visual and computer-aided pre-and post-tooth shade determination using various home bleaching procedures. J Prosthet Dent. 2009;101:92–100.
18. Kim-Pusateri S, Brewer J, Davis EL, Wee AG. Reliability and accuracy of four dental shade-matching devices. J Prosthet Dent. 2009;101:93–9.
19. http://www.xrite.com/product_overview.aspx?ID=339
20. Blaes J. Today's technology improves the shade-matching problems of yesterday. J Indiana Dent Assoc. 2002–2003;81:17–9.
21. http://www.clearmatch.com/index.htm
22. Akira H, Ikuo I, Satoshi K. Color and translucency of in vivo natural central incisors. J Prosthet Dent. 2000;83:418–23.
23. Bruce M. Using tooth and color guides together. J Prosthet Dent. 2001;86:322–3.
24. Allyson AB, Nicholas JG, Kenneth JA, Mark CY. Influence of tab and disk design on shade matching of dental porcelain. J Prosthet Dent. 2002;88:591–7.
25. Rade DP, John MP, Rose-Marie. Color comparison of two shade guides. Int J Prosthodont. 2002;15:73–8.
26. Rade DP. Evaluation of a newly developed visual shade-matching apparatus. Int J Prosthodont. 2002;15:528–34.
27. Chu SJ, Trushkowsky RD, Rade D. Paravina. Dental color matching instruments and systems. Review of clinical and research aspects. J Dent. 2010;38s:e2–e16.
28. Berns RS. Billmeyer and Saltzman's principles of color technology: John Wiley & Sons; 2000.
29. Kim-Pusateri S, Brewer JD, Dunford RG, Wee AG. In vitro model to evaluate reliability and accuracy of a dental shade-matching instrument. J Prosthet Dent. 2007;98:353–8.

30. Karamouzos A, Papadopoulos MA, Kolokithas G, Athanasiou AE. Precision of in vivo spectrophotometric color evaluation of natural teeth. J Oral Rehabil. 2007;34:613–21.
31. Baltzer A. Shading of ceramic crowns using digital tooth shade matching devices. Int J Comput Dent. 2005;8:129–52.
32. Lee KY, Derric S, Stockes A. Brightness (value) sequence for the vita lumin classic shade guide reassessed. J Prosthodont Restor Dent. 2005;13:115–8.
33. Klemetti E. Shade selection performed by novice dental professionals and colorimeter. J Oral Rehabil. 2006;33:31–5.
34. Coachman C, Van Dooren E, Gürel G, Landsberg CJ, Calamita MA, Bichacho N. Smile design: from digital treatment planning to clinical reality. In: Cohen M, editor. Interdisciplinary treatment planning. Vol 2: comprehensive case studies. Chicago: Quintessence; 2012. p. 119–74.
35. Goldstein RE. Esthetics in dentistry. Vol 1: principles, communication, treatment methods. 2nd ed. Ontario: BC Decker; 1998.
36. Tarantili VV, Halazonetis DJ, Spyropoulos MN. The spontaneous smile in dynamic motion. Am J Orthod Dentofac Orthop. 2005;128(1):8–15.
37. Omar D, Duarte C. The application of parameters for comprehensive smile esthetics by digital smile design programs: A review of literature. Saudi Dent J. 2018;30(1):7–12.
38. Naini FB, Gill DS. Facial aesthetics: 2. Clinical assessment. Dent Update. 2008;35(3):159–70.
39. Jafri Z, Ahmad N, Sawai M, Sultan N, Bhardwaj A. Digital smile design-an innovative tool in aesthetic dentistry. J Oral Biol Craniofac Res. 2020;10:194–8.
40. Cervino G, Fiorillo L, Arzukanyan AV, Spagnuolo G, Cicciù M. Dental restorative digital workflow: digital smile design from aesthetic to function. Dent J (Basel). 2019;7(2):30.
41. Zanardi PR, Zanardi RL, Stegun RC, Sesma N, Costa BN, Laganá DC. The use of the digital smile design concept as an auxiliary tool in aesthetic rehabilitation: a case report. Open Dent J. 2016;10:28.
42. Meereis CT, De Souza GB, Albino LG, Ogliari FA, Piva E, Lima GS. Digital smile design for computer-assisted aesthetic rehabilitation: two-year follow-up. Oper Dent. 2016;41(1):E13–22.
43. Halley E. The future—3D planning but with the face in motion. Br Dent J. 2015;218:326–7.

Virtual Reality in Dentistry

14

Mansi Gupta

14.1 Introduction

In the present day, it is impossible to imagine daily life without digital technology. Every aspect of our lives is dependent on digital support, from computers to mobile phones. One of the milestones considered in the medical field is the introduction of 3D radiological techniques such as CBCT in dentistry. Other digital advancements used in dentistry are CAD/CAM, intraoral scans, digital shade selection, etc. all of which have been covered in detail in this book. All this digital information facilitates data availability and storage and can further be utilized to create a special computer-simulated patient casts, the so-called virtual patients. In one sense, virtual patients can be considered digital simulations of real human beings and their findings [1].

This chapter will provide the reader with information about virtual reality and its more recent variant, augmented reality along with the differences between them, clinical applications of these techniques and their advantages and disadvantages. Future prospects will also be discussed briefly.

The reader must keep in mind that the purpose of this chapter is not to give detailed information behind the principles of information technology and knowledge; rather, it is designed to give an overview of the newer terms such as virtual patient (can also be referred to as the digital patient), augmented reality and its application in the field of dentistry. For more information about the background of the described technologies and their widespread use in other areas, the reader is referred to the existing literature of information technology, health informatics, medicine and physics.

M. Gupta (✉)
Department of Prosthodontics, Indraprastha Dental College, Ghaziabad, India

© Springer Nature Switzerland AG 2021
P. Jain, M. Gupta (eds.), *Digitization in Dentistry*,
https://doi.org/10.1007/978-3-030-65169-5_14

14.2   A Virtual Patient

The idea of a virtual patient can be explained by dividing it into three main parts. The *first part* concerns with the concept of creating a database with patient's medical and dental information/history popularly known as electronic health records (EHRs). EHRs are a part of teledentistry, which can be defined as "the practice of using video conferencing technologies to diagnose and to provide advice about the treatment over a distance". It combines telecommunications and dentistry, with the exchange of information, both clinical data and images, over remote distances for consultations and treatment options [2]. Teledentistry, patient care and education can be delivered as live video (synchronous), store and forward (asynchronous) and remote patient monitoring (RPM) [3].

It aids in distant learning via web-based self-instruction and interactive video conferencing in addition to interprofessional communications where the specialist observes the procedure in one part of the world and, in the other part, another dentist makes a digital project of complete implant and prosthetic construction and route the direction for the placement of implant or extraction of wisdom teeth through navigation.

OrthoCAD and models are two popular systems that help orthodontists achieve success with distant patient's treatments [4]. Another advantage of teledentistry is that these cumulative audio/visual data or live consultations can reduce fear and anxiety among children and people living in rural areas.

Electronic health records with standardized diagnostics and universally accepted data formats help in collecting data from different clinics. These data can vary from routine treatment to specific surgeries. These cumulative data not only minimize storage space but also help further in research especially diagnosing rare diseases. An example is the universal dental diagnostic coding system (the Standard Nomenclature for Dentistry (SNODENT)) [5].

The *second part* is digitally connecting diseases with their symptoms, EHRs and treatments. Thus, while electronic case scenarios can be created for education and training purposes, this information can be used as a source for research as well. Lastly, the *third part* comprises a 3D computer-based reconstruction of human body parts, for example, head, neck or even the entire human body.

From a dental perspective, this 3D visualization is very significant as it is based on previously captured digital dental findings such as CBCT radiographs and facial and intraoral 3D scans. The digital assembly of all this information requires the presence of an ordinary analogue (non-digital) information transformed to digital information. A specially developed software is then used to bring these data together and to create a digital simulation of a patient—a virtual patient.

14.3   Understanding the Difference between "Virtual Reality" (VR) and "Augmented Reality" (AR)

Virtual reality (VR) or "near reality" *technology* is defined as a method by which, an environment is three-dimensionally simulated, giving the user a sense of being inside it, controlling it and personally interacting with it [6]. It uses artificial scenes that are computer generated with no connection to reality. The user is exposed to a realistic multidimensional visual stimulus which creates a virtual environment for the assessment of various anatomical regions of the body for the diagnosis, planning and surgical training [7]. This is experienced via head-mounted goggles and wired clothing.

The concept of virtual reality requires the development of specialized software to manipulate the recorded 3D images of the dental and orofacial morphology. Four main types of 3D imaging systems that are currently in use and essential for virtual planning are cone-beam computed tomography (CBCT), laser scanner, structured light scanner and stereophotogrammetry [8].

Augmented reality (AR) is a variant of VR, an emerging technology. It was first developed by Ivan Edward Sunderland in 1968 with a binocular system "kinetic depth effect" made of two cathode-ray tubes. It wasn't until 1991 that the definition of "augmented reality" was first described by Tom Caudell of the Boeing Company as "a technology that superimposes a computer-generated image on a user's view of the real world, thus providing a composite view" [9, 10] (Fig. 14.1). AR is to "virtualize" the virtual image into the real space, creating a completely virtual space around the user's eyes to replace the real space. Thus, it combines virtual reality with a 3D real environment specific to an individual patient to achieve an integral image, using semi-transparent glasses, to augment the virtual scene with the real one [11]. Hence, the user feels in the real environment instead of being engaged in a computer-generated world (like in VR).

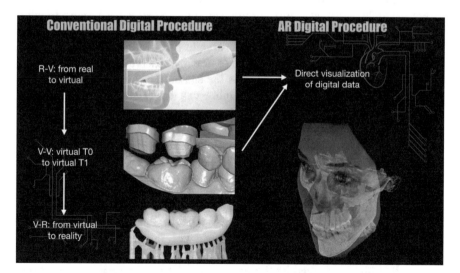

Fig. 14.1 Conventional vs Augmented reality—The direct visualization of virtual informations *(Adapted from Farronato* et al. *Current state of the art in the use of augmented reality in dentistry: a systematic review of the literature. BMC Oral Health (2019) 19:135)* (The digital image is acquired by a scanning device; the changes are performed digitally from T0 to T1 and finally the new information is transferred back to solid state. The use of augmented reality permits direct visualization bypassing the last transfer step, thus avoiding data and time loss)

Virtual reality can either be interactive (user can modify the virtual environment) or immersive (sense of being in a non-real virtual environment). Based on the level of presence experienced by a user, virtual reality technology can be further classified into immersive and non-immersive virtual reality.

Immersive reality experience includes interaction and involvement of the user within the virtual environment to create a sense of being "present" in the environment. It combines virtual reality with the added characteristics of the captured environment to provide the operator with the sense of being in the scene, able to visualize the recorded image in 3D, 3D audio direction and interact using a wearable device that detects eye movements and tracks leap motions of the hands. The user is detached from the real world and gets a feeling of being completely surrounded by a virtual computer (psychophysical experience). Non-immersive virtual reality involves computer-generated experiences on a desktop, while the user interacts with a mouse, in a virtual environment [12]. Immersive reality is similar to augmented reality but the user is interacting with a digital 3D world recreated through 360° real records. The 360 records recreate the continuity of the surrounding with no interruptions.

Augmented reality is commonly confused with virtual reality since both have many components in common, in spite of the completely different outcome. Virtual reality, as explained, is a virtual immersive environment where the user's senses are stimulated with computer-generated sensations and feedbacks and generates an "interaction". Augmented reality, on the other hand, generates an interaction between the real environment and virtual objects.

For example, a virtual reality system would be a head-worn helmet stimulating navigation inside the human body and permits the user to explore it on the base of virtual three-dimensional reconstruction. A similar example with the augmented reality would permit the user to directly observe a human body and to see virtual objects on it, or through it as the anatomy of the body was superimposed [9, 10]. Another way of explaining can be in surgical trainings and procedures.

The 3D acquired images of the head and neck region will provide a platform for education and training, whereas the recorded images can also be superimposed into the patient for a surgical procedure to be carried out in an environment of augmented virtual reality.

The use of AR (with the use of special glasses and an integrated screen) is a fairly new development in the field of medicine and dentistry. However, substituting virtual reality with augmented reality means to superimpose virtual objects to the reality in a precise and reproducible way keeping in mind, the dimensions of space as well as the users and patient's movements. This is still a controversial topic as it is highly affected by the system used. The most commonly used systems are head-mounted displays and half, silvered mirror projections, both of them are valid systems for augmented reality and different settings as described by Azuma et al. [9].

14.4   Uses of VR

14.4.1 Education and Training (Preclinical and Clinical)

Historically, dental education has been restricted to phantom heads and artificial teeth mimicking different case scenarios. Nowadays, virtual 3D simulators are available (Fig. 14.2). This virtual environment comprises of one visual display on which a mouth or even an entire patient's head is projected. These displays can be integrated into special eyewear in order to enhance the perception of reality and haptic input devices can be utilized to provide the user with the opportunity to receive feedback in terms of tactile sensations. A study done by *Buchanan* concluded that students trained with virtual reality simulators learned faster, practised more procedures per hour, accomplished the same levels of competence as traditional preclinical laboratories and requested more evaluations through the computer thus reducing instructor-student evaluation time [13].

Initial research for using VR and AR in dental education was conducted by Kim et al. They proposed a dental training system with a multi-modal workbench providing visual, audio, and haptic feedback. Haptics is the science of studying the sense of touch [14]. This system used volume-based haptic modelling which represents a tooth as a volumetric implicit surface and permits the drilling of a tooth. However, it is limited to a spherical tool [15]. Wang et al. developed a simulator that allows probing and cutting of a tooth model, but the virtual tool implementation was limited to a spherical shape, as with Kim et al.'s 2005 system [16]. These studies were considered incomplete.

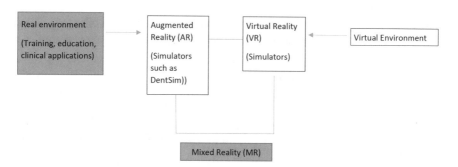

Fig. 14.2 Difference between VR and AR in Dental Education *(Modified from Paul Milgram 1994)*. The extreme left of the figure describes an environment consisting solely of real objects, and includes whatever might be observed when viewing a real-world scene either directly in person, or through some kind of a window or via some sort of a (video) display. The extreme right of the figure describes environments consisting solely of virtual objects, examples of which would include conventional computer graphic simulations, either monitor-based or immersive. Within this framework lies a generic Mixed Reality (MR) environment as one in which real-world and virtual world objects are presented together within a single display

Haptics offers an additional dimension to virtual reality or 3D environment. In combination with a visual display, haptic technology can be used to train people for tasks requiring hand-eye coordination, such as surgeries in dentistry. It creates the illusion of substances (teeth, alveolar bone, instruments, hand-pieces, burs, implants) and force within a simulated virtual world of the oral cavity. The haptic devices provide force-feedback of the virtual dental operative instruments as they come in contact with the virtual teeth and alveolar bone giving the operator a perception of manipulation of objects using the senses of touch and proprioception [14].

New technologies being developed, include "haptic" (sense of touch) and "virtual lab environments" into the simulation exercises increase motor skills and student efficiency as well as reduce the faculty time required [17].

Virtual reality for dental education holds the promise of merging educational ideas and technological capabilities thus allowing for successful use of technology in higher education; reshaping teaching and learning experiences. However, the author recommends that virtual simulation cannot solely replace the traditional teaching methods of interactive human lectures. Blended learning designs in the form of virtual reality units along with instructor teaching/feedback should be incorporated into dental education to make full use of the laboratory training time and improve fine motor skills.

Currently, there are various virtual reality simulators available (Table 14.1). By the time, this book will be released, some might be obsolete and new systems would have been introduced. Few systems will be discussed to give the reader an idea of the different technologies and how they work.

14.4.1.1 DentSim

One of the first computerized dental training simulators is the DentSim [18] virtual reality system for teaching restorative dentistry. The DentSim™ units comprise a

Table 14.1 Comparison of dental simulators

Characteristics	DentSim™	Simodont®	PerioSim®	IDEA
Ergonomic postures	Yes	Yes	No	No
Exam simulation	Yes	Yes	Yes	No
Instant feedback	Yes	Yes	No	Yes
Teeth used	Plastic	Animated	Animated	Animated
Right and left operation	Yes	Yes	Yes	Yes
Reported real life experience	Realistic experience using plastic teeth on a real manikin [24]	3D images are realistic. However, the texture of healthy decayed and restored tooth structure still needs improvement [17]	Tactile sensation is realistic for teeth and not so for gingiva [22]	Tactile sensation still needs to be tuned to simulate a genuine sensation [29]

phantom head, a set of dental instruments, infrared sensors, an overhead infrared camera with a monitor and two computers.

It enables students to practise clinical procedures on a simulated patient with on-screen visual tracking of the procedure concerned, real-time feedback and evaluation of their performance (Fig. 14.3). Studies on this indicate that it is effective in enabling students to work without the need for a supervisor to assess their performance critically, and to monitor their performance [19, 20]. This ability to mimic real-life situations allows students to train independently and enhance clinical skills, thus reducing training costs. A study by *Jasinevicius* et al. [21] reported that using virtual methods decreased faculty time by fivefold when compared to traditional preclinical teaching methods.

14.4.1.2 PerioSim©

PerioSim©, is a virtual reality simulator, for training in periodontal procedures and developed by *Luciano*. It allows the students to visualize a virtual human mouth, including teeth and surrounding gingival soft tissue, and develop skills of how to examine and detect periodontal disease in a haptic environment, without the need of preparation of teeth surfaces, with virtual dental instruments. It has the advantage that it does not require tooth surface alteration, but the disadvantage that tactile sensations for the gingival tissues are not realistic [22]. A study by Steinberg et al. [23] concluded that the device can help students develop necessary tactile skills and recommended its incorporation in dental schools. However, it was found that the realism of images of instruments and oral structures as well as the realism of tactile feedback had some limitations that needed further enhancement [23, 24].

14.4.1.3 MOOG Simodont Dental Trainer

This is a simulation unit without the need for a physical phantom head. Moog Simodont Dental Trainer combines Moog's expertise in haptic technology and ACTA's (Academic Center for Dentistry in Amsterdam) experience in dental education to help students practice more efficiently and learn faster. The system consists of a display projecting the mouth and teeth of a virtual patient as a stereo image on a mirror right above a haptic handpiece (Fig. 14.4). The system consists of a display projecting the mouth and teeth of a virtual patient as a stereo image on a mirror right above a haptic handpiece. Special stereoscopic glasses help in creating spatial illusions that enables the user to apply a physical drill handle as typically done on real patients, thus creating the illusion of a real dental experience. These haptic devices while providing various dental procedures including diagnosis and treatment planning, cavity preparation, and crown and bridge preparations, also provides different haptic feedbacks depending on the material being prepared virtually (e.g. enamel, dentin, or pulp) [25, 26].

The Simodont® software includes modules for manual dexterity, cariology, crown and bridges exercises, clinical cases and a full mouth simulation experience. Endodontics modules are being developed for future release. These units provide a very unique feature, "The case editor" which allows users to scan their own instruments and clinical cases to create a new exercise. *Bakr* et al. reported a possible

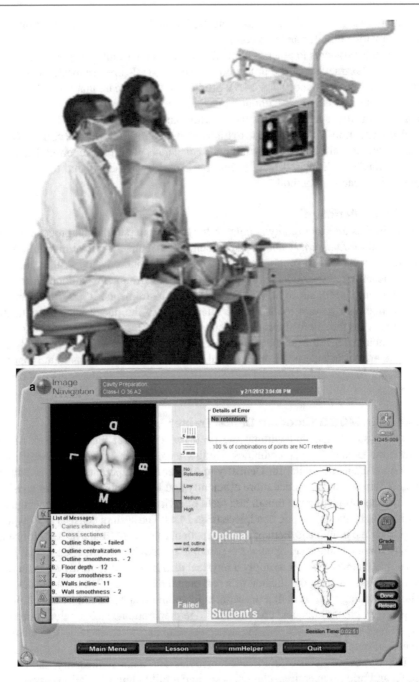

Fig. 14.3 *DentSim* simulation unit in an educational setting *(Adopted from* www.dentsimlab. com*)*. Figs. **a**, **b**, and **c** show view of evaluation screen on the simulator during different dental procedures. Upper left is the virtual image of student's preparation. Right side of screen is cross-section of optimal preparation (right middle) and student's preparation (lower right). (**a**) Retention. (**b**) Outline Shape. (**c**) Pulpal exposure

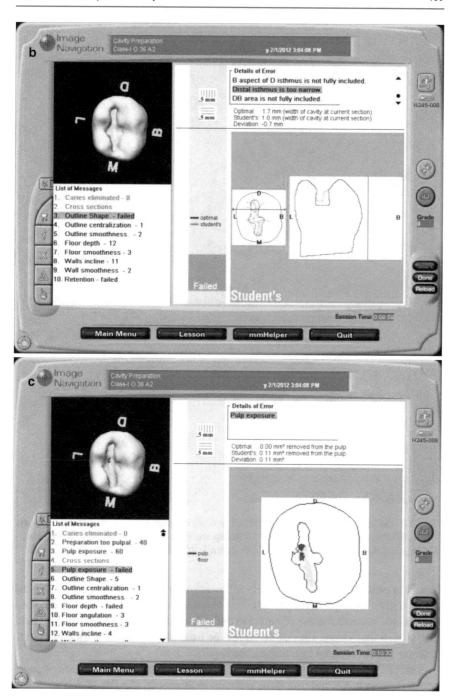

Fig. 14.3 (continued)

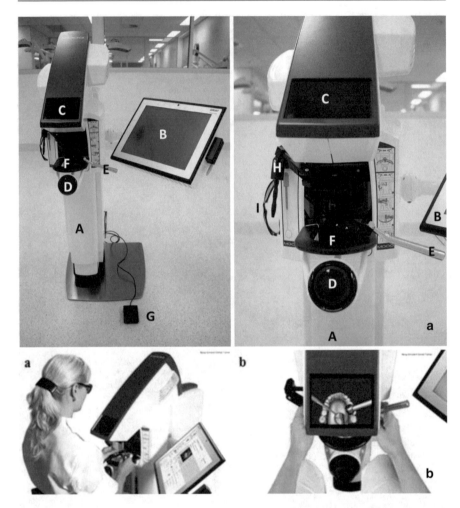

Fig. 14.4 (a) MOOG Simodont Dental Trainer showing different components (A) Simulator, (B) Screen, (C) Projection, (D) Space mouse, (E) Handpiece, (F) Hand rest, (G) Foot Pedal, (H) Mirror stick, (I) 3D Glasses (adopted from www.moog.com)). (b) A haptic tooth preparation exercise

benefit in enhancing manual dexterity following short term exposure to Simodont® dental trainer amongst undergraduate dental students. The authors reported a positive attitude towards the use of haptic to enhance the learning experience. However, they agreed that virtual simulation should be used as a supplementary tool in conjunction with traditional teaching methods [27].

Virtual Reality Dentist's Chair or *HapTEL* and 3D dental patient is another popular application in VR training [28]. Trainees wear special goggles with head tracking cameras to allow them to virtually examine teeth, sense the touch and force of the drill/tools on hard and soft tissues with realistic feedback. Like other systems, these simulators are also programmed to identify errors and assess the performance.

Since the feedback is recorded, trainees can assess their mistakes and improvise on it the next time. In surgery, these simulators help trainees visualize surgical site and practice in real mode on virtual objects.

VR has also been used in surgical training in dentistry. In a study on virtual apicoectomy procedure, Voxel Man Simulator was used. The authors stated that the majority of the trainees gave positive feedback regarding the impact of virtual simulation as an additional modality in dental education. They indicated that the integrated force feedback (e.g. simulation of haptic pressure), spatial 3D perception, and image resolution of the simulator were key features for virtual training for dental surgical procedures. Trainees were also able to develop the ability to self-assess their performance. This study also proposed that application of virtual surgery using the 3D reconstruction of patient's anatomy might help surgeons to plan complex surgical procedures [30].

Another area for use of VR in dentistry is for computer-aided cephalometry, based on haptic technology. Using haptic enabled digital cephalometric analysis and by providing a sense of touch, researchers were able to prove that the errors in cephalometric analysis can be reduced and the land-marking can become more feasible and intuitive [31]. The applicability of using 3D visualisation in dental training was also reported when a haptic dental injection was developed for inferior alveolar nerve block (Fig. 14.5) [32].

AR is also being used in temporomandibular joint motion analysis. ManMos (Mandibular motion tracking system) developed in Japan is such an example. It synchronizes the dental cast model movements via the 3D model of a patient [33, 34]. Suenaga et al. evaluated AR navigation system for providing markerless registration system using stereo vision in orthognathic surgery. They concluded that 3D contour matching is best for Teeth information viewing even with complex anatomies [35].

Advances in hardware and software technology could allow for enhancements in virtual reality experience and better adaptation of this technology into modern education. Additional features such as virtual water spray, virtual tongue and cheeks for retraction could further enhance virtual reality learning experiences. Table 14.2 summarizes the benefits and drawbacks of VR in dental education and training.

At present, there are limited clinical studies to assess the impact of virtual reality with the standard methods of delivering education. Most of the existing research on simulators focuses on the technical skills of the trainees which gives a holistic learning experience to the trainees. However, non-technical skills such as cognitive development, interpersonal communication, teamwork, and emergency management are hardly touched upon except in few studies. Further studies are required to compare the impact of augmented reality in imparting education and training.

14.4.2 Clinical Applications

In dentistry, technological advances in virtual and augmented reality systems are used in different specialities such as oral and maxillofacial surgery, dental

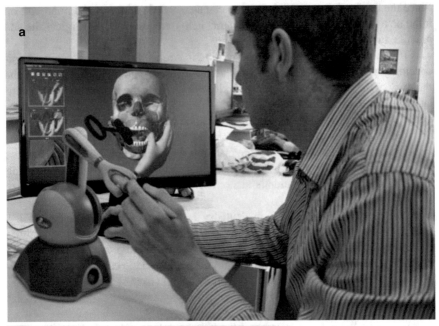

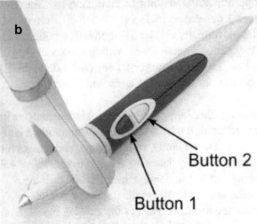

Fig. 14.5 (a) Haptic interaction for training the injection of a local anaesthetic [32]. (b) The two PHANTOM Omni pen buttons: one is for injection, and the other for reset

implantology and orthognathic surgery. They have also been used to controlling pain and anxiety during a dental procedure in recent times.

AR is also applied in orthodontics for guided bracket placement and in the field of endodontics to detect root canals and for educational and training purposes, as explained in the previous section.

Table 14.2 Advantages and disadvantages of VR in dental education and training

Advantages	Disadvantages
Working with VR provides correct ergonomic posture and positioning. Incorrect operator and/or patient positioning results in a warning signal that prevents the user from continuing (xxix)	Most of these virtual of augmented reality dental simulators are still at an early or experimental stage and not enough literature/research is available
VR helps in honing the psychomotor skills by training in direct/indirect vision and spatial orientation in a controlled setting (xxx)	Current VR systems are mainly programmed to evaluate tooth preparations only. In addition, hand instrumentation cannot be performed (with the exception of a cavity for an amalgam filling)
Self-evaluation: Students have immediate, unlimited, and objective access to detailed feedback of their work	Current VR systems are limited to using spherical tools that are simple to implement, but it also limits the realism in a simulated dental clinic, where several types of instruments are needed in different shapes and sizes
Positive student perception	The initial cost of this advanced technology can be substantial
It is not essential for faculty to supervise students while they are using the systems, thus saving staff costs	VR systems are difficult to maintain and repair and require extensive training on how to use and supervision the work

14.4.2.1 VR in Implantology

The accurate positioning of dental implants is essential to meet the functional and aesthetic demands. Currently, various soft-wares are available for the virtual planning of dental implants. This 3D virtual planning is then transferred onto the surgical field via either the static guide or the dynamic navigated approach [36]. The static transfer of the surgical plan is based on the virtual designing followed by fabrication of a surgical guide using CAD/CAM. Various static guiding systems are available based such as EasyGuide, InVivoDental, Implant 3D, Nobel Bioguide and VIP (Implant Logic System) [37]. Literature and evidence of using static guided surgery as a means of creating surgical templates to accurately position implants are ample.

Another method for computer-assisted surgery in dental implantology is image-guided surgery through dynamic navigation. Although literature previously published on this have reported comparable accuracy between dynamic and static surgical navigation [38, 39], dynamic navigation could overcome some of the disadvantages associated with static guided surgery. These included reducing costs and time needed for the impression and laboratory procedures of a static guided system.

Dynamic navigation allows the real-time adjustment of the direction of the dental implant during surgery based on virtual surgical planning and also has the ability to have a direct view of the surgical field. It also provides the clinician with the flexibility to make changes in implant planning at the time of surgery. This helps in avoiding any compromised bony foundation and anatomical structures that may have not be detected during the pre-surgical planning phase. This level of flexibility is possible with statically derived surgical guides as they are fixed and cannot be altered once they are planned and manufactured. Another advantage of using dynamic navigation is that single-tooth edentulous ridge areas can be fully guided as a dynamic guide is not restricted by drill tube size (i.e. in the anterior mandibular incisor sites). The use of VR computerized implant dentistry has opened new possibilities in managing complex cases where the anatomy of the bones is altered.

The size of the implant is also not limited with dynamically guided systems, as they are with static guides and CBCT, planning and surgery can be achieved in a single day [40].

With a dynamic navigation system, the operator can track the position of a surgical device in real time (e.g. endodontic file, implant placement, scalpel). The device position projects onto the digital image of the anatomic area of interest, providing guidance to the clinician/surgeon, helping him/her in real-time to follow the anticipated path-ways and recognize possible interference with tissue adjacent to the treatment area. In a systematic review, positioning accuracy of both dental implant horizontal apical and angular deviation was shown to improve with surgical navigation [41]. Augmented reality navigation results in smaller horizontal, vertical and angular errors in central incisors and canines than was achieved with traditional 2D image-guided navigation [42]. In endodontics, surgical navigation is safe, minimally invasive for root canal location and prevention of technical failure, especially in anterior teeth with pulp canal calcifications [43].In computer-assisted maxillofacial surgery, positioning accuracies have been reported to be <1 mm in an ideal setting and between 2 and 4 mm in a real-life surgical setting [44]. A logical extension to dynamic surgical navigation is made possible with mixed reality, integrating aspects of both virtual and augmented reality technologies, further enhancing human visualization. Virtual reality makes images seem real, even though the environment is synthetic, created through the combination of virtual reality equipment (e.g. Google Glasses) and a computer. Mixed reality integrates the real environment into the virtual space, fusing the two [45].

However, it must be emphasized that the technology is expensive in addition to requiring a significant amount of training and a rigorous intra-operative referencing and orientation process. Moreover, a disrupted surgical procedure may be encountered due to sensors being blocked during the navigation process, or difficulty in simultaneously paying attention to the patient as well as the output from the navigation system display.

The application of augmented reality for the placement of dental implants was recently tested in two cases in a pilot study [46]. The study explored the feasibility of a virtual display for dynamic navigation for the implant position, using specific glasses, on the surgical field for in augmented reality (Fig. 14.6). The two virtual environments did not affect the accuracy of the surgical procedure.

14.4.2.2   VR in Oral and Maxillo-Facial Surgery and Orthognathic Surgery

VR is being used in many aspects of oral surgery. A study demonstrated the 3D virtual plane mandibular and maxillary reconstructions achieving an excellent match. The study used 30 complex cases of head and neck reconstruction including

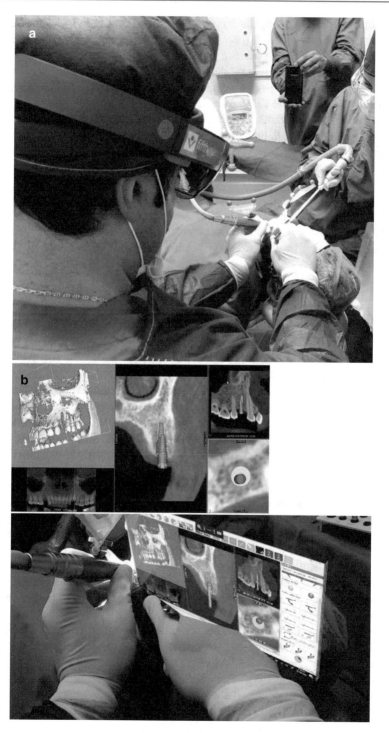

Fig. 14.6   (**a**) Overview of the glasses and navigation system [46] with Hololens Glasses [30]. (**b**) The real and the virtual implant position on the navigation system screen which is the view of the surgeon during the surgery wearing AR Hololens glasses

the planes of the resection, the length of the segmental defect and the distance between the transplanted segments and the remaining bone and concluded that there was an excellent match between the virtual plans and the achieved results [47].

Another series of case reports demonstrated the virtual surgical planning and hardware fabrication for open reduction and internal fixation of atrophic edentulous mandibular fractures were demonstrated [48, 49].

Navigation within a virtual environment also has been successfully used during orthognathic surgical [50], and for the repositioning of the maxilla to correct facial asymmetry [51]. In a study working on the same concept, the authors concluded that navigation surgery is useful as it improved the accuracy of the performed procedure and reduced operational risks.

Customized augmented reality systems seem to provide great results in clinical applications although there is a lack of randomized clinical trials with a proper sample. But its technological benefits of superimposition of digital images making it easier on bony structures are soon gaining popularity in the field of small to medium-sized surgeries.

14.4.2.3   VR in Reducing Pain and Anxiety during Dental Procedures

Despite advances in dental technologies and treatment, many people still avoid or delay dental care because of the fear and anxiety of pain. Recently, advanced technologies have moved toward using distraction and hypnosis techniques to treat pain [52]. Different therapies have been proposed for the prevention and treatment of pain and dental anxiety with virtual reality distraction system as one of them [53]. Virtual reality (VR) utilizes advanced technologies to create virtual environments (VE) that allow patients to be immersed in an interactive, simulated world [54]. These advanced systems interact at many levels with the VE, stimulating sights, sounds, and motion to encourage immersion in the virtual world to enhance distraction from pain [55].

Moreover, VR can be advantageous to patients who reject pain and anxiety control through anti-anxiety drugs because of their disadvantages or side effects. A clinical study observed that dental patients undergoing sub-gingival scaling procedure experienced considerable reduction in pain when using VR compared to participants that watched a movie and to participants that did not have any type of distraction [56]. Kumar et al. demonstrated the use of VRET (virtual reality exposure therapy) in the treatment of dental anxiety [34]. It provides a good non-real environment which objectively assesses the behavioural and rehabilitative cognitive and functional abilities.

The physiological results of another research suggest that the use of the VR distraction system (VRDS) may be a beneficial option for patients with mild to moderate fear and anxiety associated with dental treatments. This system may be a useful adjunct to help reduce anxiety, discomfort, boredom, and the time required to perform routine dental procedures. It allows them to relax by allowing them to navigate to another location while still physically remaining in the dental office [57].

However, most of the research in the past has focused mainly on reducing pain and dental anxiety in paediatrics. Studies on the adult population are few. Also, parameters such as training programs, the different types of software and hardware of virtual reality devices, the temperament and patient personality, gender difference and more have not been investigated. Due to all this, the role of virtual reality in the control of anxiety and dental pain in children and adults needs further research and validation.

14.4.3 Robotic Patients for Simulation

As discussed earlier, the use of virtual patients in dental education is gaining acceptance. Robotic systems in dentistry can be divided into two categories based on their developing goals [58, 59]. One is for dentists training by simulating real human reactions during procedures [60, 61], and the other is aiming to assist dentists during dental treatments [62–65], mainly targeting at dental implant. It can be used as an adjunctive method in dental simulation training to live patient interactions for training dental students.

A robotic patient or DENTAROID has been recently introduced in Japan by Nissin Dental Products (Fig. 14.7a) [66]. This helps in providing training in students' communication competency with patients. The robot is programmed with over 20 patterns of automatic dialogues, thus allowing communication just like with an actual patient. The robot is also equipped with various lifelike bodily movements like eye blinks and different reaction movements that simulate accidents that can occur during treatment, such as reaction to pain, cough reflex, vomiting reflex and irregular pulse. These help in creating a realistic clinical training environment, with different clinical situations, thus allowing students to gain experience during their

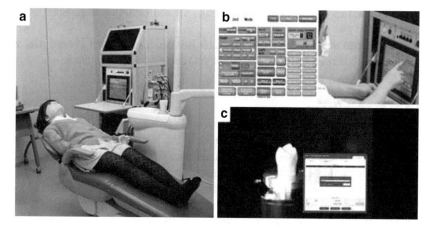

Fig. 14.7 (**a**) Robotic patient or Dentaroid; (**b**) Easy to use control panel with custom-made instructions for intuitive operation of the robot; (**c**) The Dentaroid grading system

Fig. 14.8 Technical drawing of the robot's head illustrating the range of motion. *Degrees of freedom. The head of the robot patient has 8 degrees of freedom (eyelids, eyeballs, jaw, tongue and neck)*—1/2/6 possible movements of the head, 3/4—possible movements of the eyes, 5/7/8— possible movements of the mandible (*Reproduced with permission of John Wiley & Sons, Inc.*) [60]

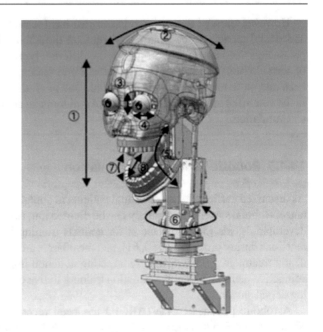

training. The robot can be operated and controlled by a clinician sitting in a separate control room (Fig. 14.7b) [67]. An easy to use control panel allows intuitive operation of the robot [68]. This new level of simulation can offer improved accuracy, predictability, safety and quality of care. In their study, Tanzawa et al. also describe a robot patient for dental education designed as a full-body replica, capable of secreting saliva and capable of communicating with users (Fig. 14.8) [69].

Wire-bending robots for orthodontic wires were introduced around the turn of the century. Recently, a mobile wire-bending machine was introduced. Using intra-oral scan data, this mobile system can create a fixed orthodontic retainer wire in only 4 min.

These systems are relatively new and their use in dentistry is still under trial and further research is required. They have not yet reached routine practice.

14.4.4 Future Prospects

Current literature indicates that virtual reality dental simulators are valuable educational tools that could be used either as an adjunct or to augment the current traditional teaching methods. Further advancement in hardware and software technology should allow for a better virtual reality experience and adaptation of this technology as an essential part of modern education.

Future developments will be focused to bring the actual technology more close to the real world. One aspect of augmented reality could be its integration where the virtual data seen is superimposed on living objects. This will give the doctor ability to look "inside" a patient (Fig. 14.9). Virtual technologies are only beginning to be

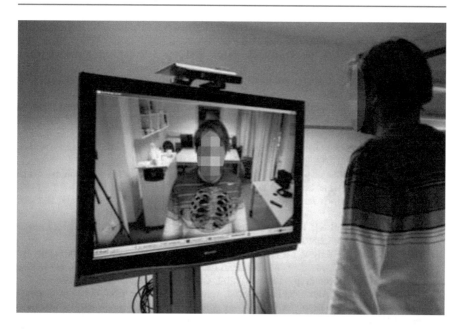

Fig. 14.9 Illustration of augmented reality. On the screen a radiological image is superimposed to a real-time capturing of a person *(Reproduced with permission from John Wiley & Sons, Inc.)* [60]

integrated into dental medicine. All forms of digital technologies will move together and it might be possible to integrate all the obtained patient data in one virtual patient model, in the near future. This integration provides the possibility of treatment planning, treatment simulation, and treatment execution on an evidence-based background in a virtual simulation. However, to bring these innovations into routine and widespread use, a close collaboration is required between the dental professionals, teachers and tutors, IT professional and entrepreneurs.

References

1. Ellaway R, Poulton T, Fors U, Mcgee JB, Albright S. Building a virtual patient commons. Med Teach. 2008;30:170–4.
2. Cook J. "ISDN videoconferencing in postgraduate dental education and orthodontic diagnosis". Learning technology in medical education conference 1997 (CTI Medicine): 111–16.
3. "ADA Guide to understanding and documenting teledentistry events". D 9995 and D 9996 ADA Guide 2017; version 1: 1–10.
4. Fernando MF, Lemos N, Roscoe M, Giraudea N. e health care in dentistry and oral medicine. A clinician's guide 2017: 99–108.
5. Louis RF, Brian ML. Periodontics: medicine, surgery and implants, vol. 2004. 1st ed: Elsevier Mosby. p. 163–71.
6. Raja'a MA, Farzaneh F. Computer-based technologies in dentistry: types and applications. J Dent (Tehran). 2016;13(3):215–22.
7. Freina L, Ott M. A literature review on immersive virtual reality in education: state of the art and perspectives; Computer science 2015.

8. Ayoub A, Xiao Y, Khambay B, Siebert P, Hadley D. Towards building a virtual human face. Int J Oral Maxillofac Surg. 2007;36(5):423–8.
9. Azuma RT. A survey of augmented reality. Presence Teleoperators Virtual Environ. 1997;6(4):355–85.
10. Bimber O, Raskar R. Spatial augmented reality: merging real and virtual worlds: Wellesley AK Peters/CRC Press; 2005.
11. Bartella AK, Kamal M, Scholl I, Steegmann J, Ketelsen D, Holzle F, et al. Virtual reality in preoperative imaging in maxillofacial surgery: implementation of "the next level". Br J Oral Maxillofac Surg. 2019;57(7):644–8.
12. Kim Y, Kim H, Kim YO. Virtual reality and augmented reality in plastic surgery: a review. Arch Plast Surg. 2017;44(3):179–87.
13. Buchanan JA. Experience with virtual reality-based technology in teaching restorative dental procedures. J Dent Educ. 2004;68:1258–65.
14. Definition of "haptics". In: Mosby's medical dictionary. 8th ed. St Louis, MO: Elsevier; 2009.
15. Kim L, Hwang Y, Park SH, Ha S. Dental training system using multi-modal interface. Comput Aided Des Appl. 2005;2:591–8.
16. Wang D, Zhang Y, Wang Y, Lu P. Development of dental training system with haptic display. In: RO-MAN: Proceedings of 12th IEEE International Workshop on Robot and Human Interactive Communication (pp. 159–164); 2003 Oct 31-Nov 2; Millbrae, CA, USA.
17. Bakr MM, Massey W, Alexander H. Students' evaluation of a 3DVR haptic device (Simodont). Does early exposure to haptic feedback during preclinical dental education enhance the development of psychomotor skills? Int J Dent Clin. 2014;6:1–7.
18. DentSim overview. Accessed (2020 July 4) at: www.denx.com/DentSim/overview.html
19. Rees JS, Jenkins SM, James T, Dummer PMH, Bryant S, Hayes SJ, et al. An initial evaluation of virtual reality simulation in teaching pre-clinical operative dentistry in UK setting. Eur J Prosthodont Restor Dent. 2007;15:92–8.
20. Gottlieb R, Buchanan JA, Berthold P, Maggio MP. Preclinical dental student' perception of the implementation of VR-based technology. J Dent Educ. 2005;69:127.
21. Asinevicius TR, Landers M, Nelson S, Urbankova A. An evaluation of two dental simulation systems: virtual reality versus contemporary non-computer-assisted. J Dent Educ. 2004;68:1151–62.
22. Luciano C, Banerjee P, DeFanti T. Haptics-based virtual reality periodontal training simulator. Virtual Reality. 2009;13(2):69–85.
23. Steinberg AD, Bashook PG, Drummond J, Ashrafi S, Zefran M. Assessment of faculty perception of content validity of PerioSim, a haptic-3D virtual reality dental training simulator. J Dent Educ. 2007;71:1574–82.
24. Mangano F, Shibli JA, Fortin T. Digital dentistry: new materials and techniques. Int J Dent. 2016;2016:5261247.
25. Sharaf B, Levine JP, Hirsch DL, Bastidas JA, Schiff BA, Garfein ES. Importance of computer-aided design and manufacturing technology in the multidisciplinary approach to head and neck reconstruction. J Craniofac Surg. 2010;21:1277–80.
26. MOOG. (2013) Haptic Technology in the Moog Simodont Dental Trainer [Online]. MOOG Inc. Available: http://www.moog.com/markets/medical-dentalsimulation/ haptic-technology-in- the-moog-simodontdental- trainer/ [Accessed july3, 2020].
27. Bakr MM, Massey WL, Alexander H. Can virtual simulators replace traditional preclinical teaching methods: a students' perspective? Int J Dent Oral Health. 2015;2(1) https://doi.org/10.16966/2378-7090.149.
28. Ta-Ko H, Chi-Hsung Y, Yu-Hsin H, Jen-Chyan W, et al. Augmented reality(AR) and virtual reality(VR) pallid in dentistry. Kaohsiung J Med Sci. 2018;34:243–8.
29. Gal GB, Weiss EI, Gafni N, Ziv A. Preliminary assessment of faculty and student perception of a haptic virtual reality simulator for training dental manual dexterity. J Dent Educ. 2011;75:496–504.

30. Pohlenz P, Grobe A, Petersik A, Von Sternberg N, Pflesser B, Pommert A, Hohne K-H, Tiede U, Springer I, Heiland M. Virtual dental surgery as a new educational tool in dental school. J Craniomaxillofac Surg. 2010;38(8):560–4.
31. Medellin-Castillo HI, Govea-Valladares EH, Perez-Guerroro CN, Gil-Valladares J, Lim T, Richie JM. The evaluation on a novel haptic-enabled virtual reality approach for computer aided cephalometry. Comput Methods Prog Biomed. 2016;130:46–53.
32. Anderson P, Chapman P, Ma M, Rea P. Real-time medical visualization of human head and neck anatomy and its applications for dental training and simulation. Curr Med Imag. 2013;9(4):298–308.
33. http://www.e-macro.ne.jp/en-macro/manmos_mandibular_motion_tracking_system.html (Accessed on May 10, 2020).
34. Fushima K, Kobayashi M. Mixed-reality simulation for orthognathic surgery. Maxillofac Plast Reconstr Surg. 2016;38(1):13.
35. Suenaga H, Tran H, Liao H, Masamune K, et al. Vision-based markerless registration using stereo vision and an augmented reality surgical navigation system: a pilot study. BMC Med Imaging. 2015;15(1):51.
36. Gulati M, Anand V, Salaria SK, Jain N, Gupta S. Computerized implant-dentistry: advances toward automation. J Indian Soc Periodontol. 2015;19(1):5–10.
37. Aichert A, Wein W, Ladikos A, Reichl T, Navab N. Image-based tracking of the teeth for orthodontic augmented reality. Med Image Comput Comput Assist Interv. 2012;15(Pt 2):601–8.
38. Ruppin J, Popovic A, Strauss M, Spüntrup E, Steiner A, Stoll C. Evaluation of the accuracy of three different computer-aided surgery systems in dental implantology: optical tracking vs. stereolithographic splint systems. Clin Oral Implants Res. 2008;19(7):709–16. https://doi.org/10.1111/j.1600-0501.2007.01430.x.
39. Somogyi-Ganss E, Holmes HI, Jokstad A. Accuracy of a novel prototype dynamic computer-assisted surgery system. Clin Oral Implants Res. 2015;26(8):882–90. https://doi.org/10.1111/clr.12414.
40. Mandelaris GA, Stefanelli LV, DeGroot BS. Dynamic navigation for surgical implant placement: overview of technology, key concepts, and a case ReportDynamic navigation for surgical implant placement: overview of technology, key concepts, and a case report. Compend Contin Educ Dent. 2018;39(9):614–21.
41. Bover-Ramos F, Vina-Almunia J, Cervera-Ballester J, Penarrocha-Diago M, Garcia-Mira B. Accuracy of implant placement with computer-guided surgery: a systematic review and meta-analysis comparing cadaver, clinical, and in vitro studies. Int J Oral Maxillofac Implants. 2018;33:101–15. https://doi.org/10.11607/jomi.5556.
42. Jiang W, Ma L, Zhang B, Fan Y, Qu X, Zhang X, et al. Evaluation of the 3D augmented reality-guided intraoperative positioning of dental implants in edentulous mandibular models. Int J Oral Maxillofac Implants. 2018;33:1219–28. https://doi.org/10.11607/jomi.6638.
43. Connert T, Zehnder MS, Amato M, Weiger R, Kuhl S, Krast IG. Microguided endodontics: a method to achieve minimally invasive access cavity preparation and root canal location in mandibular incisors using a novel computer-guided technique. Int Endod J. 2018;51:247–55. https://doi.org/10.1111/iej.12809.
44. Beumer HW, Puscas L. Computer modeling and navigation in maxillofacial surgery. Curr Opin Otolaryngol Head Neck Surg. 2009;17:270–3. https://doi.org/10.1097/MOO.0b013e32832cba7d.
45. Kubota T, Yoshimoto G. Virtual and mixed reality in clinical application. In: Rekow ED, editor. Digital dentistry: a comprehensive reference and preview of the future. Surrey: Quintessence Publishing; 2018. p. 357–64.
46. Pellegrino G, Mangano C, Mangano R, Ferri A, Taraschi V, Marchetti C. Augmented reality for dental implantology: a pilot clinical report of two cases. BMC Oral Health. 2019;19(158):1–8.
47. Hanken H, Schablowsky C, Smeets R, Heiland M, Riecke B, Nourwali I, Vorwig O, Grobe A, Al-Dam A. Virtual planning complex head and neck reconstruction results in satisfactory match between real outcomes and virtual models. Clin Oral Investig. 2015;19(3):647–56.

48. Maloney KD, Rutner T. Virtual surgical planning and hardware fabrication prior to open reduction and internal fixation of atrophic edentulous mandible fractures. Craniomaxillofac Trauma Recontr. 2019;12(2):156–62.
49. Drake VE, Rizzi CJ, Greywoode JD, Vakharia KT. Midface fracture simulation and repair: a computer-based algorithm. Craniomaxillofac Trauma Reconstr. 2019;12(1):14–9.
50. Chang HW, Lin HH, Chortrakarrnkij P, Kim SG, Lo LJ. Intraoperative navigation for single splint two-jaw orthognathic surgery. From model to actual surgery. J Craniomaxillofac Surg. 2015;43(7):1119–26.
51. Badiali G, Roncani A, Bianchi A, Taddei F, Marchetti C, Schileo E. Navigation in orthognathic surgery: 3D accuracy. Facial Plast Surg. 2015;31(5):463–73.
52. Schmitt YS, Hoffman HG, Sharar SR. A randomized, controlled trial of immersive virtual reality analgesia during physical therapy for pediatric burn injuries. Burns. 2011;37:61–8.
53. Ougradar A, Ahmed B. Patients' perceptions of the benefits of virtual reality during dental extractions. Br Dent J. 2019;227:813–6.
54. Sharar SR, Miller W, Patterson DR. Applications of virtual reality for pain management in burn-injured patients. Expert Rev Neurother. 2008;8:1667–74.
55. Wiederhold MD, Wiederhold BK. Virtual reality and interactive simulation for pain distraction. Pain Med. 2007;8:S182–8.
56. Hoffman HG, Garcia-Palacios A, Patterson DR, et al. The effectiveness of virtual reality for dental pain control: a case study. Cyberpsychol Behav. 2001;4:527–35.
57. Wiederhold MD, Gao K, Wiederhold BK. Clinical use of virtual reality distraction system to reduce anxiety and pain in dental procedures. Cyberpsychol Behav Soc Netw. 2014;17:359–65.
58. Rose JT, Buchanan JA, Sarrett DC. The DentSim system. J Dent Educ. 1999;63:421–3.
59. Imber S, Shapira G, Gordon M, et al. A virtual reality dental simulator predicts performance in an operative manikin course. Eur J Dent Educ. 2003;7:160–3.
60. Wierinck ER, Puttemans V, Swinnen SP, et al. Expert performance on a virtual reality simulation system. J Dent Educ. 2007;71:759–66.
61. Issenberg SB, McGaghie WC, Hart IR, et al. Simulation technology for health care professional skills training and assessment. JAMA. 1999;282:861–6.
62. Suvinen TI, Messer LB, Franco E. Clinical simulation in teaching preclinical dentistry. Eur J Dent Educ. 1998;2:25–32.
63. Usui T, Maki K, Toki Y, et al. Mechanical strain on the human skull in a humanoid robotic model. Am J Orthod Dentofac Orthop. 2004;126:421–31.
64. Madokoro M, Miyazaki Y, Maki K, et al. Development of a patient robot for dental clinical education. J Jpn Dent Educ. 2007;23:24–32.
65. Tanzawa T, Madokoro M, Maki K, et al. Application of humanoid robotics to management of medical emergency in dental education. J Jpn Soc Simul Sug. 2010;18:1–10.
66. Bridges S, et al. Virtual reality simulation: indications and perspectives in the field of dental education. Dental Turbines. 2015;2:6–8.
67. Pedersen SS. The use of robotics in dentistry. Today-science and practice AEEDC 2013.
68. Dalai DR, et al. Futuristic application of Nano-robots in dentistry. Int J Adv Health Sci. 2014;1(3):16–20.
69. Tanzawa, et al. Introduction of a robot patient into dental education. Eur J Dent Educ. 2012;16(1):e195–9.

Printed in the United States
by Baker & Taylor Publisher Services